Ureteroscopy

Bradley F. Schwartz • John D. Denstedt
Editors

Ureteroscopy

A Comprehensive Contemporary Guide

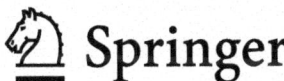 Springer

Editors
Bradley F. Schwartz
Southern Illinois University
School of Medicine
Springfield, IL
USA

John D. Denstedt
University of Western Ontario
London, ON
Canada

ISBN 978-3-030-26651-6   ISBN 978-3-030-26649-3   (eBook)
https://doi.org/10.1007/978-3-030-26649-3

This Springer imprint is published by the registered company Springer Nature Switzerland AG
The registered company address is: Gewerbestrasse 11, 6330 Cham, Switzerland

I would like to dedicate this book to my very supportive and understanding wife, Brandi, and to our four motivational and exceptional children, Steven, Olivia, Daniel, and Evan. Their unconditional loyalty, past victories, and future successes are the reasons that made this project possible. Thank you and I love you all.
        Bradley F. Schwartz, DO, FACS

To my wife, Carolyn, and my two daughters, Drs. Emily and Ellen Denstedt, without whose unqualified support and patience, my academic urologic career would have been a small fraction of what it ultimately has been.

To the pioneers of Endourology who transformed the way in which urologists worldwide deliver care to patients by way of minimally invasive techniques.
        John D. Denstedt, MD, FRCSC, FACS, FCAHS

Foreword

It has now been over 100 years since Hugh Hampton Young passed a rigid endoscope into a pediatric megaureter and over 50 years since Victor Marshall placed a nonsteerable 9F fiber-optic endoscope into a ureter during an open ureterolithotomy. In the ensuing years, we have seen unimaginable things occur from the passage of a 41 cm semirigid endoscope from the urethral meatus to the renal pelvis as detailed by Enrique Pérez-Castro Ellendt to the refinement of the flexible ureteroscope following the pioneering efforts of Demetrius Bagley and Yoshio Aso. In parallel, while alterations to stone retrieval devices have been barely incremental, the advent of laser technology has provided the urologist with 200 micron laser fibers capable of fragmenting even the hardest stones regardless of location. Despite these profound advances, it is more than 30 years since Ed Lyon, Jeff Huffman, and Demetrius Bagley published their original text on ureteroscopy and nearly a decade since Manoj Monga and colleagues provided a much-needed update. Given the recent developments in laser technology, flexible disposable endoscopes, CMOS and CCD chip technology and robotics, this book should be a welcome addition to the library of every urologist who picks up a ureteroscope.

Drs. Schwartz and Denstedt have compiled a global team of ureteroscopic experts who have in turn masterfully provided the reader with information and guidelines that will enhance one's understanding of ureteroscopy, the available instrumentation, and its effective application in a variety of scenarios from stones to tumors. Moreover, the book covers the potential complications of ureteroscopic surgery and their management as well as proper postoperative patient care and quality-of-life issues. Special patient populations are also addressed in the chapters on ureteroscopy in the pregnant and pediatric populations.

Future directions are the topic of the final chapters which focus on simulation training and robotics. In the not too distant future, residents will train on an ureteroscopic simulator to a point of competence and only then will they be provided the opportunity to transfer their simulator documented skills to the operating room. No doubt this will preclude many ureteroscopic mishaps. In addition, the evolution of robotic ureteroscopy will develop to the point at which the aching shoulders and awkward gyrations of the table side endoscopist and assistant are replaced by a seated surgeon at a console providing for effortless movement of the endoscope and its instrumentation. Indeed, many ureteroscopic procedures will one day truly be robotic rather than the master-slave technology that is the hallmark of today's computer-assisted surgery. The surgeon will sit at the console and press a button, and the procedure will ensue with the robot gently passing the selected endoscope via a previously loaded CT guidance to the patient's stone, the composition of which will be "read" by the laser allowing for automatic precise power adjustment to truly render the stone to dust, which in turn will then be effortlessly suctioned from the collecting system.

Ureteroscopy is the epitome of natural orifice surgery in Urology. For the urologist of today who is seeking to provide better, less-invasive care for stones, upper tract strictures, or urothelial tumors, this book is essential. Read well, and do well.

Ralph V. Clayman, MD
Distinguished Professor/Endowed Chair in Endourology, Dean Emeritus
University of California, Irvine, Department of Urology
Orange, CA, USA

Preface

In 1929, Dr. Young reported on a ureteroscopy he performed in 1912. Then in 1964, Dr. Marshall reported on the first flexible ureteroscopy performed in humans. Arguably, the last 100 years has seen unparalleled technological advancements in the field of endoscopy. Furthermore, the explosion in technology for this very common procedure is unprecedented in the past 20 years. According to data published by the AUA, ureteroscopy is the most common non-office procedure performed worldwide by the practicing urologist. It is not uncommon for resident trainees to have performed 200–300 by the time they are third year residents and graduate with more than 400–500 cases upon completion of their training.

We currently utilize ureterocopy for diagnosis and treatment of a wide variety of diseases from stones to cancer. We have analog and digital technology, flexible and rigid scopes, reusable and single-use scopes, and hundreds of complimentary devices to facilitate our procedures. The past 5 years has even caught the wave of robotics, and we currently have a commercially available ureteroscopic robotic platform. As it relates to training, robotic simulators, skill's laboratories, and ureteroscopic trainers are widespread in an attempt to train urologists in virtually all aspects of ureteroscopy.

Having been in practice for a total of 60 years, we are excited and enthusiastic to be part of this technical explosion to help our patients. Our hope moving forward is that the best and brightest in our field can continue to contribute to the technological advancements that have made this specialty great. The collection of world experts contributing to this textbook deserve much of the credit for many of the advancements presented in this comprehensive review. We feel this book is the most thorough and detailed account of ureteroscopy published in the world to date. We hope you enjoy it.

Springfield, IL, USA   Bradley F. Schwartz
London, ON, Canada   John D. Denstedt

Contents

Contributors

Mohammed Alfozan, MBBS, Saudi Board of Urology Department of Urology, University Hospital of Patras, Patras, Greece

College of Medicine, Prince Sattam Bin Abdulaziz University, Al Kharj, Saudi Arabia

Osama Al-Omar, MD, MBA Department of Urology, West Virginia University Medicine, Morgantown, WV, USA

Blake Anderson, MD Department of Urology, Indiana University School of Medicine, IU Health Urology Methodist Hospital, Indianapolis, IN, USA

Wesley Baas, MD Department of Urology, Southern Illinois University School of Medicine, Springfield, IL, USA

Demetrius H. Bagley, MD, FACS Department of Urology, Sidney Kimmel Medical College at Thomas Jefferson University, Philadelphia, PA, USA

John Barnard, MD Department of Urology, West Virginia University Medicine, Morgantown, WV, USA

Jennifer Bjazevic, MD, FRCSC Department of Surgery, Division of Urology, Schulich School of Medicine & Dentistry, Western University, London, ON, Canada

Brian Calio, MD Department of Urology, Sidney Kimmel Medical College at Thomas Jefferson University, Philadelphia, PA, USA

Robert C. Calvert, MA MD FRCS(Urol) Gow Gibbon Department of Urology, Royal Liverpool and Broadgreen University Hospitals NHS Trust, Kent, Lodge, Broadgreen Hospital, Thomas Drive, UK

Nikos Charalampogiannis, MD Department of Urology, SLK Kliniken Heilbronn, University of Heidelberg, Heilbronn, Baden-Württemberg, Germany

Tony Chen, MD Department of Urology, University of Washington, Seattle, WA, USA

Ben H. Chew, MD, MSc, FRCSC Department of Urologic Sciences, Vancouver General Hospital, Vancouver, BC, Canada

Vincent De Coninck, MD, FEBU Sorbonne Université, Service d'Urologie, AP-HP, Hôpital Tenon, Paris, France

Sorbonne Université, GRC n°20, Groupe de Recherche Clinique sur la Lithiase Urinaire, Hôpital Tenon, Paris, France

Chad Crigger, MD, MPH Department of Urology, West Virginia University Medicine, Morgantown, WV, USA

John D. Denstedt, MD, FRCSC, FACS, FCAHS Department of Surgery, Division of Urology, Schulich School of Medicine & Dentistry, Western University, London, ON, Canada

Mordechai Duvdevani, MD Department of Urology, Hadassah Hebrew University Medical Center, Jerusalem, Israel

Marcel Fiedler, MD Department of Urology, SLK Kliniken Heilbronn, University of Heidelberg, Heilbronn, Baden-Württemberg, Germany

Ali Hajiran, MD Department of Urology, West Virginia University Medicine, Morgantown, WV, USA

Joshua M. Heiman, MS Department of Urology, Indiana University School of Medicine, IU Health Urology Methodist Hospital, Indianapolis, IN, USA

Takaaki Inoue, MD, PhD Department of Urology and Andrology, Kansai Medical University, Osaka, Japan

Ahmet Sinan Kabakci, PhD Department of Urology, SLK Kliniken Heilbronn, University of Heidelberg, Heilbronn, Baden-Württemberg, Germany

Department of Bioengineering, Hacettepe University, Ankara, Turkey

Panagiotis Kallidonis, MD, MSc, PhD, FEBU Department of Urology, University Hospital of Patras, Patras, Greece

Ioannis Katafygiotis, MD, PhD, FEBU Department of Urology, Hadassah Hebrew University Medical Center, Jerusalem, Israel

Etienne Xavier Keller, MD, FEBU Sorbonne Université, Service d'Urologie, AP-HP, Hôpital Tenon, Paris, France

Sorbonne Université, GRC n°20, Groupe de Recherche Clinique sur la Lithiase Urinaire, Hôpital Tenon, Paris, France

Andrew Klein, BS Department of Urology, Southern Illinois University School of Medicine, Springfield, IL, USA

Jan-Thorsten Klein, MD Department of Urology, Medical School Ulm, University of Ulm, Ulm, Germany

Bodo E. Knudsen, MD, FRCSC Department of Urology, The Ohio State University Wexner Medical Center, Columbus, OH, USA

Amy Krambeck, MD Department of Urology, Indiana University School of Medicine, IU Health Urology Methodist Hospital, Indianapolis, IN, USA

Evangelos Liatsikos, MD, PhD Department of Urology, University Hospital of Patras, Patras, Greece

Jonathan R. Z. Lim Department of Urologic Sciences, Vancouver General Hospital, Vancouver, BC, Canada

Michael Lipkin, MD Department of Urology, Duke University Medical Center, Durham, NC, USA

Tadashi Matsuda, MD, PhD Department of Urology and Andrology, Kansai Medical University, Osaka, Japan

Manoj Monga, MD, FACS, FRCS (Glasgow) Glickman Urologic and Kidney Institute, The Cleveland Clinic, Cleveland, OH, USA

Michael Ost, MD, MBA Department of Urology, West Virginia University Medicine, Morgantown, WV, USA

Margaret S. Pearle, MD, PhD Department of Urology, UT Southwestern Medical Center, Dallas, TX, USA

Charles and Jane Pak Center for Mineral Metabolism and Bone Research, UT Southwestern Medical Center, Dallas, TX, USA

Dima Raskolnikov, MD Department of Urology, University of Washington, Seattle, WA, USA

Jens J. Rassweiler, MD, PhD Department of Urology, SLK Kliniken Heilbronn, University of Heidelberg, Heilbronn, Baden-Württemberg, Germany

Itay M. Sabler, MD Department of Urology, Hadassah Hebrew University Medical Center, Jerusalem, Israel

Remzi Sağlam, MD Department of Urology, Medicana International Hospital, Ankara, Turkey

Bradley F. Schwartz, DO Department of Urology, Southern Illinois University School of Medicine, Springfield, IL, USA

Kymora B. Scotland, MD, PhD Department of Urologic Sciences, University of British Columbia, Vancouver, BC, Canada

Igor Sorokin, MD Department of Urology, University of Massachusetts, Worcester, MA, USA

Michael W. Sourial, MD, FRCSC Department of Urology, The Ohio State University Wexner Medical Center, Columbus, OH, USA

Karen L. Stern, MD Department of Urology, Cleveland Clinic Foundation, Cleveland, OH, USA

Robert M. Sweet, MD Department of Urology, University of Washington, Seattle, WA, USA

Department of Surgery, WWAMI Institute for Simulation in Healthcare (WISH), University of Washington, Seattle, WA, USA

Olivier Traxer, MD Sorbonne Université, Service d'Urologie, AP-HP, Hôpital Tenon, Paris, France

Sorbonne Université, GRC n°20, Groupe de Recherche Clinique sur la Lithiase Urinaire, Hôpital Tenon, Paris, France

Brenton Winship, MD Department of Urology, Duke University Medical Center, Durham, NC, USA

Chapter 1
The History of the Development of Ureteral Endoscopy

Demetrius H. Bagley and Brian Calio

The history of human endoscopy has been based upon the need and desire to see within the next body cavity. The need to perform procedures depended upon endoscopes that could deliver devices and the development of appropriate instruments. Within the field of urology, the most obvious target is the bladder, the source of many diagnostic challenges and physical disorders residing within a very few centimeters of the surface in females and beyond a much longer urethra in the male. The need and the ability to go beyond the urethra and bladder into the ureter and even the intrarenal collecting system could only wait for the development of instruments to access each more proximal portion of the urinary tract.

The endoscopes for access to the urinary tract, from the urethral meatus to the renal papillae, all exhibit common functional and design factors. Each scope must have, by definition, a mechanism for imaging to extend the view to the end of the shaft. The next level of features includes illumination possibly by several different sources. Also needed is a mechanism for irrigation to distend the cavity being entered and inspected. As experience with endoscopes increased, the need for a channel to deliver working devices became obvious. Similarly, as flexible endoscopes became available, the need for deflection was clear. These features are common and are essential in current endoscopes. With the addition of functional features to ureteroscopes and with appropriate working instruments, the function of the endoscope could be advanced from solely visualization to stone retrieval, lithotripsy, and tumor biopsy and ablation [1, 2].

The earliest device developed for visualization within the body was Bozzini's Lichtleiter in 1806. It consisted of a tube with mirrors and a candle for illumination. Its original purpose was for the pharynx, but it could also be applied to the pelvic organs. It is notable that the original model was at the American College of Surgeons

D. H. Bagley (✉) · B. Calio
Department of Urology, Sidney Kimmel Medical College at Thomas Jefferson University, Philadelphia, PA, USA
e-mail: Demetrius.bagley@jefferson.edu

© Springer Nature Switzerland AG 2020
B. F. Schwartz, J. D. Denstedt (eds.), *Ureteroscopy*,
https://doi.org/10.1007/978-3-030-26649-3_1

in Chicago after the Second World War. It was subsequently returned to the Josephinum in Vienna, but a copy was retained in Chicago [3].

Many new designs were introduced in the nineteenth century, but one by Desormeaux (1815–1882) in Paris indicated the shape to come for instruments for the male urethra. It consisted of a long metal channel with a mirror to reflect light from the petroleum-fueled lamp. It had an angled beak at the tip like other later designs and foretold of controversial tip designs in ureteroscopes over a century later. Again, this instrument was not practical because it became very hot during use [4].

Other designs were introduced elsewhere in the world. Wales and Kern in the USA introduced a design using reflected light from an ophthalmic mirror to look down a center channel into the bladder. The tip again had an acutely angled beak. It did not get hot in use but had limited visualization.

In 1878, Nitze, working with Leiter, an Austrian instrumental maker, demonstrated the first working cystoscope. A tungsten wire was electrified to give light but it also produced heat. The endoscope included a system for water cooling. Other future cystoscopes included many of the same conceptual features in this model [5, 6].

Another major advancement came with the development of the mignon bulb by Electrosurgical Instruments in Rochester, New York [7]. These were low amperage light bulbs small enough to fit on the tip of a cystoscope. Although the bulbs did not cause problems by overheating, they could burn out causing an endoscopic blackout.

After Reinhold Wappler immigrated to New York in 1890, he set up a company to produce a cystoscope. The Tilden Brown composite cystoscope proved to be a practical and long-lasting design [7]. It consisted of different lenses, or telescopes, which could look forward, at a minor angle or at a right angle. Obturators with an angled tip were used initially to pass the sheath and then removed for subsequent placement of the lenses.

Instrument development also continued in Europe. A catheterizing cystoscope was designed by the German, Leopold Casper. Although it used a mirror system between the eyepiece and the shaft, it did allow ureteral catheterization but without deflection of the catheter.

Albarrán introduced the next instrument which could deflect the ureteral catheter. It was a purely mechanical device which could be used with the telescope and sheaths of other endoscopes. It remains in use and in production today.

A major refinement in cystoscope design dates to 1910 when Buerger in New York based his design on one by Tilden Brown. Known as the Brown-Buerger cystoscope, it remained in use for over half a century (Fig. 1.1). It included interchangeable telescopes and channels for irrigation and instruments and could accept the Albarrán deflector. The imaging system consisted of multiple thin lenses (similar to magnifying glasses or optical lenses) arranged throughout the cylindrical shaft [8].

The next major step was Harold Hopkins patent of his rod-lens system in 1959. The system essentially reversed the roles of the glass and the air in the conventional lensing system. Most of the space in the shaft of the telescope was taken up by glass rods. The short spaces between the rods served as the lensing. This provided for

Fig. 1.1 The Brown-
Buerger cystoscope
consists of several
components which are
placed and were delivered
in a wooden box

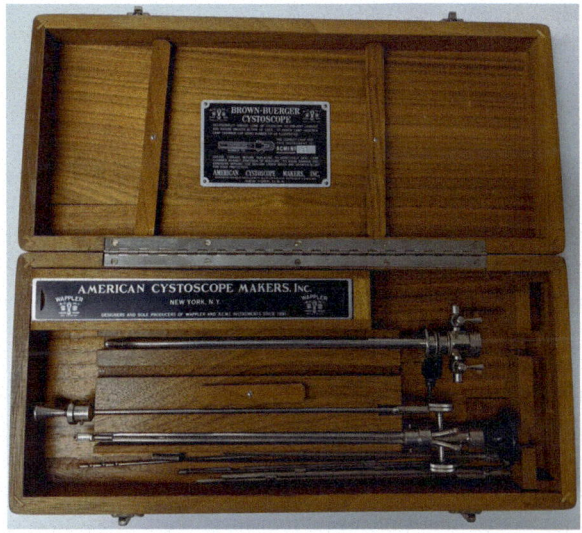

greater light transmission, better resolution, and less loss of lens alignment. Karl
Storz, setting up a new manufacturing company, obtained the patent and began producing endoscopes with clearly superior visualization. Others soon followed. [9]

Fiber optics played a major role both in rigid and flexible endoscopes. In rigid
instruments, fiber-optic bundles could provide the light for illumination in a small
package directed exactly at the area of interest. In flexible endoscopes, they would
be responsible for both illumination and visualization.

In a parallel fashion, fiber optics were first developed and then later applied to
imaging. Coladon in the 1840s demonstrated the concept of internal reflection in
"light guiding" of fiber optics [10]. An important concept, the transmission of light
through bent or angled glass fibers, was shown by Babinet. Still at that point, the
fibers were carrying only diffuse light which could be useful for illumination but not
for imaging. That step was taken in patents from Baird and Hansell in 1927 and
1930, respectively. Their fiber design provided image transmission. By 1957,
Curtiss demonstrated that fibers with another layer of glass, or a cladding, offered
better internal reflectivity and resultant light transmission. Also in 1957, Hirschowitz
developed a flexible gastroscope using glass fibers with cladding which was clinically usable as he demonstrated on himself [11, 12].

These endoscopes found interested users throughout medical fields. Both rigid
endoscopes and flexible fiber-optic imaging devices were being used anecdotally by
urologists for examination of the ureter. Hugh Hampton Young performed the first
ureteroscopy in a pediatric patient with posterior urethral valves and a severely
dilated ureter which easily accepted a rigid pediatric cystoscope in 1912. It was
reported in 1929 in a review of congenital urethral valves [13].

The next phase of ureteroscopy, still tentative, occurred in 1961. Marshall placed
a 9F flexible fiber-optic scope through a ureterotomy made during an open operation to inspect for calculi. The scope had neither channel nor deflection. Two years
later, Marshall reported the first transurethral flexible ureteroscopy performed by

MacGovern and Walzak. A 9F flexible endoscope was passed through a 26F McCarthy sheath into a ureter to visualize a calculus [14].

Efforts to develop a functional flexible ureteroscope became serious in 1968 when Takagi et al. initiated their studies of transurethral ureteroscopy with flexible endoscopes. The hurdles quickly became evident. The instrument they used was a 70 cm 8F fiber optic passively deflectable flexible endoscope. In both cadavers and patients, they could visualize the renal pelvis and papillae but could not manipulate the tip. They also found it difficult to insert the scope from the bladder into the ureter even with cystoscope sheaths and flexible introducer sheaths, each with irrigation. In these initial studies, they recognized the need for active deflection, for an irrigation channel and the limitations of instrument size [15].

The next phase started a decade later with efforts at rigid ureteroscopy. Two urologists working independently, Goodman [16] and Lyon [17], used pediatric cystoscopes for distal ureteroscopy in women. Lyon subsequently used longer, juvenile cystoscopes in men [18]. These instruments are as large as 13F and required dilation of the intramural ureter. This step alone required considerable development of techniques and instruments. Urethral dilators were first used and were followed by unguided interchangeable bougies, wire-guided bougies, and subsequently balloons. The latter proved to be the most effective device in its final form. It required a nonelastic balloon which could achieve a high pressure in the range of 20 bar.

The next version was an even longer, 41 cm, specifically designed rigid ureteroscope. This instrument could reach the renal pelvis if it could be passed through the curvature of the ureter as it courses over the iliac vessels and lumbar muscles. The scope had a removable rod-lens telescope and a working channel [19].

To be useful, ureteroscopes had to have the capability to diagnose and treat lesions, not just to visualize them. This capability matured with the addition of working channels and suitable working instruments. Simple stone retrieval was the first therapeutic procedure. Das performed the first transurethral ureteroscopic basket retrieval of a stone in 1981 [20]. The following year Huffman used the 23 cm ureteroscope to treat 16 distal ureteral calculi. Procedures were limited to the distal ureter because of the length of the endoscope and larger stones could not be treated. The success rate was 69% [21].

The next major step in stone treatment was reported by Huffman et al. in 1983 [22]. This was the first ureteroscopic ultrasonic lithotripsy of larger stones throughout the ureter and the renal pelvis. Both of these steps in stone treatment were also dependent upon the development of new working instruments. Small baskets compatible with the working channel in the ureteroscope end and an ultrasonic lithotripter probe 2.5 mm in diameter, long enough to fit through the sheath of the long ureteroscope, were essential.

This earliest technique involved approaching the stone with the long rigid ureteroscope, engaging it with a basket and pulling it tightly against the tip of the scope. The telescope was then removed, and the ultrasonic probe passed through the sheath to touch the stone. The touch of the probe onto the stone could be felt with the basket held in the operator's second hand. The ultrasonic probe was then activated, and as it removed a portion of the stone, resistance was relieved. The probe was removed, and the telescope replaced to visualize the stone and reposition a portion of it at the end of the sheath. The procedure was then repeated until the stone was small enough to remove. The procedure was considered a tactile technique or less generously as a blind technique. It was tedious but effective. Huffman stated "Do you know what this means? We can remove any stone that we can see ureteroscopically" [23] (Fig. 1.2).

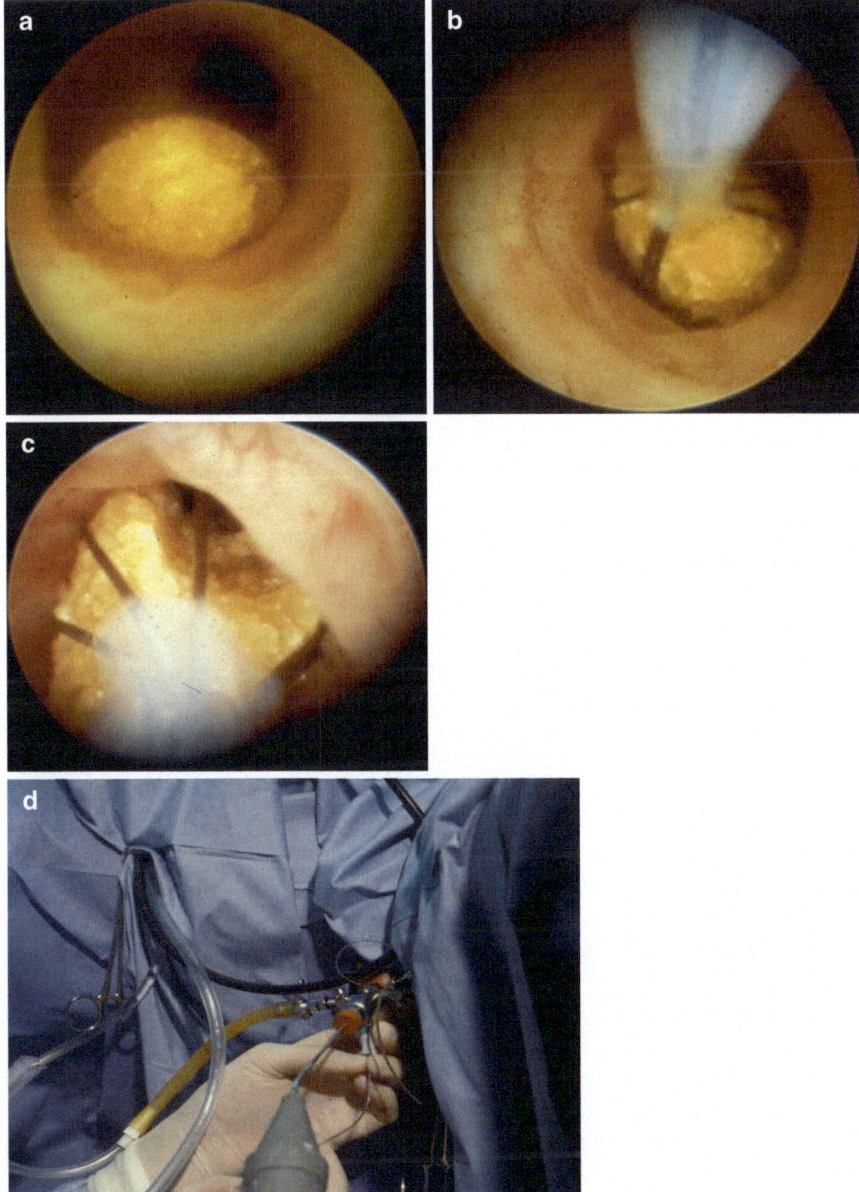

Fig. 1.2 (**a**) The stone is visualized in the ureter with the rod lens ureteroscope. (**b**) The stone is trapped with a basket. (**c**) After applying the ultrasound probe, there is a groove in the stone. (**d**) The basket is held in one hand and can feel pressure of the ultrasound probe

Fig. 1.3 The offset ureteroscope is assembled with a handle to hold the ultrasound probe and allow it to pass directly through the straight channel

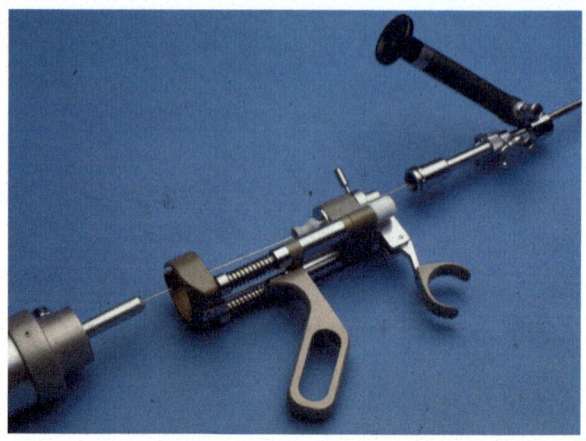

The next logical step required a change in the endoscope and the lithotripter. A long ureteroscope was designed with a straight channel which could accept a rigid instrument and an offset eyepiece. At the same time, a smaller, 4F, ultrasonic lithotripter was developed. Therefore the probe could be passed through the ureteroscope as the stone was visualized. Although the ultrasonic lithotripter was not nearly as powerful as the other designs, it was effective in reducing the size of stones and removing fragments.

A second effective offset and visualizing working ureteroscope used the solid probe ultrasonic lithotripter probe or the Goodfriend design [24] (Fig. 1.3). This was a very powerful lithotripter which could easily fragment even the hardest calcium oxalate monohydrate stones. The probe was positioned beside the stone so there was much less risk of causing proximal migration. Despite the effectiveness, at the time it suffered from the inability to remove any of the fragments during lithotripsy.

The success of rigid ureteroscopy also emphasized its limitations. Often it was not possible to access the ureter proximal to the iliac vessels or the lumbar segment. These limitations were emphasized in male patients. Flexible endoscopes could overcome these hurdles but needed the capability of irrigation and deflection to be effective. The early attempts at flexible ureteroscopy are noted above. In the 1980s, Olympus developed a deflectable flexible ureteroscope based on its pediatric bronchoscope. It was a fiber-optic instrument with a working channel. Maximal deflection was in the up direction with distal movement of the thumb lever, appropriate for a bronchoscope but possibly not a ureteroscope. Initially in the USA, there was one instrument available, used by Rob Kahn in San Francisco and D Bagley in Philadelphia, each doing 1–2 days each week with the instrument traveling by overnight carrier between the locations.

Production models of deflectable flexible ureteroscopes were introduced in the USA by ACMI. The AUR series initially included two different sized endoscopes. The larger at 9.8F had a 3.6F channel while the smaller at 8.5F had a 2.5F channel. They had 180° of deflection in one direction. This design was used to minimize the outer dimension. The one-way deflection was adequate for inspection throughout the collecting system since the endoscope could be rotated easily. The shaft was constructed of an extrusion with multiple channels for fiber optics, illuminating fibers, pull wires, and irrigation. Other flexible endoscopes at that time and even now were constructed of separate lumens for each function which were then grouped within the outer body. The size and cost savings were the basis for the extrusion design. It also eliminated the need for a separate, manually controlled vent valve. This concept arose again for the single-use endoscopes several years later.

The next in this series was the AUR7. It had two-way deflection but was remarkable for its size – 7.4F along the distal 24 cm with a 3.6F channel. The original design consisted of a shaft which tapered from the base of the handle to the tip. It proved to be resilient in clinical testing but was too difficult and expensive to manufacture. Therefore, it was changed to a step-down design at the 24 cm point. This rendered it very delicate with twisting of the shaft at that point whenever it was advanced and rotated against some resistance in the ureter. It was discontinued and subsequent models from all manufacturers were larger. The AUR7 remains the smallest fully deflectable flexible ureteroscope that became a full production model.

Deflection of the tip of a flexible ureteroscope is often limited by the instruments within the channel. These include biopsy forceps, laser fibers, and various probes. This has largely been overcome by the Storz Flex X series. This ureteroscope offers deflection of 220° in each direction (Fig. 1.4). Although this extent is very rarely used, it compensates for the loss of deflection when there are instruments within the

Fig. 1.4 The tip is deflected to approximately 220°. This extent helps to correct for loss of deflection with an instrument in the channel

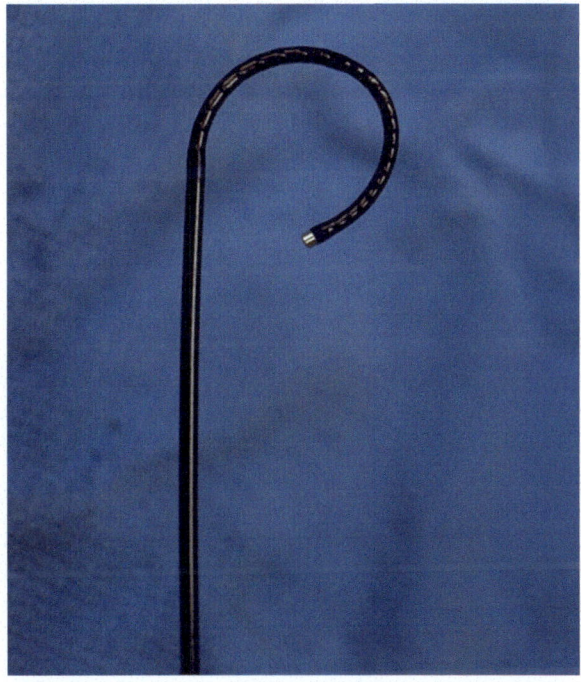

channel. This series, introduced in 2012, then added a new design feature in the digital model with a shaft which is oval in cross section. This allows more efficient packing of the channels and wiring within the shaft. The overall outer dimension is 8.3F and set a new standard for flexible ureteroscopes.

Flexible ureteroscopes have not totally replaced rigid models. Rigid endoscopes are less expensive and more durable than flexibles. It is also easier to pass them into the distal ureter for active procedures. One of the major efforts in this development has been downsizing the total outer dimension of the endoscope. The visualization system, the rod-lens telescope, was a major space-occupying factor in the shaft, and the working channel was the second major factor.

The first step taken was to change from a rod-lens system to fiber-optic imaging which had proven its value in many endoscopes in different specialties. It was used in the ACMI RigiFlex, or HTO-5, rigid ureteroscope to provide a channel which could accept a 5F ultrasound probe along with adequate irrigation. The eyepiece was offset to offer a straight channel through the shaft and was carried within a gooseneck form to allow movement and positioning. Overall the endoscope maintained an outer dimension of nearly 12F. It had a relatively short production duration since other smaller lithotripters became available allowing smaller endoscope design.

The concept of fiber-optic imaging in a rigid metal endoscope advanced rapidly to the next enduring plateau with the introduction of laser lithotripters. The pulsed dye laser was an effective lithotripter despite being a single-purpose laser which was relatively difficult to maintain and was expensive. The small fiber (<400 μm) could be passed through a channel <2F. Watson and Dretler developed a design with the laser manufacturer of a rigid 7F endoscope with two channels, each 2F [25]. The original concept was for continuous irrigation with fluid passing through one channel and draining out the other. That feature was not very effective. However, the design of a small rigid endoscope was a winner with variations existing to the present time.

The endoscope itself was not widely accepted because the laser manufacturer permitted sales only to laser owners and the channels could not accept any stone retrieval device then in existence.

A more successful version of the small rigid ureteroscope was the MR6 which had two channels, a 3.4F and a 2.3F [26]. These could be packaged along with the fiber-optic imaging and illumination system in an instrument with a 7F outer dimension at the tip by using a triangular cross section. 3F retrieval devices were available at that time and could be passed through the larger channel. Since stones tended to move during fragmentation with the pulsed dye laser, it was helpful to stabilize them in a basket. The fiber could be passed easily through the smaller channel. Like other rigid ureteroscopes, it was available in shorter versions of 33 cm for use in the distal ureter alone or 41 cm to reach the proximal ureter or renal pelvis. . This group of endoscopes has been termed "semirigid," but there is no question that they are made of metal and are rigid. They can tolerate some bending but can be pushed through tissue. The successful use of these endoscopes, which have a flat tip, demonstrates that there is no need for a beak on a ureteroscope.

Another great advance has been the change in the imaging mechanism for flexible ureteroscopes. For many years, the standard was fiber optics. The introduction of small digital chips for imaging provided an image of clarity and resolution never seen before in flexible devices. Initially referred to as "chip on a stick," digital imaging flexible ureteroscopes are available from all the major manufacturers. Both CMOS (complementary metal-oxide-semiconductor) and CCD (charge-coupled devices) chips have been used. Initially the digital instruments were approximately 2F sizes larger than fiber-optic scopes, but with a reduction in size of the chips, the tips and the shafts have reached the same size range of 8.4F. The image is rather uniformly considered superior to a fiber-optic image but may be seen to have its own deficits. There can be variations in color, highlights or burnout, and contrast. There have been concerns with scatter when there is blood in the visual field. Usually when there is failure in the system, it is total. Either there is an image or there is not. It does not have the image degradation seen with fiber optics as individual fibers break. A major barrier to the acceptance of digital imaging systems is the cost. In addition to the endoscope itself, other devices are needed to complete the imaging chain.

Driven by the high cost of flexible ureteral endoscopy, there has been increasing interest in single-use endoscopes. This is not really new but was seen in 1985 with the VanTec disposable flexible fiber-optic ureteroscope. Single-use shafts were connected to a reusable handle containing the illuminating and the optical imaging system. There was a channel with size related to the outer dimension of the shaft, adequate for irrigation and usually a working instrument. They did not have deflection, but several different versions of rigid shafts were also available. Production was discontinued when the company was acquired (Fig. 1.5).

Bard also introduced a disposable flexible ureteroscope but with deflection. Unfortunately the deflection mechanism was operated by a rotating handle which was difficult to use while holding the scope. Another fatal flaw was that the image was upside down and backward similar to the endoscopes from the nineteenth century [27] (Fig. 1.6).

Fig. 1.5 The VanTec single-use scope was a fiber-optic device with interchangeable rigid and flexible tips

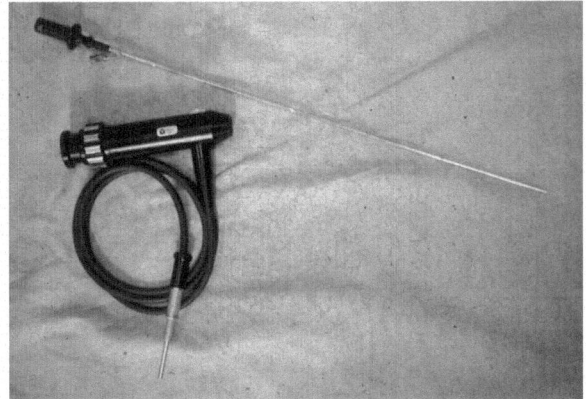

Fig. 1.6 The Bard single-use ureteroscope was deflectable, but a rotating ring was used for the deflection. It was very difficult to use with one hand

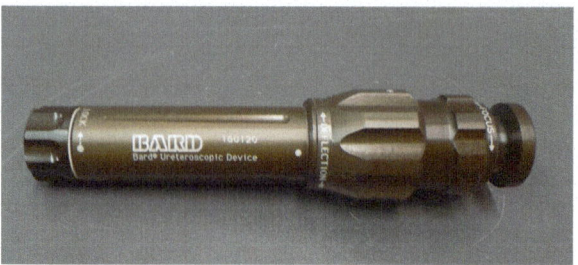

There were other attempts to introduce a single-use flexible ureteroscope all with their own failures. None were deflectable. More than one had a problem with torque stability, or a low durometer, flimsy, shaft, which was not pushable into the ureter.

The first flexible, fully deflectable single-use digital ureteroscope was the LithoVue from Boston Scientific, introduced in 2016. The shaft has a dimension of 9.6F with a 3.6F channel. It uses a proprietary video processing unit, and it is programmed to last no longer than 4 h. In vitro and clinical studies have shown the comparability of the function of this endoscope to the more standard reusable instruments [28].

Other single-use digital flexible ureteroscopes have also been introduced to the market. Pusen, from China, has a similar sized ureteroscope which is being sold worldwide. NeoScope, made in the USA, is smaller with a 9.0F tip and shaft of 8.4F and has also been sold in the USA and internationally [29–31].

The development and sales of these single-use flexible endoscopes are based on the cost and fragility of the reusable models. Several studies have found that there are major repairs after as few as 10–12 uses. Others have gone as high as 40 uses for repair [32–34]. A single report from a private clinic in Italy where the instruments are processed by the physicians themselves found that the ureteroscope was used in 100 cases before repair [35]. Overall, it appears that the more accurate rate is closer to a number between 10 and 20. The economic basis for using a single-use endoscope includes the frequent need for repair, the high cost of repair, and the high cost of initial acquisition of the reusable instrument. Various economic models have been used but must take into account the cost of handling and reprocessing the instruments in addition to the repairs. In this way, there appears to be justification for the cost of single-use instruments in some circumstances [31].

Associated Instruments

Ureteroscopes have a limited usefulness without associated instrumentation. Throughout the development of these instruments, we have seen the symbiotic relationship between the endoscope and the working device. Among the examples above, the first ultrasonic lithotripsy required securing the stone in the basket to apply pressure with the ultrasound probe. The endoscope sheath was not large enough to accept the probe, the basket, and the imaging telescope at the same time. The small rigid ureteroscopes, approximately 7F, would be of no value without the capabilities of lasers for lithotripsy and tissue ablation. The small channels can accept laser fibers and small baskets, graspers, and forceps. An endoscope of that size would have been useless in the 1980s as ureteroscopy developed. Two of the most important additions to the urologists instruments were the Holmium laser [36, 37] and the nitinol baskets [38], particularly as they were downsized to <2F. The entire complement of instruments is required.

Although much of the development of ureteroscopic instrumentation has been driven by the need for treatment of urinary calculi, diagnosis and therapy of upper tract tumors cannot be neglected. Lyon's first patient had a distal ureteral tumor which he treated and followed ureteroscopically [2]. These efforts of treatment have continued to the present-day endoscopic approach to tumors in the upper tract over 3 cm in diameter [39]. This effort has required biopsy devices, both forceps and baskets, and ablative devices including both electrodes and lasers. Neodymium and holmium:YAG lasers have been employed. Here again, better sampling and ablative devices will be helpful.

Current Development

Endoscopic Histology

Confocal microscopy offers the chance to see histology in real time in situ. This approach uses a very fine beam of light passed into the subject tissue to minimize scatter. It has been used very successfully and has become a standard technique in ophthalmology. It has been used on a study basis in the urinary tract, both the bladder and upper tract. Its role remains to be defined [40].

Diagnostic Color Imaging

There are several efforts to enlist color in endoscopic imaging to emphasize neoplasms. In general these techniques amplify the visualization of tumor vasculature with alteration of the illumination or by chemical identification of the tumor itself.

Blue light cystoscopy with hexaminolevulinate instilled into the bladder is the most thoroughly studied form. It has been shown to enhance visualization of tumors and CIS and has been recommended in published guidelines. It has not been studied in the upper tract and presents specific technical difficulties because of the need to instill the medication and maintain contact for 1 h in the study area [41, 42].

Narrow-band imaging (NBI) uses only specific wavelengths of blue and green light to enhance visualization of tumors. No medical or chemical sensitization is needed. Early studies in the upper tract have suggested value in detection of tumors when compared to white light [43].

Storz has an endoscopic visual enhancement system which can lighten dark areas of an image and can intensify color contrast to assist in differentiation of tissue types. It has been used for cystoscopy and extensively in laparoscopy but remains to be studied definitively in ureteroscopy [44].

Robotics

The first public presentation of a robotic ureteroscope was at the World Congress of Endourology in 2006. Flexible ureteroscopy is a complex procedure with a long learning curve and has become a possible target for robotic assistance. Clinical use of the instrument was not published until 2011 [45]. A specially designed flexible shaft was employed but at 14F was too large for general application. It was later considered as part of a multipurpose robotic base but has not been commercialized. A later entry was a robot which used commercially available flexible ureteroscopes with a dedicated console and manipulator [46]. This model could be produced more economically and benefited from the known and well-designed ureteroscopes. It has not reached commercialization and general acceptance. It can be expected that robotics will play a role in flexible endoscopy at some point in the future.

The Ideal Ureteroscope

Despite the developments over the past 3+ decades, we still have not achieved the perfect ureteroscope, particularly among the flexible designs. The small rigid ureteroscopes have proven their value in use and longevity, both in terms of durability and continued production. This durability must be maintained. The size should remain at 7F or less for ease of insertion. Imaging could be improved with finer fiber-optic bundles or digital chips. The number of channels required may change with the development of different working instruments.

Flexible ureteroscopes remain far from the ideal. The shaft size should be no larger than 7.5F. The ideal would be closer to 6F [47]. The length is satisfactory at 65–70 cm. The channel has become standardized at 3.6F, but a smaller lumen may be adequate as working instruments become smaller. The overall weight should be as light as possible to minimize operator fatigue and long-term hand and arm injury. Similarly, the handle can be changed and should be ergonomically designed for comfort and usability to minimize thumb fatigue [48]. High-resolution imaging is essential. These endoscopes should be affordable for all settings (Table 1.1).

Table 1.1   Features of an ideal flexible ureteroscope

Working length	65–70
Shaft size	≤7.5F [46]
Channel	3.6F possibly smaller
Weight	As light as possible
Handle	Ergonomically designed for comfort and usability to minimize thumb fatigue
Imaging	High-resolution video
Cost	Broadly affordable

References

1. Leone NT, Garcia-Roig M, Bagley DH. Changing trends in the use of ureteroscopic instruments from 1996 to 2008. J Endourol March. 2010;24(3):361–5.
2. Lyon ES. The birth of modern ureteroscopy: the Albona Jaybis story. J Endourol. 2004;18(6):525–6.
3. Hanlan CR. Bozzini: endoscope returns. Bull of Am Coll Surg. 2002;87:39–40.
4. Desmoreaux AJ. The endoscope and its application to the diagnosis and treatment of affections of the genitourinary passages. Chicago Medizinhist J. 1867;24:177–94.
5. Reuter MA, Reuter HJ. The development of the cystosocope. J Urol. 1997;159:638–40.
6. Herr HW. Max Nitze, the cystoscope and urology. J Urol. 2006;176:1313–6.
7. Moran ME. The light bulb, cystoscopy and Thomas Alva Edison. J Endourol. 2010;24(9):1395–7.
8. Buerger L. A new indirect irrigating observation and double catheterizing cystoscope. Ann Surg. 1909;49:225–37.
9. Hopkins HH. Optical principles of the endoscope in: endoscopy (Berci G ed). New York: Appleton Century Crafts; 1976. p. 3–26.
10. Coladon D. On the reflections of a ray of light inside a parabolic liquid stream. Comptes Rendus. 1842;15:800.
11. Hecht J. City of lights: the story of fiber optics. New York: Oxford University Press; 1999. p. 13–27.
12. Hirschowitz BI, Curtiss LE, Peters CW, Pollard HM. Gastroenterology. 1958;35:50. rlow DE. Fiberoptic instrument technology. In: Small animal endoscopy. St. Louis: C.V. Mosby; 1990. p.1.
13. Nesbit RM. Congenital valvular obstruction of the prostatic urethra. J Urol. 1944;48:509.
14. Marshall VF. Fiber optics in urology. J Urol. 1964;91:110.
15. Takayasu H, Aso Y. Recent development for pyeloureteroscopy: guide tube method for its introduction into the ureter. J Urol. 1974;112:176.
16. Goodman TM. Ureteroscopy with pediatric cystoscope in adults. Urology. 1977;9(4):394.
17. Lyon ES, Kyker KS, Shoenberg HW. Transurethral ureteroscopy in women: a ready addition to the urological armamentarium. J Urol. 1978;119:35.
18. Lyon ES, Banno JJ, Shoenberg HW. Transurethral ureteroscopy in men using juvenile cystoscopy equipment. J Urol. 1979;122:152.
19. Perez-Castro EE, Martinez-Piniero JA. Transurethral ureteroscopy-a current urological procedure. Arch Esp Urol. 1980;33(5):445–60.
20. Das S. Transurethral ureteroscopy and stone manipulation under direct vision. J Urol. 1981;125:112.
21. Huffman JL, Bagley DH, Lyon ES. Treatment of distal ureteral calculi using rigid ureteroscope. Urology. 1982;20(6):574.

22. Huffman JL, Bagley DH, Schoenberg HW, Lyon ES. Transurethral removal of large ureteral and renal pelvic calculi using ureteroscopic ultrasonic lithotripsy. J Urol. 1983;130:31–4.
23. Huffman J. Personal communication.
24. Chaussy C, Fuchs G, Kahn R, Hunter P, Goodfriend R. Transurethral ultrasonic ureterolithotripsy using a solid-wire probe. Urology. 1987;29:531–2.
25. Dretler SP. An evaluation of ureteral laser lithotripsy: 225 consecutive patients. J Urol. 1990;143:267–72.
26. Abdel-Razzak OM, Bagley DH. The 6.9F semi-rigid ureteroscope in clinical use. Urology. 1993;41(1):45–8.
27. Bagley DH. Flexible ureteropyeloscopy with a modular, "disposable" endoscope. Urology. 1987;29:296–300.
28. Tom WR, Wolllin DA, Jiang R, Radvak D, Simmons WN, Preminger GM, Lipkin ME. Next generation single use ureteroscopes: an in vitro comparison. J Endourol. 2017;12:1301–6.
29. Emiliani E, Traxer O. Single use and disposable flexible ureteroscopes. Curr Opin Urol. 2017;27:176–81.
30. Scotland KB, Chan JYH, Chew BH. Single use flexible ureteroscopes: how do they compare with reusable ureteroscopes? J Endourol. 2019;33:71–8.
31. Hennessey DB, Fojecki GL, Papa NP, et al. Single use disposable digital flexible uretero-scopes: an exvivo assessment and cost analysis. BJU Int. 2018;121(Suppl 3):55–61.
32. Traxer O, Dubosq F, Jamali K, et al. New generation flexible ureterorenoscopes are more durable than previous ones. Urology. 2006;68(2):276–9.
33. Kromolowksy E, McDowell Z, Moore B, et al. Cost analysis of flexible ureteroscope repairs: evaluation of 655 procedures in a community based practice. J Endourol. 2016;30:254–6.
34. Carey RI, Gomez CS, Maurizi G, et al. Frequency of ureteroscope damage seen at a tertiary care center. J Urol. 2006;176:607–10.
35. Defidio L, DeDominicis M, DiGianfrancesco L, Fuchs G, Patel A. Improving flexible uretero-renoscope durability up to 100 procedures. J Endourol. 2012;26(10):1329–34.
36. Webb DR, Kockelberg R, Johnson WF. The Versapulse holmium:YAG laser in clinical urol-ogy: a pilot study. Minim Invas Ther. 1993;2:23–6.
37. Johnson DE, Cromeens DM, Price RE. Use of the holmium:YAG laser in urology. Lasers Surg Med. 1992;12:353–63.
38. Honey RJ. Assessment of a new tipless nitinol stone basket and comparison with an existing flat-wire basket. J Endourol. 1998;12:529–31.
39. Scotland KB, Kleinmann N, Cason D, Hubbard L, Tanimoto R, Healy KA, Hubosky SG, Bagley DH. Ureteroscopic management of large ≥ 2 cm upper tract urothelial carcinoma: a comprehensive twenty-three year experience. Urology. 2018;121:66–73.
40. Chen SP, Liao JC. Confocal laser endomicroscopy of bladder and upper tract urothelial carci-noma: a new era of optical diagnosis? Curr Urol Rep. 2014;15(9):437.
41. Chou R, Selph S, Buckley DI, et al. Comparative effectiveness of fluorescent versus white light cystoscopy for initial diagnosis or surveillance of bladder cancer on clinical outcomes: systematic review and meta-analysis. J Urol. 2017;197:548–58.
42. Smith AB, Daneshmand S, Patel S, et al. Patient-reported outcomes of blue-light flexible cys-toscopy with hexaminolevulinate in the surveillance of bladder cancer: results from a prospec-tive multicentre study. BJU Int. 2019;123(1):35–41.
43. Traxer O, Geavlete B, deMedina SG, et al. Narrow band imaging digital flexible ureteros-copy in detection of upper urinary transitional cell carcinoma: initial experience. J Endourol. 2011;25(1):19–23.
44. Kamphius GM, deBruin DM, Brandt MJ, et al. Comparing image perception of bladder tumors in four different Storz professional image enhancement system modalities using the íSPIES app. J Endourol. 2016;30(5):602–8.
45. Desai MM, Aron M, Gill IS, et al. Flexible robotic retrograde renoscopy: description of novel robotic device and preliminary laboratory experience. Urology. 2008;72(1):42–6.

46. Rassweiler J, Fiedler M, Charalampogiannis N, et al. Robot-assisted flexible ureteroscopy: an update. Urolithiasis. 2018;46(1):69–77.
47. Hudson RG, Conlin MJ, Bagley DH. Ureteric access with flexible ureteroscopes: effect of the size of the ureteroscope. BJU Int. 2005;95(7):1043–4.
48. Healy KA, Pak RW, Cleary RC, Colon-Herdman A, Bagley DH. Hand problems among Endourologists. J Endourol Dec. 2011;25(12):1915–20.

Chapter 2
Indications for Ureteroscopy: Guidelines

Igor Sorokin and Margaret S. Pearle

Introduction

Historically, shock wave lithotripsy (SWL) was the preferred treatment modality for proximal ureteral and small renal calculi. However, with expanded indications for ureteroscopy (URS), URS utilization has increased such that it has now equaled or surpassed SWL as the most common stone procedure in many countries around the word [1]. Indeed, the cost of URS remains the lowest among stone procedures, especially in developed countries.

With the increasing prevalence of stone disease worldwide, the American Urological Association (AUA) [2, 3] and the European Association of Urology (EAU) [4] have developed guidelines for the surgical management of kidney stones that are based on outcomes derived from the literature. These two Guidelines differ in the classifications utilized for level of evidence and strength of recommendations (Table 2.1) [5], although overall the treatment recommendations from the two Associations are similar, with slight differences in the indications for URS and SWL. We explore these differences in the two Guidelines and review the literature, focusing on the specific indications for URS.

I. Sorokin
Department of Urology, University of Massachusetts, Worcester, MA, USA

M. S. Pearle (✉)
Department of Urology, UT Southwestern Medical Center, Dallas, TX, USA

Charles and Jane Pak Center for Mineral Metabolism and Bone Research,
UT Southwestern Medical Center, Dallas, TX, USA
e-mail: margaret.pearle@utsouthwestern.edu

© Springer Nature Switzerland AG 2020
B. F. Schwartz, J. D. Denstedt (eds.), *Ureteroscopy*,
https://doi.org/10.1007/978-3-030-26649-3_2

Table 2.1 Recommendations from AUA and EAU Guidelines on surgical management of renal and ureteral calculi

		AUA Guideline	EAU Guideline
Ureteral stones			
Ureteral stones – general recommendations		Size >10 mm	Size >6 mm
		Treat after 4–6 weeks if failed conservative management	No specific observation time period recommended
Distal ureteral stones	<10 mm	1st line = URS	SWL or URS
		2nd line = SWL	
	>10 mm	1st line = URS	1st line = URS
		2nd line = SWL	2nd line = SWL
Proximal ureteral stone	<10 mm	No specific 1st line recommendations[a]	SWL or URS
	>10 mm	No specific 1st line recommendations[a]	1st line = URS
			2nd line = SWL
Renal stones			
Asymptomatic renal stones		No specific size criteria	Size >15 mm
			If no treatment follow periodically (initially 6 months then yearly imaging)
Renal stones, non-lower pole	<10 mm	SWL or URS	1st line = SWL or URS
			2nd line = PCNL
	10–20 mm	SWL or URS	SWL or URS or PCNL
	>20 mm	1st line = PCNL	1st line = PCNL
		*SWL not recommended	2nd line = URS or SWL
Renal stones, lower pole	<10 mm	SWL or URS	1st line = SWL or URS
			2nd line = PCNL
	10–20 mm	URS or PCNL	URS or PCNL or SWL
		*SWL not recommended	
	>20 mm	URS or PCNL	1st line = PCNL
		*SWL not recommended	2nd line = URS or SWL
Other recommendations			
Stone composition		URS for cystine or uric acid stones (that failed MET or desire intervention)	URS/PCNL for cystine, brushite, calcium oxalate monohydrate
Residual fragments		No specific size criteria	Size >5 mm
Calyceal diverticulum		URS/PCNL/lap/robotic depending on situation	SWL, PCNL (if possible), or URS
		*SWL not recommended	Patients may become asymptomatic after SWL, but stone may remain
Horseshoe kidney		Consider PCNL over URS for lower pole stone >10 mm	Acceptable SFR can be achieved with URS
Kidney transplant		No specific recommendation	Offer patients SWL, URS, or PCNL as management options
Pediatric urolithiasis		SWL or URS 1st line for ≤20 mm renal stone burden	SWL 1st line for <20 mm stone burden

URS ureteroscopy, *SWL* shock wave lithotripsy, *PCNL* percutaneous nephrolithotomy, *SFR* stone-free rate
[a]Overall URS has greater SFR in single procedure, and SWL has lower morbidity

Ureteral Calculi

Ureteroscopy can be utilized for stones in any location in the ureter. The 2016 AUA Surgical Management of Stones Guideline [3] reported higher overall stone-free rates (SFR) for URS compared to SWL for treatment of patients with ureteral stones (median SFR 90% for URS versus 72% for SWL, RR SWL/URS 0.294, 95% CI 0.214–0.404, $p < 0.001$). Although URS SFRs increased the more distally in the ureter the stone is located, SWL SFRs did not show location-dependence. Size-stratified outcomes demonstrated that for ≤10 mm ureteral stones, URS SFRs were superior to SWL SFRs at all locations in the ureter (85% versus 66.5%, respectively, for proximal; 91% versus 75%, respectively, for middle; and 94% versus 74%, respectively, for distal ureteral stones). On the other hand, while URS SFRs were superior to SWL SFRs in the middle and distal ureter for stones >10 mm in size (82.5% versus 67%, respectively, for middle ureter and 92% versus 71%, respectively, for distal ureter), there was little difference between the two treatment modalities for larger stones in the proximal ureter (79% for URS and 74% for SWL) [3]. A large, prospective, international URS registry from the Clinical Research Office of the Endourological Society (CROES) comprised of 9681 patients with ureteral stones demonstrated similar SFRs of 84.5%, 89%, and 94% for stones in the proximal, middle, and distal ureter, respectively [6]. SFRs were lower overall (77%) for patients with stones in multiple ureteral locations.

The recommendation of one treatment modality over another for management of patients with ureteral stones depends not only on SFRs but also complication rates. Analysis by the AUA Guideline Panel [3] revealed no significant differences in complication rates between URS and SWL with regard to urinary tract infection (UTI), sepsis, or ureteral stricture, but URS was associated with a higher rate of ureteral perforation than SWL (3.2% versus 0%, respectively). Consequently, the Panel stated that URS is the procedure associated with the highest SFR in a single procedure but that SWL is associated with lower morbidity.

The 2017 EAU Guidelines on Urolithiasis [4] also found higher SFRs up to 4 weeks for URS compared to SWL, although at 3 months the difference was not statistically significant. Likewise, the Panel reported less need for re-treatment and secondary procedures compared to SWL. However, complication rates and need for adjuvant procedures were higher, and hospital stay was longer for URS compared to SWL. Consequently, the EAU recommendation for the management of ureteral stones, which were classified as proximal or distal only, differs slightly from the AUA recommendations. For <10 mm proximal or distal ureteral stones, the EAU Guideline recommends either URS or SWL as first-line therapy. However, for >10 mm ureteral stones, the Panel recommends URS as first-line and SWL as second-line therapy.

It is noteworthy that most of the data on which both Guidelines are based are derived from retrospective studies, with few prospective and/or randomized trials. Furthermore, many of the studies assessing outcomes in patients with proximal ureteral stones were based on semirigid URS. Indeed, among 2656 patients with proximal ureteral stones from the CROES global ureteroscopy study, 72% were treated

with semirigid ureteroscopy alone [6]. Although SFRs were not significantly different between semirigid and flexible URS (84% versus 85.5% respectively), failure
(3.2% versus 1%, respectively, $p < 0.05$) and retreatment (14% versus 8%, respectively, $p < 0.01$) rates were significantly higher with semirigid URS [6]. A recent
multicenter, prospective study evaluating outcomes of flexible URS for the management of proximal ureteral calculi (mean stone size 7.4 mm) reported an overall SFR
of 95% among 71 patients, although stone clearance was assessed by plain abdominal radiography (KUB) and renal ultrasound (US) at 4–6 weeks rather than the more
sensitive computed tomography (CT) [7]. Notably, all ten patients with residual
stones had an initial stone size >10 mm. This study further validates the endorse-
ment of flexible URS for the treatment of patients with proximal ureteral stones.
Although the CROES study demonstrates that semirigid URS can be successfully
used to treat proximal ureteral stones, particularly in woman, the higher failure and
retreatment rates with semirigid URS validate the AUA Guideline statement that
"clinicians performing URS for proximal ureteral stones should have a flexible ureteroscope available" [3].

Renal Calculi

The indications for treatment of renal calculi are multifold. The EAU Guidelines on
Urolithiasis cite the following specific indications for active stone removal: growth
of stones, symptomatic stones, stones >15 mm in size, stones <15 mm in size for
which observation is not optimal, infection, stones in patients at high risk of stone
growth, obstruction, patient preference for treatment, comorbidities, and patient circumstances (occupation, travel) [4]. Acknowledging that the need for treatment of
calyceal stones is not well-defined, the EAU Guideline specifically recommends
treatment of calyceal calculi that are associated with obstruction, infection, and
acute and/or chronic pain.

The AUA Guideline also supports the treatment of patients with symptomatic,
non-obstructing, calyceal stones in whom no other etiology of the pain is identified
[3]. In addition, the Panel recommends intervention for asymptomatic stones in
cases of stone growth, associated infection, and specific situations such as voca-
tional requirements or poor access to medical care [2, 3]. While the AUA Guideline
did not specify a stone size threshold for treatment, the EAU Guideline recommends
active stone removal for renal stones exceeding 15 mm[4].

For patients with asymptomatic stones that are not associated with infection or
obstruction, the need for intervention is less clear. Natural history studies indicate a
cumulative likelihood of developing symptoms or requiring intervention of nearly
50% at 5 years after diagnosis [8–10]. As such, the AUA Panel offers that patients with
asymptomatic, non-obstructing calyceal stones may be offered active surveillance [3].

For patients in whom intervention is indicated and/or desired, both the AUA [3]
and EAU [4] Guidelines support the use of URS for the treatment of <20 mm non-
lower pole renal calculi, although the EAU Panel additionally considers SWL an

acceptable first-line therapy for <10 mm stones and percutaneous nephrolithotomy (PCNL) an acceptable first-line therapy for 10–20 mm stones. The AUA Guideline recommends either URS or SWL for <20 mm non-lower pole renal calculi.

For stones exceeding 20 mm in size, there is consensus that PCNL is the recommended first-line therapy for renal calculi regardless of location in the kidney. However, reports of URS treatment of >20 mm renal calculi have generally indicated favorable outcomes, with a weighted mean SFR of 79% in selected series (Table 2.2) [11–18]. Geraghty and co-workers [18] performed a systematic review of 12 series comprising 651 patients who underwent URS for treatment of large (>2 cm) renal calculi and reported a 91% SFR. However, nearly half the patients required more than one procedure to achieve that SFR; in nearly all series, plain abdominal radiographs and renal ultrasound were used to determine stone-free status, and "stone-free" in many series included <4 mm residual fragments. Given the high single procedure SFRs for PCNL for stones of this size, URS is not recommended for routine treatment of large renal calculi by either Guideline.

For the purpose of treatment recommendations, the lower pole of the kidney is distinguished from non-lower pole locations because of the lower SFRs reported with SWL of lower pole stones compared to other locations. For ≤10 mm lower pole stones, both URS and SWL are considered acceptable first-line treatment options. Indeed, a multicenter, randomized controlled trial (RCT) in which 78 initial patients with ≤10 mm lower pole stones were randomized to SWL or URS found no significant difference in SFRs between the two modalities, despite a 15% difference in SFRs favoring URS (35% for SWL and 50% for URS) [19]. However, for lower pole stones 10–20 mm in size, the AUA Guideline recommend URS but not SWL because of poor SFR for SWL of >10 mm stones [20]. This recommendation is additionally supported by retrospective data from a matched cohort of 99 patients with 1–2 cm lower pole stones who underwent SWL or flexible URS which found significantly higher SFRs by CT imaging (86.5% versus 68%, respectively, $p = 0.038$) and lower retreatment rate (8% versus 60%, respectively, $p < 0.001$) for URS than SWL [21].

The development of improved ureteroscopes, small laser fibers, and nitinol baskets resulted in less impact on ureteroscope deflectability, thereby allowing more reliable entry of the ureteroscope into difficult-to-access lower pole locations and successful stone treatment [19]. As such, URS has become a viable treatment option for lower pole stones. Although introduction of a laser fiber can result in loss of 10–15° of deflection of a flexible ureteroscope leading to failure of access into the lower pole [22], repositioning of a lower pole stone to a less dependent calyx can salvage a ureteroscopic procedure and improve SFR. Relocation of 1–2 cm lower pole stones during URS resulted in higher SFRs compared to in situ URS (100% versus 29%, $p < 0.001$) in one comparative retrospective study [23].

While historically, series of URS for intrarenal calculi demonstrated high SFRs, ranging from 77% to 91% [24–26], these early URS series relied on KUB and/or US to assess stone-free status. More contemporary series utilizing CT have shown substantially lower SFRs, ranging from 50% to 62% [19, 27–29]. The consequences of residual fragments include stone growth, stone passage, or need for surgical

Table 2.2 Flexible ureteroscopy for >20 mm renal stones

Study	Type	No. Pts	Mean stone size (mm)	SFR	SFR definition	Imaging	Complications	Mean no. proc
El-Anany et al. (2001) [11]	Retrospective	30	>20	77% (23/30)	<2 mm	US/KUB	6.6%	1.0
Ricchiuti et al. (2007) [12]	Retrospective	23	30.9	74% (17/23)	<2 mm	CT/KUB	0%	1.4
Hyams et al. (2010) [13]	Retrospective	120	24	83% (100/120)	≤4 mm	CT/US/KUB	6.7%	1.2
Takazawa et al. (2011) [14]	Retrospective	20	31	85% (22/26)	≤4 mm	CT/KUB	5%	1.4
Cohen et al. (2012) [15]	Retrospective	145	29	87% (143/164)	≤4 mm	US/KUB	1.9%	1.6
Karakoyunlu et al. (2015) [16]	Prospective	30	27	30% (9/30)	≤2 mm	US/KUB	3.6%[a]	1.8
Karakoç et al. (2015) [17]	Retrospective	57	>20	67% (38/57)	–	CT	3.5%	–
Geraghty et al. (2016) [18]	Retrospective	43	29	84% (36/43)	≤2 mm	US/KUB	8.8%	1.6
Total	–	468	–	79% (388/493)	–	–	–	–

Pts patient, *SFR* stone-free rate

[a]Clavien ≥2

intervention. The incidence of a stone-related event attributable to residual fragments has been reported in 20–44% of patients, with need for surgical intervention in up to 29% [30–32]. Although the AUA Guideline does not specify a size threshold above which intervention is recommended for RFs, the Panel did recommend that patients be offered an endoscopic procedure to remove RFs [2]. On the other hand, the EAU Guideline recommends intervention for fragments >5 mm [4]. Neither Guideline takes into account the imaging modality used to determine stone-free status.

The need for retreatment after URS for renal calculi increases with stone size. Karakoyunlu and colleagues [16] performed a single-center RCT comparing PCNL ($n = 30$) to staged URS ($n = 30$) for >2 cm renal pelvic stones (mean stone size 27 mm for URS and 26 mm for PCNL). Repeat URS was performed until patients were left with no RF or with RFs ≤ 4 mm. PCNL was performed only once. URS patients underwent a mean of 1.83 sessions per patient (one session in 9 patients, two sessions in 17 patients, and three sessions in 4 patients) and also required a mean of 2 weeks of treatment time to become stone-free. SFR was statistically comparable between the two treatment modalities despite lower SFR for URS (67% for URS and 87% for PCNL, $p = 0.067$), and therefore the authors concluded that if patients are willing to accept longer overall treatment and operative times and a greater number of procedures, then staged URS is an effective and safe modality.

Bilateral Stones

Bilateral stones occur frequently, and many patients desire same-session bilateral treatment to prevent future stone events. Neither Guideline specifically endorses nonurgent, simultaneous, bilateral treatment of renal calculi, although there are substantial published data addressing bilateral URS. Review of the CROES global URS registry identified 2153 patients treated for multiple renal and/or ureteral calculi, of whom 1880 (87.3%) and 273 (12.7%) underwent unilateral and same-session bilateral URS, respectively [33]. Although there was no significant difference in complication rates between unilateral and bilateral URS groups, univariate analysis demonstrated lower SFRs (OR 0.7, 95% CI 0.49–1.00, $p = 0.048$), higher re-treatment rates (OR 1.52, 95% CI 1.13–2.05, $p = 0.006$), and longer operative times (OR 1.41, 95% CI 1.11–1.80, $p = 0.005$) for same-session bilateral URS compared to unilateral URS.

Ingimarsson and associates [34] identified 113 patients who underwent 117 bilateral same-session URS for renal and/or ureteral calculi. SFR assessed by KUB/US at 6 weeks was 91%. Ureteral injuries occurred in 2.1% of renal units (5/234), of which 3 were superficial (grade I) and 1 each were grade II and grade III, all of which were managed with stent placement for 2 weeks. Short-term complications were largely Clavien-Dindo I–II ($n = 15$) and the remainder were Clavien-Dindo III ($n = 4$). At 6 weeks follow-up, no patients demonstrated evidence of stricture, new-onset hydronephrosis, or significant change in creatinine from baseline. Of note, 11% of patients required immediate, unplanned admission after surgery, and another

12% were seen in the emergency department within 30 days of the procedure with pain, fever, or other symptoms. An additional 19% of patients called with stent pain or renal colic post-stent removal. The authors admit these numbers may indicate a higher rate of discomfort after bilateral same-session URS than after unilateral URS. Indeed, in a retrospective study of 1798 patients undergoing URS, Tan and co-workers [35] found on multivariate analysis that bilateral URS was one of the factors associated with a higher likelihood of unplanned admission (OR 2.88, 95% CI 1.19–6.99, $p = 0.019$).

A number of bilateral same-session ureteroscopy series have been reported [34, 36–41] (Table 2.3). SFRs after one therapeutic session ranged from 52% to 90%. Mild ureteral injuries were not uncommon, and one study [37] with long-term follow-up showed that 4.5% of patients developed ureteral strictures after 6–12 months. Major postoperative complications were uncommon, with most complications classified as Clavien grades I–II. Despite demonstrated safety and efficacy of bilateral same-session URS, however, many surgeons are still reluctant to perform bilateral URS. Rivera and colleagues [42] conducted a survey of 153 members of the Endourological Society querying them on their preferred management of bilateral stone disease. Although a higher proportion of urologists were willing to perform same-session bilateral URS (48%) than bilateral PCNL (38%), still less than half of urologists surveyed indicated that they are comfortable treating stones in both kidneys and ureters in the same setting ureteroscopically.

Although stones in both kidneys and/or ureters that otherwise fall within established guidelines for ureteroscopic management may be treated ureteroscopically under the same anesthetic, no guidelines for operative time limits or total stone burden have been established for same-session bilateral procedures. Furthermore, patients should be informed that bilateral procedures and/or stents may result in greater discomfort and/or a higher likelihood of emergency department visits or hospital admission. Without further guidance, treatment of bilateral renal and/or ureteral calculi should be left to the discretion of the surgeon.

Stones in Patients with a Solitary Kidney

The indications for URS in patients with renal or ureteral calculi in a solitary renal unit generally follow the same guidelines as for unilateral stones in a patient with two kidneys. A recent systematic review comprising 12 papers and 696 patients who underwent URS for stones in a solitary kidney (mean stone size 10–27 mm) revealed a mean SFR of 72% [43]. Although complications occurred in 16.4% of patients, major complications (Clavien ≥ 3) occurred in only 2%, including ureteral perforation ($n = 6$) and avulsion ($n = 4$). Of note, the AUA Guideline states that one of the criteria that must be satisfied in order to safely omit ureteral stenting after URS is a *normal contralateral kidney* [3]. As such, placement of a ureteral stent after URS in a solitary kidney is strongly advised.

Table 2.3 Bilateral same-session ureteroscopy for calculi series

Study	No. Pts/no. renal units	Total stone burden	Stone-free rate[a]	Intra-op complications	Post-op complications	Long-term complications	ER visits and/or readmission
Hollenbeck et al. (2003) [36]	23/46[b]	Mean 16.1 mm	52% (11/21)	4% (1/24)	29% (7/24)	–	17% (4/23)
El-Hefnawy et al. (2011) [37]	89/178	–	86% (153/178)	6.2% (11/178)	3% (3/89)[c]	4.5% (4/89)[d]	–
Gunlusoy et al. (2012) [38]	55/110	Mean 11.0 mm	90% (99/110)	7.3% (4/55)	29% (16/55)	–	–
Mushtaque et al. (2012) [39]	60/120	Range 6–20 mm	85% (51/60)	10% (6/60)[e]	27% (16/60)[e]	–	–
Huang et al. (2012) [40]	25/50	Mean 24 mm	70%	0% (0/25)	16% (4/25)[c]	0% (0/25)	–
Drake et al. (2015) [41]	21 (25 procedures)	Mean 21 mm	80% (34/42)	0% (0/25)	14% (3/21)[c]	0% (0/21)	–
Ingimarsson et al. (2017) [34]	117/234	Median renal stone = 6.9 mm Median ureteral stone = 7.0 mm	87% (134/154)	2.1% (5/234)[f]	16.2% (19/117)	0% (0/117)	23% (27/117)

Pts patients, *ER* emergency room
[a]After one single therapeutic session
[b]One patient required stent placement initially without treatment thus 23 patients with 24 procedures
[c]Clavien (I–II) only
[d]Four patients (4.5%) developed ureteral strictures at 6–12-month follow-up
[e]Minor ureteral perforations or false passages from impacted stones
[f]Three superficial ureteral injuries, one grade II, one grade III

Stones in Patients with Bleeding Diatheses

The AUA Guideline specifically addressed the management of patients with stones and uncorrected bleeding diatheses, recommending URS as first-line therapy when bleeding diatheses cannot or should not be corrected [2]. In the global URS study from CROES, among 11,719 patients undergoing URS, 6% were on medications that increase bleeding risk at the time of surgery, with the most common medication being aspirin [44]. Among these patients, 1.1% experienced a bleeding complication compared with 0.4% of patients on no therapy ($p < 0.01$). Furthermore, those on medications that carry a bleeding risk demonstrated higher complication rates overall compared to those on no such medications (7% versus 3.3%, $p < 0.001$).

A recent systematic review and meta-analysis of eight URS series (seven retrospective and one prospective from CROES) compared outcomes in patients on medications that increase bleeding risk versus those on no such medication [45]. The at-risk cohort demonstrated a 2.2% incidence of bleeding complications, and pooled analysis revealed a more than threefold increased bleeding risk in the treatment arm ($n = 1075$) over the control arm ($n = 11,687$) (RR 3.59, 95% CI, 1.81–5.73, $p < 0.0001$). Major complications included 4 patients with clot retention, 2 with clot colic, 16 with mild hematuria, 1 with of epistaxis, 2 with retroperitoneal hemorrhage requiring transfusion, and another with hemorrhage requiring arterial embolization. Of note, pooled analysis of total complications, including thrombotic events, did not show a statistically significant difference between the groups.

Based on these data, URS in patients on anticoagulation therapy should be approached with caution, but the procedure can be performed with relatively low risk. The use of an access sheath and judicious use of pressurized irrigation to minimize intrarenal pressure may constitute measures that can be taken to reduce bleeding risk, although there is no evidence to support this. In the general population, subcapsular hematoma associated with URS occurs with an incidence of 0.45%, and predisposing factors include moderate-to-severe hydronephrosis, thin renal parenchyma, long operative time, hypertension, and preoperative urinary tract infection [46]. As such, clinicians should be especially cautious when considering URS in patients with any of these characteristics who are on medications that increase bleeding risk, and operative time should be minimized.

Stones in Obese Patients

The increasing prevalence of obesity as well as the association of obesity with stone disease has resulted in an increasing need to surgically treat obese patients with stones [47]. URS is an attractive option for treatment of obese patients because it requires very little alteration of standard procedure or need for specialized instrumentation as is required for PCNL. Furthermore, SWL may be prohibited by long skin-to-stone distances that exceed the distance between F1 and F2, thereby reducing

SWL success. The EAU Guidelines recommend URS over SWL as a more successful therapeutic option in morbidly obese patients [4].

A systematic review by Ishii and co-workers of 15 studies comprising 835 patients with a mean BMI of 40.5 kg/m² and a mean stone size of 14.2 mm found an overall SFR of 82.5% and a complication rate of 9.2%, outcomes that are comparable to those reported for URS in the general population [48]. Although the complication rate for morbidly obese patients was 17.6% in this review, twice that of obese patients at 8.4%, all complications in the morbidly obese group were Clavien grade II. While the sample size of this systematic review is large, the impact of the review is limited by the low quality of evidence and variable definitions of stone-free among the studies.

Krambeck and colleagues [49] analyzed data from the CROES study which included 10,099 patients undergoing URS with recorded BMI. Among this group, 17.4% of patients ($n = 1758$) were obese and 2.2% ($n = 223$) were morbidly obese. While the overall SFR was 87% with a 16.8% retreatment rate, multivariable analyses revealed that higher BMI was associated with lower SFR. On the other hand, no association was found between BMI and intraoperative complications, which overall occurred in 5.1% of patients.

The AUA Panel did not specifically address the role of URS in obese patients, but they did acknowledge the impact of obesity and skin-to-stone distance on the success of SWL and the need to consider endoscopic therapies when SWL is unlikely to be successful [2]. Consequently, URS should be considered first-line therapy in obese patients with stones who are not candidates for SWL and in whom stone size does not preclude URS.

Stones in Patients with Calyceal Diverticula

Because of distal obstruction from the narrow diverticular neck, SWL is generally not recommended for treatment of stones in calyceal diverticula. Meta-analysis by the AUA Guideline Panel demonstrated SFRs of only 13–21% for SWL, and consequently the Panel recommended endoscopic therapy for the optimal management of stones in calyceal diverticula, reporting SFRs of 18–90% for URS and 62.5–100% for PCNL [3]. Although the EAU Guidelines acknowledge that stone fragments are unlikely to clear after SWL of diverticular stones, SWL is still considered an option because in some patients, despite retained stone fragments, symptoms resolve [4]. Among endoscopic options, URS is usually best reserved for management of moderate-sized (<15 mm) mid-calyceal and upper pole diverticular stones or for stones in anterior calyceal diverticula. Challenges may arise in identifying the ostium in approximately 30% of cases via a ureteroscopic approach [50].

A retrospective review by Bas and colleagues [51] compared management of stone-bearing calyceal diverticula in 29 patients undergoing PCNL with 25 patients undergoing URS. Although mean stone size was significantly smaller for URS than

PCNL (211 mm^2 versus 154 mm^2, respectively, $p = 0.023$), both treatment modalities had high overall success, symptom-free, and complication rates. Major complications and need for blood transfusions occurred only with PCNL, and hospital length of stay was 2 days longer for PCNL than URS. While selection bias is likely at play in this nonrandomized comparison, it does demonstrate that URS in properly selected cases may appropriately represent first-line therapy for stone-bearing calyceal diverticula.

Stones in Patients with Horseshoe Kidneys

Horseshoe kidney is a common anatomical variant with an estimated incidence of 1 in 400–666 individuals that is associated with stones in 21–60% of those affected [52, 53]. The high rate of stone disease is likely multifactorial, due to both abnormal drainage causing urinary stasis and metabolic predisposition [54, 55]. Because of relative obstruction at the ureteropelvic junction caused by malrotation of the kidney and draping of the ureter over the isthmus, SWL SFRs are often poor [56]. However, URS can be challenging as well because of the high insertion and often narrow ureteropelvic junction and the acute infundibulopelvic angle associated with the medial lower pole calyces. Nonetheless, series of URS in horseshoe kidneys have demonstrated SFRs ranging from 78% to 84% [55, 57]. A systematic review of 3 studies encompassing 41 patients undergoing URS for stones in horseshoe kidneys (mean stone size 16 mm) revealed a SFR of 78% with a 32% complication rate (Clavien 1 and II only) [57]. As such, the EAU Guideline recommends URS as one of the treatment options in this setting, while the AUA Guideline cautions against URS for stones >10 mm in the lower pole calyces of a horseshoe kidney. PCNL remains a good salvage option for URS or SWL failures or as first-line therapy for large or complex stones in a horseshoe kidney.

Stones in Patients with a Transplant Kidney

Stones in transplant kidneys may impact graft function and cause significant morbidity if they obstruct. While smaller stones may be reasonably treated with SWL in the prone position, antegrade or retrograde URS and PCNL are viable treatment options. Successful retrograde URS depends on the degree of tortuosity of the ureter and the position of the ureteral orifice. Access to ureters implanted on the dome of the bladder can be challenging if not impossible, and access may require a variety of guidewires, angiographic catheters, and sheaths. The AUA Guideline does not address the treatment of stones in transplant kidneys, while the EAU advises that all treatment modalities including flexible URS, PCNL, and SWL are viable options, but acknowledge that SWL may result in poor SFR due to difficulty localizing the stone. A small retrospective series by Hyams and associates [58] evaluated outcomes of URS from a retrograde ($n = 7$) or antegrade ($n = 5$) approach. With a mean stone size of 8 mm and 11 of 12 patients with adequate follow-up, all patients were rendered stone-free except one patient who was left with a 2 mm RF that ultimately cleared with observation. While data is limited and technical challenges exist, an attempt at URS for smaller stone burdens in transplant kidneys is reasonable. The use of a ureteral access sheath to optimize maneuverability of the flexible ureteroscope is advisable but should be used with caution due to the compromised blood supply of the ureter.

Stones in Pregnant Patients

It is estimated that a stone event occurs in 1 out of every 200–1500 pregnancies and is the most common cause of hospitalization in pregnant women from non-obstetric causes [59, 60]. Although the incidence of stones has been reported to be no higher than in the general nonpregnant female population, stones in pregnant women can be a challenging and anxiety-provoking situation for both the patient and clinician. Historically stones in pregnant women that failed conservative management were typically treated with serial stent or nephrostomy tube changes. However, URS has recently become a widely acceptable treatment option, with multiple reports demonstrating stone-free and complication rates comparable to those in nonpregnant women [60–63]. As such, both the EAU and AUA Guidelines endorse URS as an acceptable alternative to long-term stenting/drainage in pregnant women who fail observation [2, 4]. Because SWL is contraindicated for the treatment of stones during pregnancy and PCNL is generally avoided due to the need for fluoroscopy in most cases, URS is generally the only definitive stone procedure offered during pregnancy [2, 4]. It is important to note that most data on URS in pregnant patients is derived from experienced surgeons at high-volume academic centers. Consequently, the recommendation of URS for the treatment of moderate-sized (<15 mm) obstructing ureteral stones presupposes the availability of adequate obstetric backup and an experienced ureteroscopist. Furthermore, URS for large or complex stones is best delayed until after delivery.

Symptomatic Patients with Non-obstructing Calyceal Stones

While most patients with non-obstructing, calyceal stones do not experience pain, some patients report symptoms of atypical renal colic characterized by non-radiating, persistent pain directly over the kidney [64]. Some investigators have hypothesized that these symptoms may be the result of the stone acting as an irritant to the collecting system leading to abnormal peristalsis or from increased localized renal pressure due to collecting duct obstruction [64, 65]. While the exact etiology of the pain has yet to be elucidated, eradication of flank pain after treatment of non-obstructing calyceal stones has been reported [3, 65, 66]. URS offers a good treatment option in these patients and may reduce the uncertainty of retained fragments associated with SWL, but patient selection should follow the same recommendations with regard to stone size and location as for symptomatic renal calculi. The AUA Guideline endorses treatment of the symptomatic, non-obstructing calyceal stones if other etiologies for the pain have been ruled out. However, it is important to have an honest discussion with the patient prior to intervention so he/she understands that removal of the stone may not necessarily alleviate their symptoms.

Pediatric Urolithiasis

Mirroring the trends of adult urolithiasis, a growing body of literature suggests the prevalence of pediatric urolithiasis, and consequently the need for surgical intervention for stones in children, is on the rise [67, 68]. SWL is an attractive option for treatment of stones in children as stents are unnecessary in most cases, and fragments tend to pass more readily in children than in adults, with long-term SFRs in the range of 57–92% [4]. However, miniaturization of ureteroscopes and instrumentation has made URS an increasingly viable treatment option for shock wave-resistant stones in the pediatric population, largely obviating the need for pre-stenting to passively dilate the ureter prior to URS.

The AUA and EAU Guidelines offer specific recommendations for the management of stones in children that take into account the higher SFRs for SWL in children compared to adults. The AUA meta-analysis demonstrated SFRs for URS of 95% and 78%, respectively, for ureteral stones ≤10 mm and >10 mm [2]. With comparable SWL SFRs, either treatment option is acceptable for ureteral stones in children. Of note, the AUA Panel recommends *against* the routine use of pre-stenting prior to URS because of the high success rate of ureteroscopic access in most cases.

Similar to the recommendations in adults, while the AUA Panel considers both URS and SWL acceptable first-line treatment options for ≤20 mm renal calculi in children, URS is not offered as recommended treatment for >20 mm renal calculi [2, 3]. In contrast, recognizing the higher success rates for SWL of larger stones in children, the EAU Guideline recommends SWL as first-line therapy for all stones <20 mm, while URS is considered a good alternative for SWL failures or if SWL is not anticipated to be successful [4]. Neither the AUA nor EAU Guideline used stone location as a deciding factor for the selection of optimal therapy for renal calculi.

Conclusions

Indications for URS in the management of urolithiasis have expanded from treatment of ureteral stones only to include increasingly larger stones and renal calculi. Furthermore, with improved instrumentation and technique, URS now provides an effective treatment option for stones in variety of circumstances where SWL is contraindicated and PCNL is considered too invasive, such as for stones in patients with horseshoe kidneys or calyceal diverticula, in pregnant women, and in patients with bleeding diatheses. Current guideline recommendations from both the AUA and EAU reflect a preference for URS over SWL for ureteral stones and the acceptance of URS as a first-line treatment option for <20 mm renal calculi. While current guidelines are limited by few published RCTs, lack of standardized definitions of stone-free, and nonuniformity in postoperative imaging practices, nonetheless they provide guidance for practitioners attempting to select appropriate treatment strategies for patients with renal and ureteral calculi. It is clear from the evolution of these guidelines that URS will continue to play an increasing role in the management of upper tract stones.

References

1. Raheem OA, Khandwala YS, Sur RL, et al. Burden of urolithiasis: trends in prevalence, treatments, and costs. Eur Urol Focus. 2017;3:18.
2. Assimos D, Krambeck A, Miller NL, et al. Surgical management of stones: American Urological Association/Endourological Society Guideline. PART I J Urol. 2016;196:1153.
3. Assimos D, Krambeck A, Miller NL, et al. Surgical management of stones: American Urological Association/Endourological Society Guideline. PART II J Urol. 2016;196:1161.
4. Turk C, Neisius A, Petrik A. et al. EAU guidelines on urolithiasis. 2017. Available at https://uroweb.org/guideline/urolithiasis.
5. Pradere B, Doizi S, Proietti S, et al. Evaluation of guidelines for surgical management of urolithiasis. J Urol. 2018;199:1267.
6. Perez Castro E, Osther PJ, Jinga V, et al. Differences in ureteroscopic stone treatment and outcomes for distal, mid-, proximal, or multiple ureteral locations: the Clinical Research Office of the Endourological Society ureteroscopy global study. Eur Urol. 2014;66:102.
7. Hyams ES, Monga M, Pearle MS, et al. A prospective, multi-institutional study of flexible ureteroscopy for proximal ureteral stones smaller than 2 cm. J Urol. 2015;193:165.
8. Burgher A, Beman M, Holtzman JL, et al. Progression of nephrolithiasis: long-term outcomes with observation of asymptomatic calculi. J Endourol. 2004;18:534.
9. Hubner W, Porpaczy P. Treatment of caliceal calculi. Br J Urol. 1990;66:9.
10. Inci K, Sahin A, Islamoglu E, et al. Prospective long-term followup of patients with asymptomatic lower pole caliceal stones. J Urol. 2007;177:2189.
11. El-Anany FG, Hammouda HM, Maghraby HA, et al. Retrograde ureteropyeloscopic holmium laser lithotripsy for large renal calculi. BJU Int. 2001;88:850.
12. Ricchiuti DJ, Smaldone MC, Jacobs BL, et al. Staged retrograde endoscopic lithotripsy as alternative to PCNL in select patients with large renal calculi. J Endourol. 2007;21:1421.
13. Hyams ES, Munver R, Bird VG, et al. Flexible ureterorenoscopy and holmium laser lithotripsy for the management of renal stone burdens that measure 2 to 3 cm: a multi-institutional experience. J Endourol. 2010;24:1583.
14. Takazawa R, Kitayama S, Tsujii T. Successful outcome of flexible ureteroscopy with holmium laser lithotripsy for renal stones 2 cm or greater. Int J Urol. 2012;19:264.
15. Cohen J, Cohen S, Grasso M. Ureteropyeloscopic treatment of large, complex intrarenal and proximal ureteral calculi. BJU Int. 2013;111:E127.
16. Karakoyunlu N, Goktug G, Sener NC, et al. A comparison of standard PCNL and staged retrograde FURS in pelvis stones over 2 cm in diameter: a prospective randomized study. Urolithiasis. 2015;43:283.

17. Karakoc O, Karakeci A, Ozan T, et al. Comparison of retrograde intrarenal surgery and percutaneous nephrolithotomy for the treatment of renal stones greater than 2 cm. Turk J Urol. 2015;41:73.
18. Geraghty R, Abourmarzouk O, Rai B, et al. Evidence for Ureterorenoscopy and Laser Fragmentation (URSL) for large renal stones in the modern era. Curr Urol Rep. 2015;16:54.
19. Pearle MS, Lingeman JE, Leveillee R, et al. Prospective, randomized trial comparing shock wave lithotripsy and ureteroscopy for lower pole caliceal calculi 1 cm or less. J Urol. 2005;173:2005.
20. Albala DM, Assimos DG, Clayman RV, et al. Lower pole I: a prospective randomized trial of extracorporeal shock wave lithotripsy and percutaneous nephrostolithotomy for lower pole nephrolithiasis-initial results. J Urol. 2001;166:2072.
21. El-Nahas AR, Ibrahim HM, Youssef RF, et al. Flexible ureterorenoscopy versus extracorporeal shock wave lithotripsy for treatment of lower pole stones of 10-20 mm. BJU Int. 2012;110:898.
22. Bach T, Geavlete B, Herrmann TR, et al. Working tools in flexible ureterorenoscopy--influence on flow and deflection: what does matter? J Endourol. 2008;22:1639.
23. Schuster TG, Hollenbeck BK, Faerber GJ, et al. Ureteroscopic treatment of lower pole calculi: comparison of lithotripsy in situ and after displacement. J Urol. 2002;168:43.
24. Fuchs GJ, Fuchs AM. Flexible endoscopy of the upper urinary tract. A new minimally invasive method for diagnosis and treatment. Urologe A. 1990;29:313.
25. Fabrizio MD, Behari A, Bagley DH. Ureteroscopic management of intrarenal calculi. J Urol. 1998;159:1139.
26. Grasso M. Ureteropyeloscopic treatment of ureteral and intrarenal calculi. Urol Clin North Am. 2000;27:623.
27. Portis AJ, Rygwall R, Holtz C, et al. Ureteroscopic laser lithotripsy for upper urinary tract calculi with active fragment extraction and computerized tomography followup. J Urol. 2006;175:2129.
28. Macejko A, Okotie OT, Zhao LC, et al. Computed tomography-determined stone-free rates for ureteroscopy of upper-tract stones. J Endourol. 2009;23:379.
29. Rippel CA, Nikkel L, Lin YK, et al. Residual fragments following ureteroscopic lithotripsy: incidence and predictors on postoperative computerized tomography. J Urol. 2012;188:2246.
30. Rebuck DA, Macejko A, Bhalani V, et al. The natural history of renal stone fragments following ureteroscopy. Urology. 2011;77:564.
31. Portis AJ, Laliberte MA, Heinisch A. Repeat surgery after ureteroscopic laser lithotripsy with attempted complete extraction of fragments: long-term follow-up. Urology. 2015;85:1272.
32. Chew BH, Brotherhood HL, Sur RL, et al. Natural history, complications and re-intervention rates of asymptomatic residual stone fragments after ureteroscopy: a report from the EDGE research consortium. J Urol. 2016;195:982.
33. Pace KT, Kroczak T, Wijnstok NJ, et al. Same session bilateral ureteroscopy for multiple stones: results from the CROES URS Global Study. J Urol. 2017;198:130.
34. Ingimarsson JP, Rivera M, Knoedler JJ, et al. Same-session bilateral ureteroscopy: safety and outcomes. Urology. 2017;108:29.
35. Tan HJ, Strope SA, He C, et al. Immediate unplanned hospital admission after outpatient ureteroscopy for stone disease. J Urol. 2011;185:2181.
36. Hollenbeck BK, Schuster TG, Faerber GJ, et al. Safety and efficacy of same-session bilateral ureteroscopy. J Endourol. 2003;17:881.
37. El-Hefnawy AS, El-Nahas AR, El-Tabey NA, et al. Bilateral same-session ureteroscopy for treatment of ureteral calculi: critical analysis of risk factors. Scand J Urol Nephrol. 2011;45:97.
38. Gunlusoy B, Degirmenci T, Arslan M, et al. Is bilateral ureterorenoscopy the first choice for the treatment of bilateral ureteral stones? An updated study. Urol Int. 2012;89:412.
39. Mushtaque M, Gupta CL, Shah I, et al. Outcome of bilateral ureteroscopic retrieval of stones in a single session. Urol Ann. 2012;4:158.
40. Huang Z, Fu F, Zhong Z, et al. Flexible ureteroscopy and laser lithotripsy for bilateral multiple intrarenal stones: is this a valuable choice? Urology. 2012;80:800.

41. Drake T, Ali A, Somani BK. Feasibility and safety of bilateral same-session flexible ureteroscopy (FURS) for renal and ureteral stone disease. Cent European J Urol. 2015;68:193.
42. Rivera ME, Bhojani N, Heinsimer K, et al. A survey regarding preference in the management of bilateral stone disease and a comparison of Clavien complication rates in bilateral vs unilateral percutaneous nephrolithotomy. Urology. 2018;111:48.
43. Pietropaolo A, Jones P, Whitehurst L, et al. Efficacy and safety of ureteroscopy for stone disease in a solitary kidney: findings from a systematic review. Urology. 2018;119:17–22.
44. Daels FP, Gaizauskas A, Rioja J, et al. Age-related prevalence of diabetes mellitus, cardiovascular disease and anticoagulation therapy use in a urolithiasis population and their effect on outcomes: the Clinical Research Office of the Endourological Society Ureteroscopy Global Study. World J Urol. 2015;33:859.
45. Sharaf A, Amer T, Somani BK, et al. Ureteroscopy in patients with bleeding diatheses, anticoagulated, and on anti-platelet agents: a systematic review and meta-analysis of the literature. J Endourol. 2017;31:1217.
46. Whitehurst LA, Somani BK. Perirenal hematoma after ureteroscopy: a systematic review. J Endourol. 2017;31:438.
47. Taylor EN, Stampfer MJ, Curhan GC. Obesity, weight gain, and the risk of kidney stones. JAMA. 2005;293:455.
48. Ishii H, Couzins M, Aboumarzouk O, et al. Outcomes of systematic review of ureteroscopy for stone disease in the obese and morbidly obese population. J Endourol. 2016;30:135.
49. Krambeck A, Wijnstok N, Olbert P, et al. The influence of body mass index on outcomes in ureteroscopy: results from the Clinical Research Office of Endourological Society URS Global Study. J Endourol. 2017;31:20.
50. Canales B, Monga M. Surgical management of the calyceal diverticulum. Curr Opin Urol. 2003;13:255.
51. Bas O, Ozyuvali E, Aydogmus Y, et al. Management of calyceal diverticular calculi: a comparison of percutaneous nephrolithotomy and flexible ureterorenoscopy. Urolithiasis. 2015;43:155.
52. Weizer AZ, Silverstein AD, Auge BK, et al. Determining the incidence of horseshoe kidney from radiographic data at a single institution. J Urol. 2003;170:1722.
53. Yohannes P, Smith AD. The endourological management of complications associated with horseshoe kidney. J Urol. 2002;168:5.
54. Raj GV, Auge BK, Assimos D, et al. Metabolic abnormalities associated with renal calculi in patients with horseshoe kidneys. J Endourol. 2004;18:157.
55. Blackburne AT, Rivera ME, Gettman MT, et al. Endoscopic management of urolithiasis in the horseshoe kidney. Urology. 2016;90:45.
56. Ray AA, Ghiculete D, RJ DAH, et al. Shockwave lithotripsy in patients with horseshoe kidney: determinants of success. J Endourol. 2011;25:487.
57. Ishii H, Rai B, Traxer O, et al. Outcome of ureteroscopy for stone disease in patients with horseshoe kidney: review of world literature. Urol Ann. 2015;7:470.
58. Hyams E, Marien T, Bruhn A, et al. Ureteroscopy for transplant lithiasis. J Endourol. 2012;26:819.
59. Ishii H, Aboumarzouk OM, Somani BK. Current status of ureteroscopy for stone disease in pregnancy. Urolithiasis. 2014;42:1.
60. Semins MJ, Matlaga BR. Kidney stones during pregnancy. Nat Rev Urol. 2014;11:163.
61. Semins MJ, Trock BJ, Matlaga BR. The safety of ureteroscopy during pregnancy: a systematic review and meta-analysis. J Urol. 2009;181:139.
62. Polat F, Yesil S, Kirac M, et al. Treatment outcomes of semirigid ureterorenoscopy and intracorporeal lithotripsy in pregnant women with obstructive ureteral calculi. Urol Res. 2011;39:487.
63. Travassos M, Amselem I, Filho NS, et al. Ureteroscopy in pregnant women for ureteral stone. J Endourol. 2009;23:405.
64. Coury TA, Sonda LP, Lingeman JE, et al. Treatment of painful caliceal stones. Urology. 1988;32:119.

65. Taub DA, Suh RS, Faerber GJ, et al. Ureteroscopic laser papillotomy to treat papillary calcifications associated with chronic flank pain. Urology. 2006;67:683.
66. Jura YH, Lahey S, Eisner BH, et al. Ureteroscopic treatment of patients with small, painful, non-obstructing renal stones: the small stone syndrome. Clin Nephrol. 2013;79:45.
67. VanDervoort K, Wiesen J, Frank R, et al. Urolithiasis in pediatric patients: a single center study of incidence, clinical presentation and outcome. J Urol. 2007;177:2300.
68. Dwyer ME, Krambeck AE, Bergstralh EJ, et al. Temporal trends in incidence of kidney stones among children: a 25-year population based study. J Urol. 2012;188:247.

Chapter 3
Flexible Ureteroscope Technology

Kymora B. Scotland, Jonathan R. Z. Lim, and Ben H. Chew

Abbreviations

ALA   Aminolevulinic acid
CCD   Charge-coupled device
CMOS   Complementary metal oxide semiconductor
FDA   Food and Drug Administration
LED   Light-emitting diodes
OCT   Optical coherence tomography
UTUC   Upper tract urothelial carcinoma
YAG   Yttrium aluminum garnet

Introduction

Development of the Early Flexible Ureteroscopes

The first documented ureteroscopic procedure was of a 1912 procedure performed by Hugh Hampton Young. Dr. Young inadvertently introduced a pediatric cystoscope into the enormously dilated ureter of a pediatric patient with posterior urethral valves [1]. However, the development of flexible endoscopy really began decades earlier in the 1840s with the work of Daniel Colladon [2] who introduced the concept of internal reflection and "light guiding," which is predicated on the principle of refraction (Fig. 3.1). This ability of light to change direction on moving from one material to another is the foundation for contemporary fiberoptics [3]. The principles of fiberoptic imaging depend on total internal reflection which occurs

K. B. Scotland
Department of Urologic Sciences, University of British Columbia, Vancouver, BC, Canada

J. R. Z. Lim · B. H. Chew (✉)
Department of Urologic Sciences, Vancouver General Hospital, Vancouver, BC, Canada
e-mail: ben.chew@ubc.ca

© Springer Nature Switzerland AG 2020   35
B. F. Schwartz, J. D. Denstedt (eds.), *Ureteroscopy*,
https://doi.org/10.1007/978-3-030-26649-3_3

Fig. 3.1 Light bending

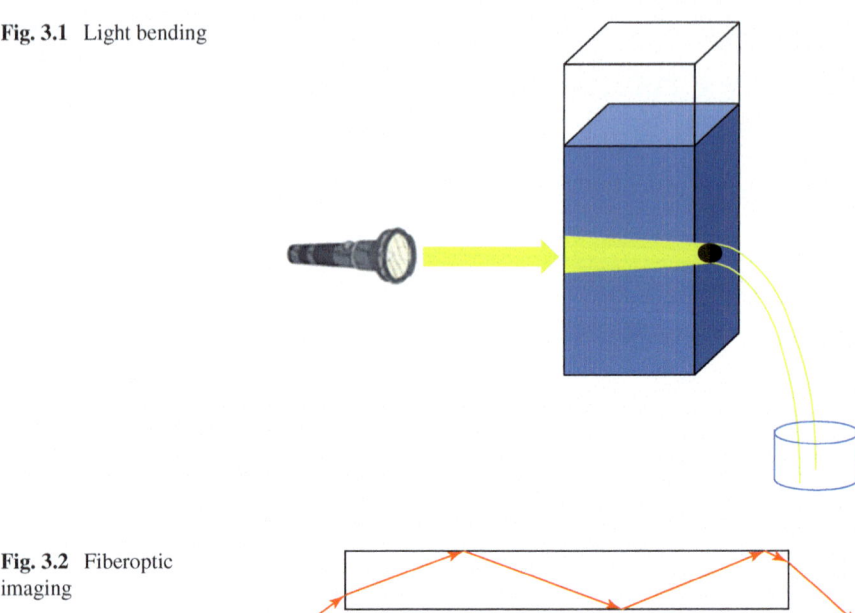

Fig. 3.2 Fiberoptic
imaging

when light travels between materials of very different densities where light is refracted back into the much denser material. In the case of ureteroscopes, this involves the "bending" of light within flexible glass [3].

Subsequent discoveries in the field of light transmission over the next several decades led to the field of fiberoptics. Documentation of these advancements was undertaken by Curtis and colleagues who incorporated fiber-optic technology into medical instruments, thus allowing image conduction [4]. Curtis and Hirschowitz first built fiberoptic scopes for use in gastroenterology. They were the first to arrange coherent bundles of fibers while protecting adjacent fibers from image mixing [5]. Their work sparked the interest of others in the potential of flexible endoscopy for use in separate fields. To understand how flexible ureteroscopes were devised, one must first understand the mechanics of fiberoptic imaging. The light from the object of interest travels in a glass fiber surrounded by a cladding with a lower refractory index. Through the phenomenon of total internal reflection, this light is transmitted over the length of the ureteroscope with minimal degradation (Fig. 3.2). The fiber-optic strands are clad with a material of a lower index of refraction, thus preventing leakage of light. A standard fiberoptic bundle will contain several hundred thousand individual fibers, each of which has a diameter of approximately 10 μm. Each fiber in a given coherent bundle essentially accepts one pixel of information about the specific image. That information is then transmitted to the other end of the bundle to allow for visualization of that image. Since the fibers have an identical orientation at the ends of each bundle, the exact image is transmitted to the eyepiece. The simple eyepiece then presents a magnified view to the eye [6]. The image obtained by fiberoptic bundles is not a single image but a composite matrix of each fiber within the bundle, giving it the classic "honeycomb" appearance. The fibers are only fixed to each other at the ends; thus, much of the length of the endoscope is able to be flexed allowing significant maneuverability and the capacity to navigate tortuous ureters and previously difficult to access calyces. It is this flexibility that was revolutionary and a significant advance over rigid ureteroscopes, thus allowing access to the entire urinary system.

The performance of flexible ureteroscopy was first reported by Marshall with the use of their 9 French endoscope first during an open ureterostomy and subsequently during a transurethral procedure by his colleagues [7]. In 1968, Takagi and Asi reported on their work in developing flexible fiberoptic access to the upper tract of the urinary system [8]. They reported their successful attempts at visualizing the renal collecting system including pelvis and papillae utilizing an 8 French fiberoptic endoscope and evaluated its performance in both cadavers and patients. The Takagi group was the first to present their findings using still photographs of the renal papillae with their newly developed pyelo-ureteroscope [8]. Takayasu subsequently was the first to show video evidence of renal pelvis visualization with the ureteroscope in 1970 [9].

This group did much of the earliest work of flexible ureteroscope development, devising strategies for addressing various limitations. They also recognized difficulty in inserting the ureteroscope from the bladder into the ureter and initially addressed this by employing the cystoscope sheath before later developing a flexible polytetrafluoroethylene introducer sheath [10]. This difficulty was largely due to the struggle to successfully manipulate the endoscope tip. Passing the flexible ureteroscope through a catheter served to provide axial rigidity and transmitted torque along the length of the endoscope. This technique enabled the ability to maneuver the tip in the chosen direction. This experience led to the realization that a flexible tip was required for a successful endoscope.

In another breakthrough, Takayasu et al. realized that the lack of irrigation was problematic, and their first attempt at irrigation utilized the 12 Fr sheath as a means of ureteral luminal distension and better visualization. Continued innovation led to their group being the first to introduce a channel for irrigation and working instruments [9].

Ureteroscopes initially utilized optical lenses arranged sequentially in series for imaging (Fig. 3.3), resulting in large external diameters. Additionally, with even minor flexion, these lenses would become improperly aligned with subsequent instrument failure [11], thus strictly relegating them to use in rigid endoscopes. The advantage of a fiberoptic bundle lens was that even upon circumferential deflection, it would continue to clearly illuminate the field. The early fiberoptic lenses were fashioned from equally spaced packed quartz bundles which produced a completely flexible optical imager [6]. The progress of fiberoptic imaging allowed for the

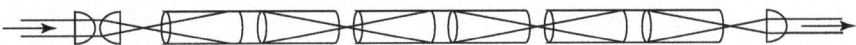

Fig. 3.3 Rod-lens imaging

introduction of the flexible ureteroscope which eventually revolutionized the way urologists approached ureteral and renal stones. However, widespread adoption of flexible ureteroscopy at that time was deterred by its limitation as a strictly diagnostic procedure. Additionally, urologists were initially hesitant to embrace flexible ureteroscopes because of the very valid concern that scope diameters were prohibitively large, which introduced the significant risk of ureteral damage.

Over the next two decades, advances in rigid ureteroscope technology allowing for the fragmentation of ureteral and even renal pelvis calculi in some cases emphasized the need for ureteroscopes that could navigate the renal collecting system [12]. Changes to the original flexible ureteroscope began in the 1980s first with a passively deflectable instrument which was only able to access limited regions of the intrarenal collecting system. In 1983, Bagley and colleagues reported their experience with a new pyeloscope designed with a flexible tip that was able to be deflected 160° in one direction and 90° in the opposite direction all in the same plane [13]. This ureteroscope was also of a small enough diameter that it was able to be placed through the sheath of a rigid telescope on removing the actual telescope. This strategy of fitting the flexible ureteroscope through the rigid sheath mitigated two problems previously encountered with flexible ureteroscopy: difficulty in maneuvering the flexible ureteroscope in the renal pelvis and obtaining sufficient irrigation for visualization. The Lyon group later attempted to address the problem of ureteral access by using both a rigid and a flexible endoscope. This practice of using complimentary ureteroscopes, a semirigid ureteroscope for access to the distal ureter, and more proximal endoscopy with an actively deflectable flexible scope [13] has proven useful.

Urologists quickly recognized the need to visualize the entire collecting system which would require a steerable scope with a small deflectable tip [14]. Bagley and Rittenberg performed investigations to determine the tip deflection required for total visualization of the renal collecting system [15]. On evaluating patient radiographs, they found that the average angle between the major axis and the lower pole infundibulum was 140° and a maximum of 175°. Hence, they proposed a ureteroscope that would deflect 175°. However, on clinical use, the endoscope manufactured to these parameters often could not access the lower pole since deflection was frequently limited by instruments in the working channel and/or by variations of the collecting system itself. As such, active deflection angles continued to increase until they reached 270°, now considered the industry standard [16].

Also by the late 1980s, miniaturization and tighter packing of fiberoptic fibers produced smaller bundles, resulting in smaller-diameter flexible ureteroscopes. Eventually, several different flexible ureteroscope designs offered in sizes ranging from 8.1 to 10.8 Fr were introduced, all of which could be inserted over a wire and used to provide panoramic visualization of the intrarenal architecture without the need for a stabilizing sheath [17].

While access to portions of the lower pole could still be challenging, visualization was often able to be achieved using active (primary) and passive (secondary) deflection of the ureteroscope tip. Primary deflection up and down is controlled by the lever, while secondary deflection is a further degree of deflection that can be accomplished with an already deflected ureteroscope tip. This was achieved by introducing a more bendable segment approximately 6 cm proximal to the tip which allowed for passive endoscope buckling when the ureteroscope was maximally deflected. Secondary deflection proved particularly helpful in not only gaining access to the lower pole calyces but in allowing for the treatment or retrieval of calculi located there [18]. It has since become a standard component of flexible ureteroscope design.

Innovations in ureteroscope technology were inextricably connected to the development of working instruments. In fact, one might argue that the crucial phenomenon that made the use of ureteroscopes feasible was the development of smaller, functional instruments. In many cases the introduction of new or improved working instruments spurred the development of endoscopes to more appropriately take advantage of the advances allowed by the new or updated ancillary equipment. Many of the improvements in ureteroscope design paralleled advances in intracorporeal lithotripsy. In particular, the potential opportunity presented by the development of ever smaller electrohydraulic lithotripsy probes of 2.5, 1.9, and 1.7 French [19] encouraged the design of increasingly smaller ureteroscopes.

The introduction of the 3.6 French endoscope working channel facilitated placement of an ancillary instrument while still allowing the passage of irrigant. This design allowed the use of a wide assortment of working instruments, including guide wires, baskets and other stone retrieval implements, laser fibers, and electrohydraulic lithotripter probes. Most currently available flexible ureteroscopes continue to have a single 3.6 Fr working channel. One notable exception is the Wolf Cobra™ dual-channel ureteroscope with two 3.3 Fr channels [20]. This allows for simultaneous ancillary instrument use or for increased irrigation flow rate. However, the compromise for having two channels is a 9 Fr sheath diameter.

A successful strategy for stone treatment is the use of a small diameter ureteroscope along with an effective small diameter lithotrite. This has largely been achieved with the combination of flexible ureteroscopes with laser fibers. The first documented use of lasers was in 1966 as a result of work by Bush and coworkers who used a bovine renal model to evaluate the effect of a focused argon laser beam on renal calculi [21]. However, this and several subsequent lasers were inadequate or inappropriate for kidney calculus fragmentation [22, 23]. The development of pulsed lasers, where the energy is emitted in pulses of a given duration instead of in a continuous mode, was a major breakthrough for laser lithotripsy [24]. This type of laser allows for precision in control of the laser beam while minimizing lateral heat conduction and subsequent overheating of nearby tissue. The holmium: yttrium-aluminum-garnet (YAG) laser, first championed for use in urology by Johnson and colleagues in the early 1990s [25, 26], has proven quite versatile and rapidly became the laser fiber of use for stone fragmentation [16]. As the laser becomes more accepted in ureteroscopy for its ability to fragment any stone with minimal tissue damage, ureteroscopes were devised to work in concert with this working instrument. Depending on fiber size, lasers can be advanced to the stone through flexible ureteroscopes with little loss of deflection capability of the scope [27].

Ureteroscope tip design has also undergone enhancements over the years. The earliest flexible ureteroscopes had flush "tin-can" tips. However, several subsequent scope iterations were introduced with beveled tips. The rationale for this engineering change was that these tips would better facilitate insertion of the scope into the ureteral orifice, thus decreasing injury. Most flexible ureteroscopes have a 0° angle of view.

There were several attempts in the 1990s to decrease ureteroscope diameter from approximately 10 Fr [28]. One of the more impactful offerings was from the Storz company in 1994; they produced an optical quality small diameter fiberoptic bundle. The miniaturization of the fiberoptic cable facilitated a substantial decrease in the size of the resulting ureteroscope's outer diameter. Along with a corresponding increase in tip deflection, these innovations facilitated enhanced ureteral intubation and scope maneuverability throughout the upper tract. The collective work of several instrument makers that has since effected a decrease in ureteroscope diameter from 10 Fr to what is now 7.5 Fr has enabled the surgeon to gain routine endoscopic access to the intrarenal calyceal system often without a need for ureteral dilation, thus noticeably increasing treatment efficacy.

Limitations of Flexible Ureteroscopes

One of the major issues that has proven an enduring challenge for urologists is the ability to access the lower pole of the kidney using a flexible ureteroscope. While countless hours have undoubtedly gone into attempts at improving ureteroscope deflectability, natural variations in intrarenal architecture continue to make unimpeded access to all areas of the collecting system a challenge.

In their initial experiments with the flexible endoscope, Takayasu and colleagues noted significant challenges manipulating the tip. As such, they identified the need for a deflectable ureteroscope tip. The angle of scope deflection has increased over time from an initial 130° in the early 1990s [18] to a now-standard 270° two-way active deflection (upward and downward). Degree of deflection decreases, often dramatically, with the introduction of instruments via the working channel. The challenge of maintaining deflection is currently being addressed with the use of smaller instruments such as 200 μm laser fibers and 1.8 Fr baskets (as compared to 3 Fr baskets) which cause less of a change in deflection ability. Deflection occurs via movement of a lever on the ureteroscope handle. This movement can be intuitive (the tip deflects in the direction the lever is moved) or counterintuitive. While intuitive scopes are more common, there has been no consensus, and thus both options are available in current ureteroscopes. Passive or secondary deflection is available in all flexible ureteroscopes due to a flexible segment several centimeters proximal to the active deflectable segment. This allows for further maneuverability of the ureteroscope, particularly when attempting to reach difficult regions such as the lower pole of the kidney. Despite the improvements in deflection, there continues to be incomplete accessibility to the entirety of the intrarenal collecting system, often due to insufficient deflecting ability of the flexible ureteroscope with an associated working instrument.

Another limitation of current flexible ureteroscopes is the irrigant flow rate. Most current flexible ureteroscopes have a single working channel which must consequently be used for both passage of instruments and irrigation. Thus, an instrument in the channel will reduce the irrigant flow rate. The decreased flow may be offset somewhat by pressurizing the irrigant fluid and the use of smaller, less than 1.9-Fr-caliber instruments. However, maneuvering the ureter and visualizing the upper tract particularly in the event of bleeding continue to be challenging for ureteroscopists.

To this day, urologists continue to intermittently have difficulty entering the ureter directly with a flexible ureteroscope. Despite advancements by several device manufacturers, ureteroscope size continues to be a challenge; in narrow ureters advancement of the ureter may be challenging, with the urologist forced either to dilate the ureter or to place a stent and return for a subsequent procedure.

Finally, as flexible ureteroscopes become increasingly more widespread, ergonomic concerns have been more commonly discussed. Ureteroscope manufacturers addressed some of these issues by developing lighter scopes as well as improving maneuverability. However, there continue to be several ergonomic concerns (Table 3.1). Continued work has been focused on improving the ergonomics of flexible ureteroscopes [29].

An ideal ureteroscope would have a smaller diameter while still maintaining a large working channel(s) so that instruments and irrigation can both be accommodated. Irrigation will remain necessary for the intubation and distension of the ureter as well as for access to and full inspection of the intrarenal collecting system.

Table 3.1 Comparison of ergonomics of robot-assisted and traditional ureteroscopy

Operative maneuver	Roboflex™ Avicenna	Traditional ureteroscopy
Insertion of ureteroscope	Fine control with joystick and numeric display of horizontal movement	Surgeon uses fingers of both hands (at glans and instrument)
Deflection of ureteroscope	Deflection via wheel for right hand with display of grade and direction of deflection	Surgeon holds the handpiece of the scope and uses his finger to control deflection
Rotation of ureteroscope	Fine-tunable by sophisticated left joystick	Surgeon holds the handpiece of the scope with the fingers of his other hand at the meatus
Irrigation	Integrated irrigation pump activated by touchscreen	Assistant controls irrigation using hand, foot, or fingers, depending on mode of irrigation
Laser lithotripsy	Integrated control of laser fiber by touchscreen; activation by foot pedal	Assistant inserts the fiber into the scope and controls the settings from the control panel; surgeon uses foot pedal to activate laser
Use of basket/ grasper	No function for basket or grasper integrated	Assistant inserts the basket or grasper and is in charge of closing the basket or grasper, while the surgeon manually manipulates the implement within the patient

Digital Ureteroscopes

The next major breakthrough in imaging technology after the development of fiber-optics was the introduction of digital imaging. Compared to fiberoptic cables, digital sensors are composed of millions of photodiodes, which convert photons into electric current that is subsequently converted into voltage then amplified and changed into a digital form (Table 3.2).

The first digital ureteroscopes utilized the charge-coupled device (CCD) chip technology which employed two miniature light-emitting diodes (LEDs) as the light source. They are positioned adjacent to the distal lens (Table 3.3), allowing images

Table 3.2 Comparison of technology behind digital and fiberoptic ureteroscopes

Parameters	CCD and CMOS chip (digital)	Fiberoptic bundle
Initial reception of field of vision	"Chip on the tip": CCD or CMOS chip positioned on distal tip of the ureteroscope with LED	Objective lens at distal end of the ureteroscope with a light diode receives the reflected light rays and focuses them onto a fiberoptic bundle
Reception of initial image	Convert photons of light to a series of electrons	Reflected light rays focused onto a fiberoptic bundle
Transmission of image through the scope	Wires within ureteroscope transmit the flow of electrons to the image processor	Light received from the objective lens and transmitted through the fiberoptic bundle
Reception of final image and display	Image processor receives the electric signal and converts it into an image for real-time display	Camera located at the proximal end of the scope receives the light rays from the fiberoptic bundle and displays the image on-screen

Table 3.3 Comparison of digital and fiberoptic ureteroscopes

Parameters	Digital ureteroscope	Fiberoptic ureteroscope
Head (proximal end of scope)	External camera head not required, single cord for camera and light	External camera head with two cords (camera and light) connected to the scope head
Weight[a]	320 g	576 g
Image resolution[a]	3.17 lines/mm from 10 mm; Resolution determined by sensitivity of distal sensor (CMOS or CCD chip) and can reach 60,000 pixels	1.41 lines/mm from 10 mm; Resolution determined by number of individual fiberoptic strands in a bundle and limited by shaft diameter
Image quality	Superior color representation, clarity, and magnification	Honeycomb lattice superimposed on the image
Diameter	8.4–9.9 F	5.3–8.7 F
Cost	Newer technology and consequently higher costs	Mature technology with minimized costs
Durability	60–150 uses before repair is needed, depending on model and surgical techniques [37, 56]	Fiberoptic strands are fragile, with an average of 27 uses before repair is needed [57]

[a]Based on comparison between Flex-X^2 (fiberoptic) and Flex XC (digital) ureteroscopes

to be transmitted from a digital sensor on the ureteroscope tip to a proximal point via a single wire. This was advantageous because it offered greater image clarity with the capability for digital magnification in a system that was also able to autofocus. The digital image appears on a standard monitor with a clear image that no longer included the honeycomb effect associated with the image produced by fiberoptic quartz bundles [30]. The improvement in image quality has implications not only for the treatment of calculi but also for the diagnosis and possible treatment of upper tract urothelial carcinoma as well as multiple other pathologies. An early comparative study revealed parity of the digital and fiberoptic ureteroscopes [31], while later studies have reported superior visibility with digital ureteroscopes [32].

Digital ureteroscopes have other advantages compared to fiberoptic scopes including substantial weight reductions due to decreased cabling and the loss of the light cord and camera head, thus minimizing hand fatigue and improving ergonomics (Table 3.3). However, the digital endoscopes continue to be slightly larger in diameter compared to most fiberoptic ureteroscopes currently on the market. Most newer digital ureteroscopes employ complementary metal oxide semiconductor (CMOS) chips. These chips allow for very high resolution compared to traditional fiberoptic ureteroscopes. Image enhancement, background noise removal, and color modification were able to be applied to digital flexible ureteroscopes [30]. However, it is these same chips that are currently the limiting factor in producing smaller diameter digital ureteroscopes due to their size and location at the tip of the scope.

The first commercially available digital ureteroscope, the Invisio DUR-D from Olympus (Gyrus ACMI), was introduced in 2006 [33]. The initial imaging chip was the charge-coupled device (CCD) chip designed by Boyle and Smith [34]. This chip was able to store data in the form of electric charges within a grid for later retrieval. This capacity to transfer electric charges made it ideal for the recording of images as a grid of pixels. However, the complementary metal oxide semiconductor (CMOS) chip, first patented in 1967, was found to offer a lower cost alternative to CCD devices while also allowing for reductions in cost and chip size [35]. Several manufacturers have apparently deemed this a cost-effective option, since most currently available digital ureteroscopes utilize CMOS chips.

One of the first ureteroscope innovations stemming from the introduction of digital imaging was the production of the endoscope protection system software by Gyrus ACMI in 2008 [36]. This utilized the capability of the CMOS sensor to differentiate individual colors in specific portions of the optical field to identify the laser fiber. The associated computer control unit could then halt the system if a laser fiber was retracted into the field while being actively used. However, there was a high false shutdown rate of 60% on clinical testing [36]. Most systems do not employ this type of laser safety, but rely on the urologist to ensure the tip of the laser fiber extends enough beyond the ureteroscope tip as to avoid damage to the ureteroscope.

Distal sensor ureteroscopes have been noted clinically to have superior image resolution than was possible with the fiberoptic endoscope [32]. Due to this optical advantage, this and similar technologies may hold promise in the identification of upper tract urothelial carcinoma. Work is underway to continue miniaturizing digital scopes so that they can be of comparable or even smaller diameter compared to fiberoptic ureteroscopes currently on the market.

Single-Use Ureteroscopes

As flexible ureteroscopes have become more widely and more extensively used, becoming the premier tool in a urologist's armamentarium for the management of upper tract calculi and pathology, their durability has come into question. Despite superior durability of digital ureteroscopes as compared to fiberoptic equipment [37], reusable flexible ureteroscopes continue to be noted for their fragility with a high repair rate [38]. This fragility is a matter of concern not only intraoperatively but in the pre- and postoperative period as damage has been noted during storage as well as the cleaning and sterilization process [39]. In addition, various reports of serious ureteroscope-associated outbreaks of infection have been a cause of concern [40]. The idea of single-use ureteroscopes had been discussed since the early 2000s with some preliminary prototypes being eventually abandoned due to technologic constraints. The first commercially available disposable ureteroscope was the PolyScope introduced by Lumenis. It consisted of a reusable fiberoptic bundle which could be attached to disposable flexible catheters [41]. However, the second disposable ureteroscope, the LithoVue™ introduced by Boston Scientific in 2016, is now in widespread use [42]. This and other recently offered single-use uretero-scopes continue to be larger in diameter compared to the typical fiberoptic scope and even some reusable digital ureteroscopes (Table 3.4).

The authors recently performed a comprehensive comparison of two single-use digital flexible ureteroscopes and a reusable digital scope, investigating bench parameters including deflection and tip and shaft diameter (Tables 3.5 and 3.6). Color representation and imaging characteristics such as distortion, resolution, and field of view were also evaluated. The two single-use flexible digital ureteroscopes are comparable to an existing reusable ureteroscope in maneuverability, visualization

Table 3.4 Manufacture's parameters

Feature	LithoVue	Uscope	Flex XC
Deflection up/down	270°/270°	270°/270°	270°/270°
Tip diameter (outer)	9.5 Fr	9 Fr	8.5 Fr
Working channel	3.6 Fr	3.6 Fr	3.6 Fr
Imager technology	CMOS	CMOS	CMOS
Light source	Handle	Handle	Handle

Table 3.5 Ureteroscope deflection

Deflection	LithoVue	Uscope	Flex XC
Empty (up)	295	290	285
Empty (down)	285	280	270
200 μm laser (up)	295	280	280
200 μm laser (down)	275	265	255
2.4 Fr basket (up)	295	280	270
2.4 Fr basket (down)	275	260	260

Table 3.6 Measured scope diameter

Shaft dimension (mm)	LithoVue	Uscope	Flex XC
Tip	3.09 (9.27 Fr)	3.16 (9.48 Fr)	2.5 (7.5 Fr)
Distal shaft	3.1 (9.3 Fr)	3.18 (9.54 Fr)	2.8 (8.4 Fr)
Mid shaft	3.1 (9.3 Fr)	3.18 (9.54 Fr)	2.8 (8.4 Fr)
Proximal shaft	3.1 (9.3 Fr)	3.18 (9.54 Fr)	2.8 (8.4 Fr)

of the collecting system, and ease of use of accessories. These ureteroscopes have only recently been introduced to the market, and there is now an ever-growing number of single-use digital flexible ureteroscopes available. They allow the surgeon to treat stones in challenging areas without fear of the costs associated with ureteroscope damage. However, cost and other considerations will determine whether and how widely they will be embraced long term.

Robot-Assisted Ureteroscopy

The first report of a robotic system for flexible ureteroscopy was in 2007 with the Sensei-Magellan system by Hansen Medical [43]. This system was not originally developed for ureteroscopy and only allowed passive manipulation of the ureteroscope [44]. A flexible digital ureteroscopy-specific robot has been developed and introduced by ELMED in 2010 [45]. The Roboflex Avicenna is similar to other robots used in urology in that it has the surgeon's console as well as a robotic arm to which the instrument – in this case the ureteroscope – can be attached for manipulation. The arm is controlled at the console which also has two foot pedals for laser and fluoroscopy. Use of the robot requires a 12/14 French ureteral access sheath through which the ureteroscope is manually docked before subsequent advancement from the console. Several reports have provided data showing a wide range of movement and ease of deflection all while improving surgeon ergonomics (Table 3.1), and decreasing radiation exposure for the surgeon [44, 45]. Ureteroscopists may sometimes have to perform significant contortions of the hand or even the body in order to access certain regions of the renal collecting system; the robot dispenses with the need for any such uncomfortable and potentially injury-causing compensatory movements.

This system awaits FDA approval. However, questions persist about the disadvantage associated with the lack of tactile feedback inherent in any robotic system and whether there is even a need for a robot in flexible ureteroscopy, particularly in light of the costs of any such system. Other robots are currently in development and look to overcome the limitations of today's ureteroscopes in deflectability, irrigation, and visualization while providing excellent imaging and ergonomics.

Current Innovations

Flexible ureteroscopy revolutionized the treatment of upper tract urothelial carcinoma (UTUC), allowing for the biopsy and eventually the treatment of upper tract pathology in a minimally invasive fashion [46]. The growing enthusiasm for flexible ureteroscopy stems from its ease of use. Moreover, it allows urologists to safely treat patients such as those who are obese and have spinal cord abnormalities or bleeding diatheses which would previously have been quite challenging, and can often achieve this on an outpatient basis. Notwithstanding this, there is a need for improved visualization for upper tract urothelial carcinoma. A more recent adaptation of technology to ureteroscopy has been the use of various imaging techniques for the diagnosis and potential management of upper tract urothelial carcinoma. Optical coherence tomography (OCT) is a cross-sectional microscopic imaging technique that shows promise in providing histologic structure in addition to identifying likely upper tract urothelial carcinoma [47]. Proponents of OCT maintain that it can distinguish between low-grade and high-grade tumors in real time [48, 49]. A related image enhancement technique is confocal laser endomicroscopy which uses a low-energy laser light source to identify urothelial carcinoma also in real time [50]. Prospective clinical trials evaluating this technique have been proposed.

Another ureteroscopy-related imaging technology is narrow band imaging (NBI) which uses optical interference filters to enhance tumor detection with the CCD chip [51]. It does so by reducing the overall light spectrum to those of its blue and green components. These components are absorbed by hemoglobin [52]. As such, viewers can detect a marked contrast between blood vessels (presumed to be associated with tumor) and normal mucosal tissue. The manufacturers propose that this will improve neoplastic tissue identification. It has yet to be universally embraced by the wider urologic community. A somewhat different technology in this area of urothelial carcinoma detection is photodynamic diagnosis. This is a fluorescence-based optical enhancement technique that allows for the detection of potentially malignant tissue [53]. It utilizes the ability of the drugs delta-aminolevulinic acid (also referred to as 5-ALA) and hexaminolevulinate to produce an end product that preferentially emits red fluorescence in malignant tissue when subjected to blue light. While this is generally used for cystoscopic evaluation of non-muscle invasive bladder cancer, a prospective pilot study did show feasibility for detection of UTUC in four patients administered an oral formulation of 5-ALA [54]. There have since been several small studies showing superior UTUC detection with photodynamic diagnosis versus white light ureteroscopy [55].

Future Innovations

Indications for flexible ureteroscopy have broadened with innovations and improvements to the instruments over the last five decades. Dedicated efforts by investigators worldwide have continued to address the limitations of working flexible ureteroscopes. One major concern of urologists is the inability to know intraoperatively what the pressure in the kidney is due to pressurized irrigation. This is a significant issue due to concerns that persistent excess pressures in the kidney may be reached during ureteroscopy, increasing the risk of postoperative complications such as infection. A way to enable consistent and reliable decompression of the upper urinary tract is necessary. In addition to this, ureteroscope developers would do well to devise a means of providing constant pressure monitoring of the inflow and outflow pressure within the renal pelvis.

The abilities of CCD and CMOS chips to stratify and manage information have prompted a revolutionary change in the expectations for the functioning of newer iterations of the flexible ureteroscope. New or improved digital chips are anticipated; it is hoped that these improved imaging tools will come with improved visual processing algorithms and even three-dimensional imaging.

There is a continued need for additional technical improvements to ureteroscopes. It can sometimes be challenging to enter the ureter solely using a flexible ureteroscope. This can be particularly frustrating if one is attempting to use the "notouch" technique to thoroughly investigate the upper tract on suspicion of carcinoma. A ureteroscope that can be made sufficiently rigid to intubate the ureter but then continues to be flexible in order to advance up the ureter would be welcome in the urologic community.

Gaining access to difficult regions of the collecting system such that renal calculi can be treated while maintaining torque stability continues to be an elusive quest. This may be helped in particular by robot-assisted ureteroscopy since it removes the ergonomic barriers to treating stones in challenging positions. Robot-assisted ureteroscopy will add further innovations. For example, the robot could be devised to identify respiratory movements of the kidney and even compensate for them so that the ureteroscope remains centered on the stone while performing laser lithotripsy. Another welcome innovation would be the addition of technologies such as pressure or temperature sensors as well as the ability to measure the size of stone fragments to determine if they are small enough to pass spontaneously. Finally, several groups are currently working on algorithms that will help surgeons to better judge stone size and composition. This will assist surgeons in better planning of ureteroscopic procedures.

References

1. Young HH, McKay R. Congenital valvular obstruction of the prostatic urethra. Surg Gynecol Obstet. 1929;48:509–12.
2. Colladon D. On the reflections of a ray of light inside a parabolic liquid stream. Comptes Rendus. 1842;15:800.
3. Smith AD, Preminger G, Badlani G, Kavoussi L. Smith's textbook of endourology. 3rd ed. USA: Wiley; 2012.
4. Curtiss LE, Hirschowitz B, Peters CW. A long fiberscope for internal medical examination. J Opt Soc Am. 1957;47:117.

5. Hirschowitz BI, Curtiss LE, Peters CW, Pollard HM. Demonstration of a new gastroscope, the fiberscope. Gastroenterology. 1958;35(1):50; discussion 1–3.
6. Hecht J. City of light: the story of fiber optics. New York: Oxford University Press; 1999.
7. Marshall VF. Fiber optics in urology. J Urol. 1964;91:110–4.
8. Takagi T, Go T, Takayasu H, Aso Y, Hioki R. Small-caliber fiberscope for visualization of the urinary tract, biliary tract, and spinal canal. Surgery. 1968;64(6):1033–8.
9. Takayasu H, Aso Y, Takagi T, Go T. Clinical application of fiber-optic pyeloureteroscope. Urol Int. 1971;26(2):97–104.
10. Takayasu H, Aso Y. Recent development for pyeloureteroscopy: guide tube method for its introduction into the ureter. J Urol. 1974;112(2):176–8.
11. Berci. Endoscopy. New York: Prentice- Hall; 1976.
12. Huffman JL, Bagley DH, Schoenberg HW, Lyon ES. Transurethral removal of large ureteral and renal pelvic calculi using ureteroscopic ultrasonic lithotripsy. J Urol. 1983;130(1):31–4.
13. Bagley DH, Huffman JL, Lyon ES. Combined rigid and flexible ureteropyeloscopy. J Urol. 1983;130(2):243–4.
14. Bagley DH, Huffman JL, Lyon ES. Flexible ureteropyeloscopy: diagnosis and treatment in the upper urinary tract. J Urol. 1987;138(2):280–5.
15. Bagley DH, Rittenberg MH. Intrarenal dimensions. Guidelines for flexible ureteropyeloscopes. Surg Endosc. 1987;1(2):119–21.
16. Alexander B, Fishman AI, Grasso M. Ureteroscopy and laser lithotripsy: technologic advancements. World J Urol. 2015;33(2):247–56.
17. Basillote JB, Lee DI, Eichel L, Clayman RV. Ureteroscopes: flexible, rigid, and semirigid. Urol Clin North Am. 2004;31(1):21–32.
18. Grasso M, Bagley D. A 7.5/8.2 F actively deflectable, flexible ureteroscope: a new device for both diagnostic and therapeutic upper urinary tract endoscopy. Urology. 1994;43(4):435–41.
19. Willscher MK, Conway JF Jr, Babayan RK, Morrisseau P, Sant GR, Bertagnoll A. Safety and efficacy of electrohydraulic lithotripsy by ureteroscopy. J Urol. 1988;140(5):957–8.
20. Haberman K, Ortiz-Alvarado O, Chotikawanich E, Monga M. A dual-channel flexible ureteroscope: evaluation of deflection, flow, illumination, and optics. J Endourol. 2011;25(9):1411–4.
21. Bush IMWW, Lieberman PH, Paananen R, Whitehouse D, editors. Experimental surgical applications of the laser. Presented at the Association for the Advancement of Medical Instrumentation. Boston: Association for the Advancement of Medical Instrumentation; 1966.
22. Zarrabi A, Gross AJ. The evolution of lasers in urology. Ther Adv Urol. 2011;3(2):81–9.
23. Sandhu AS, Srivastava A, Madhusoodanan P, Sinha T, Gupta SK, Kumar A, Sethi GS, Khanna R. Holmium: YAG Laser for intra corporeal lithotripsy. Med J Armed Forces India. 2007;63(1):48–51.
24. Dretler SP, Watson G, Parrish JA, Murray S. Pulsed dye laser fragmentation of ureteral calculi: initial clinical experience. J Urol. 1987;137(3):386–9.
25. Johnson DE, Cromeens DM, Price RE. Use of the holmium: YAG laser in urology. Lasers Surg Med. 1992;12(4):353–63.
26. Sayers RD, Thompson MM, Underwood MJ, Graham T, Hartshorne T, Spyt TJ, et al. Early results of combined carotid endarterectomy and coronary artery bypass grafting in patients with severe coronary and carotid artery disease. J R Coll Surg Edinb. 1993;38(6):340–3.
27. Busby JE, Low RK. Ureteroscopic treatment of renal calculi. Urol Clin North Am. 2004;31(1):89–98.
28. Hudson RG, Conlin MJ, Bagley DH. Ureteric access with flexible ureteroscopes: effect of the size of the ureteroscope. BJU Int. 2005;95(7):1043–4.
29. Ludwig WW, Lee G, Ziemba JB, Ko JS, Matlaga BR. Evaluating the ergonomics of flexible ureteroscopy. J Endourol. 2017;31(10):1062–6.
30. Haleblian GE, Springhart W, Maloney ME. Digital video ureteroscope: a new paradigm in ureteroscopy. J Endourol. 2005;19:a80.
31. Cohen JH, Traxer O, Rao P, Desai M, Grasso M, editors. Small diameter, digital flexible ureteroscopy: initial experience. Turin: Videourology; 2011.

32. Multescu R, Geavlete B, Georgescu D, Geavlete P. Conventional fiberoptic flexible uretero-scope versus fourth generation digital flexible ureteroscope: a critical comparison. J Endourol. 2010;24(1):17–21.

33. Binbay M, Yuruk E, Akman T, Ozgor F, Seyrek M, Ozkuvanci U, et al. Is there a difference in outcomes between digital and fiberoptic flexible ureterorenoscopy procedures? J Endourol. 2010;24(12):1929–34.

34. Boyle WS, Smith G. Charge coupled semiconductor devices. Bell Syst Tech J. 1970;49:587–93.

35. Golden JP, Ligler FS. A comparison of imaging methods for use in an array biosensor. Biosens Bioelectron. 2002;17(9):719–25.

36. Xavier K, Hruby GW, Kelly CR, Landman J, Gupta M. Clinical evaluation of efficacy of novel optically activated digital endoscope protection system against laser energy damage. Urology. 2009;73(1):37–40.

37. Multescu R, Geavlete B, Georgescu D, Geavlete P. Improved durability of flex-Xc digital flex-ible ureteroscope: how long can you expect it to last? Urology. 2014;84(1):32–5.

38. Kramolowsky E, McDowell Z, Moore B, Booth B, Wood N. Cost analysis of flexible ure-teroscope repairs: evaluation of 655 procedures in a community-based practice. J Endourol. 2016;30(3):254–6.

39. Sooriakumaran P, Kaba R, Andrews HO, Buchholz NP. Evaluation of the mechanisms of dam-age to flexible ureteroscopes and suggestions for ureteroscope preservation. Asian J Androl. 2005;7(4):433–8.

40. Ofstead CL, Heymann OL, Quick MR, Johnson EA, Eiland JE, Wetzler HP. The effective-ness of sterilization for flexible ureteroscopes: a real-world study. Am J Infect Control. 2017;45(8):888–95.

41. Bansal H, Swain S, Sharma GK, Mathanya M, Trivedi S, Dwivedi US, et al. Polyscope: a new era in flexible ureterorenoscopy. J Endourol. 2011;25(2):317–21.

42. Proietti S, Dragos L, Molina W, Doizi S, Giusti G, Traxer O. Comparison of new single-use digital flexible ureteroscope versus nondisposable fiber optic and digital ureteroscope in a cadaveric model. J Endourol. 2016;30(6):655–9.

43. Desai MM, Grover R, Aron M, Ganpule A, Joshi SS, Desai MR, et al. Robotic flexible ure-teroscopy for renal calculi: initial clinical experience. J Urol. 2011;186(2):563–8.

44. Rassweiler J, Fiedler M, Charalampogiannis N, Kabakci AS, Saglam R, Klein JT. Robot-assisted flexible ureteroscopy: an update. Urolithiasis. 2018;46(1):69–77.

45. Saglam R, Muslumanoglu AY, Tokatli Z, Caskurlu T, Sarica K, Tasci AI, et al. A new robot for flexible ureteroscopy: development and early clinical results (IDEAL stage 1–2b). Eur Urol. 2014;66(6):1092–100.

46. Grasso M. Ureteroscopic management of upper urinary tract urothelial malignancies. Rev Urol. 2000;2(2):116–21.

47. Bus MT, Muller BG, de Bruin DM, Faber DJ, Kamphuis GM, van Leeuwen TG, et al. Volumetric in vivo visualization of upper urinary tract tumors using optical coherence tomog-raphy: a pilot study. J Urol. 2013;190(6):2236–42.

48. Wang H-W, Chen Y. Clinical applications of optical coherence tomography in urology. IntraVital. 2014;3(1):e28770.

49. Zlatev DV, Altobelli E, Liao JC. Advances in imaging technologies in the evaluation of high-grade bladder cancer. Urol Clin North Am. 2015;42(2):147–57, vii.

50. Breda A, Territo A, Guttilla A, Sanguedolce F, Manfredi M, Quaresima L, et al. Correlation between confocal laser endomicroscopy (Cellvizio((R))) and histological grading of upper tract urothelial carcinoma: a step forward for a better selection of patients suitable for conservative management. Eur Urol Focus. 2018;4(6):954–9.

51. Traxer O, Geavlete B, de Medina SG, Sibony M, Al-Qahtani SM. Narrow-band imaging digi-tal flexible ureteroscopy in detection of upper urinary tract transitional-cell carcinoma: initial experience. J Endourol. 2011;25(1):19–23.

52. Asge Technology C, Song LM, Adler DG, Conway JD, Diehl DL, Farraye FA, et al. Narrow band imaging and multiband imaging. Gastrointest Endosc. 2008;67(4):581–9.

53. Burger M, Grossman HB, Droller M, Schmidbauer J, Hermann G, Dragoescu O, et al. Photodynamic diagnosis of non-muscle-invasive bladder cancer with hexaminolevulinate cystoscopy: a meta-analysis of detection and recurrence based on raw data. Eur Urol. 2013;64(5):846–54.

54. Somani BK, Moseley H, Eljamel MS, Nabi G, Kata SG. Photodynamic diagnosis (PDD) for upper urinary tract transitional cell carcinoma (UT-TCC): evolution of a new technique. Photodiagn Photodyn Ther. 2010;7(1):39–43.

55. Osman E, Alnaib Z, Kumar N. Photodynamic diagnosis in upper urinary tract urothelial carcinoma: a systematic review. Arab J Urol. 2017;15(2):100–9.

56. Al-Qahtani SM, Geavlette BP, Gil-Diez de Medina S, Traxer OP. The new Olympus digital flexible ureteroscope (URF-V): initial experience. Urol Ann. 2011;3(3):133–7.

57. Pietrow PK, Auge BK, Delvecchio FC, Silverstein AD, Weizer AZ, Albala DM, Preminger GM. Techniques to maximize flexible uretero-scope longevity. Urology. 2002;60(5):784–8.

Chapter 4
Radiation Safety During Surgery for Urolithiasis

Takaaki Inoue and Tadashi Matsuda

Abbreviations

ALARA	As low as reasonably achievable
BMI	Body mass index
ED	Effective dose
FT	Fluoroscopy time
ICRP	International Commission on Radiological Protection
KUB	Kidney-ureter-bladder
LDCT	Low-dose NCCT
NCCT	Non-contrast CT
PCNL	Percutaneous nephrolithotomy
URS	Ureteroscopy
US	Ultrasonography

Background

On April 26, 1986, the Chernobyl nuclear power plant in Ukraine experienced an accident. On May 11, 2011, the nuclear power plant in Fukushima, Japan, was similarly affected. These accidents resulted in a tremendous fallout of radioactive materials, which greatly influenced the environment, food sources, and local populations for many years. The extended low-dose radiation exposure resulting from these accidents also greatly affected human health. There was an increased incidence of malignancies, including thyroid cancer, leukemia, and breast cancer, among others [1].

Generally, the effects of radiation exposure on human health are referenced as deterministic and/or stochastic. Deterministic effects mean that the severity of certain effects on humans will increase with increasing radiation doses. Below a certain

T. Inoue (✉) · T. Matsuda
Department of Urology and Andrology, Kansai Medical University, Osaka, Japan
e-mail: inouetak@hirakata.kmu.ac.jp; matsudat@takii.kmu.ac.jp

© Springer Nature Switzerland AG 2020
B. F. Schwartz, J. D. Denstedt (eds.), *Ureteroscopy*,
https://doi.org/10.1007/978-3-030-26649-3_4

exposure level, the "threshold," the effect is absent. Therefore, the severity of deterministic effects depends on the accumulating radiation dose. There is a threshold for deterministic effects in the skin, lens of the eye, testis, and bone marrow. For example, skin erythema occurs with exposure of 2–5 Gy, hair loss with 2–5 Gy, cataracts with 5 Gy, lethality (whole body) at 3–5 Gy, and fetal abnormalities at 0.1–0.5 Gy. Conversely, stochastic effects have no thresholds. The severity of the threat is independent of the absorbed radiation dose. Thus, the probability of damage (e.g., radiation-induced cancer) is based on the individual's genetics.

In just a few decades, interventional radiology (IR) has developed as a useful adjunct in the fields of radiology, cardiology, gastroenterology, orthopedic surgery, and urological surgery. It has become a minimally invasive approach to treating various diseases, including both benign and malignant lesions. The great advantages of interventional radiology for patients are that it is less invasive than conventional surgery, including the degree of pain, complications, and cosmetic scarring.

Procedures performed under fluoroscopic guidance for diagnosis and therapy are commonly used in the urological field as well. Endoscopic surgery for treating urolithiasis generally comprises fluoroscopy-guided real-time imaging to add to the safety and success of procedures by avoiding complications and confirming the location of stones, the endoscope, the percutaneous puncture needle, and the anatomical pattern of the urinary tract. The fluoroscopy-guided techniques markedly improve many perisurgical parameters, such as the operation time, blood loss, postsurgical pain, hospital stay, and complication rate.

More sophisticated radiological equipment has contributed to expanding the use of fluoroscopy-guided interventional radiological therapy. During this expansion, however, radiation exposure of patients and medical personnel including the surgeon, assistant surgeon, surgical nurse, and anesthesiologist has increased. Therefore, even if radiation exposure dose is relatively small for medical personnel, urologists must be aware of the risk of the harmful effects of such exposure. Knowledge about the safe use of fluoroscopy may be a less important concern to urologists than to radiologists and cardiologists involved in interventional radiology. Nevertheless, with the worldwide increase in the prevalence of urolithiasis, the influence of radiation exposure must not be ignored. All urologists using fluoroscopy should know about the risk as well as the techniques available to prevent radiation exposure, thereby endeavoring to minimize adverse events following radiation exposure.

The International Commission on Radiological Protection (ICRP) is an international academic organization that developed, maintained, and elaborated on the International System of Radiological Protection used worldwide as the common basis for radiological protection standards, legislation, guidelines, programs, and practice [2]. The System of Radiological Protection is anchored in three fundamental principles according to the ICRP recommendations: justification, protection, and dose limits.

- Principle of justification: Any decision that alters the radiation exposure should do more good than harm.

- Principle of optimization of protection: The likelihood of incurring exposure, the number of people exposed, and the magnitude of their individual doses should all be kept as low as reasonably achievable, taking into account economic and societal factors.
- Principle of application of dose limits: The total dose to any individual from regulated sources during planned exposure situations other than medical exposure of patients should not exceed the appropriate limits specified by the ICRP.

Preoperative evaluation and endourological procedures for upper urinary tract stones are mostly performed under fluoroscopy. Patients with urolithiasis and the surgeons and medical staff involved in the management of upper urinary tract stones have numerous opportunities to undergo radiation exposure. Radiation exposure in endourological fields is mainly divided into two parts: (1) the medical exposure for patients and (2) the occupational radiation exposure for surgeons and the medical staff. Although the dose limit for patients' radiation exposure has not been established, the National Council on Radiation Protection and Measurements defined the occupational radiation exposure dose limit as 50 mSV per year [3].

Ionizing radiation exposure is considered a risk factor for malignancies such as thyroid cancer, leukemia, and breast cancer. It is still uncertain, however, how harmful the radiation exposure is in the long term as low-dose irradiation has been extrapolated to estimate the radiation-related cancer risk. Therefore, the linear, nonthreshold hypothesis is applied as basic to considering the biological effect of radiation exposure. Some investigators reported that chronic occupational exposure to low levels of ionizing radiation caused an increased frequency of micronuclei in chromosomes, which is a biomarker of chromosomal damage, genome instability, and cancer risk [4]. Also, according to some studies, thyroid cancer increased among Australian orthopedic surgeons as a direct result of constant exposure to low-level ionizing radiation [5]. Protracted low-dose exposure to ionizing radiation has been associated with solid-cancer-related mortality [6]. Occupational radiation to the breast was positively associated with breast cancer risk [7]. Currently, there is great concern about occupational radiation exposure having an influence on the lens of the eye. The ICRP recommends not to exceed a mean eye lens dose of 20 µSv/year.

Here, the issue of long-term low-dose radiation exposure for medical personnel arises. Even if the risk of harmful effects of occupational radiation exposure is relatively small, doses exceeding the standard limits likely carry a small, short-term health risk. The ICRP has recommended the principle of limiting radiation exposure to "as low as reasonably achievable" (ALARA) [8, 9].

Medical radiation protection principles should be applied for both patients and medical staff members involved in imaging (e.g., surgeons, nurses, medical engineers). The general factors that should be addressed to optimize protection against radiation are as follows:

- Time: Radiation time should be minimized for the fluoroscopy duration and the number of X-ray-related photographs obtained.
- Distance: Medical staff should be positioned as far as possible from the X-ray source.
- Shielding: Medical staff should use adequate shielding material—e.g., lead apron, lead glasses, lead glass (radiation-shielding glass), and a shield plate.

It is also important to recognize that the measures taken to reduce the patient's radiation exposure almost always decreases that of the medical staff—but the reverse is not always true [1]. To protect the patients and oneself from radiation exposure—even that as low as possible—physicians must perform the surgery based on these three factors. Hence, the advances needed to create radiation-free techniques for imaging stones are needed. This chapter is focused on preventive methods currently available to minimize radiation exposure for patients and medical personnel.

Radiation Protection for Patients During Diagnosis and Surgery

Radiation exposure during procedures is generally due to either direct or scattered radiation. A major source of radiation exposure for patients during procedures is direct radiation generated in the fluoroscopy field between an X-ray tube and an image intensifier (Fig. 4.1). Direct irradiation provides about 1000 times stronger radiation exposure for patients than scattered radiation. Overall doses of medical exposure are not limited because many patients undergo radiological examinations and treatment, although the amount of radiation exposure per patient depends on their disease. However, decreasing the radiation exposure for patients as much as possible is of great concern according to the ALARA principle. Patients with nephrolithiasis (upper urinary tract stones) suffer radiation exposure from diagnostic, treatment, and follow-up imaging. Children with suspected urolithiasis are a special concern regarding radiation exposure because they may require irradiation over an extended period of time.

Standard diagnostic imaging for nephrolithiasis is mostly performed with non-contrast computed tomography (NCCT). Currently, the effective dose (ED) for NCCT of the abdomen and pelvis is 4.5–5.0 mSv [10]. The use of low-dose NCCT (LDCT) offers the advantage of less radiation exposure for the patients. A meta-analysis of LDCT studies revealed sensitivity and specificity of 96.6% and 94.9%,

Fig. 4.1 Schema of radiation exposure from direct and scattered radiation for the surgeon and surgical assistant

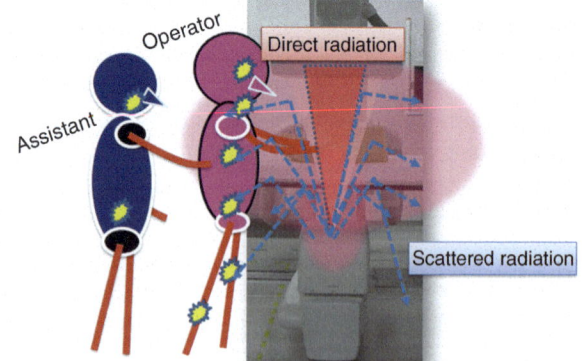

respectively, for diagnosing urolithiasis, which was comparable to that of NCCT [11]. The mean ED for patients undergoing LDCT was reported at 1.40 mSV in men and 1.97 mSV in women. When body mass index (BMI) was considered, however, the sensitivity and specificity decreased to 50% and 89%, respectively, for those with BMI >30 kg/m^2 [12]. The American Urological Association currently recommends the standard NCCT value over the LDCT value when planning to address stones in obese patients (BMI >30 kg/m^2) [13]. Furthermore, current imaging advances have enabled the development of ultralow-dose iterative reconstruction algorithms, which preserve image quality at low doses, making it possible to evaluate urolithiasis. Ultralow-dose NCCT delivers an ED of <1 mSV, which is a lower ED than that with LDCT [14, 15].

The follow-up of patients on medical expulsive therapy or after procedures for nephrolithiasis have shown that standard imaging studies—plain radiography of the kidney-ureter-bladder (KUB) and ultrasonography (US)—are better modalities than NCCT in terms of radiation exposure and cost. The mean ED for KUB imaging is 0.5–1.0 mSv [16], and the patient is not exposed to any radiation when using US. Current guidelines recommend initial US for children with suspected urolithiasis to avoid being sensitized to ionizing radiation [17].

During procedures for managing nephrolithiasis, including retrograde intrarenal surgery and percutaneous nephrolithotomy (PCNL), almost all patients are exposed to radiation by way of fluoroscopy. The radiation exposure associated with PCNL is generally higher than that with ureteroscopy (URS) for nephrolithiasis because of the prolonged fluoroscopy time (FT). A retrospective study revealed that the mean FT during PCNL was 7.09 ± 4.8 min and the mean ED of patients undergoing PCNL was 8.66 mSV [18]. Furthermore, an increasing number of risk factors—radiation exposure during PCNL, high BMI, high stone burden, and more percutaneous tracts—were significantly associated with an increased radiation ED. Obese patients (BMI >30 kg/m^2) required a more than twofold higher dose than normal weight patients (BMI <25 kg/m^2) (6.49 vs 2.66 mSV, $p < 0.001$) [19].

Various techniques can be used to decrease radiation exposure during PCNL. Air retrograde pyelography with the patient in a prone position can clarify the calyceal anatomy of the puncture site. Consequently, the mean adjusted ED during PCNL was 4.45 mSV for air retrograde pyelography compared with 7.67 mSV for contrast retrograde pyelography. This finding is likely due to the increased density of the contrast medium, leading to automatic adjustment of the C-arm tube and tube voltage (lower tube voltage is needed when air is in the field) [20]. Compared with fluoroscopic guidance to assist PCNL, US guidance reduces radiation exposure and is particularly beneficial for treating obese patients with renal stones [21]. Furthermore, combined US/URS-assisted access for PCNL reduces the mean FT compared with that for conventional PCNL under fluoroscopy-guided access [22].

Generally, radiation exposure of patients with nephrolithiasis is significantly less during URS than during PCNL. One study found a median FT of 46.9 s and a median ED of 1.13 mSV per procedure [23]. Another study found, in an anthropomorphic adult phantom, that during PCNL the mean ED rate (mSV/s) was significantly increased during URS in the obese model (BMI >30 kg/m^2) compared with that of the nonobese model [24].

Typically, the surgeon's experience influences fluoroscopic use during URS. Surgeons having extensive experience with fluoroscopic surgery have less radiation exposure than trainees due to the shorter FT during URS [25]. Weld et al. investigated whether added training in safety, minimization, and awareness during radiation training for urology residents reduced the FT during URS for urolithiasis. The authors found that the residents exposed to this dedicated training had a 56% shorter mean FT than the same residents had shown earlier during their first 6 months of training (before the dedicated training) [26]. Therefore, proper education about fluoroscopy and its protocols (e.g., tactile and visual feedback) reduces their radiation exposure [27]. Similarly, for URS, the mean FT and entrance skin dose from before the radiation safety training protocols to afterward were −0.5 min and −0.1 mGy (34%), respectively [28]. Other points of which to be aware include the fluoroscopy beam, which should be collimated with the area of interest. In addition, the image intensifier should be placed as close to the patient as possible, and a pulsed fluoroscopy mode should be used to minimize radiation exposure during PCNL and URS for nephrolithiasis [29, 30]. For URS, urologists found that pulsed fluoroscopy images were adequate and equivalent for most tasks during the surgery compared with continuous fluoroscopy images [31]. Furthermore, a drape placed over or under the patient may help reduce radiation scatter. The key point for reducing patients' radiation exposure, however, is the promotion of physician awareness of the risk of radiation exposure and the importance of radiation protection.

Radiation Protection for Surgeons and Medical Staff During Surgery

The major source of occupational radiation exposure for surgeons and the medical staff is the scattered radiation produced from interaction of the primary radiation beam with the patient's body and the operating table during procedures (Fig. 4.1). Rarely, these personnel may also be exposed to direct radiation when their hands move into the fluoroscopy field between the X-ray tube and image intensifier.

Radiation scattering is divided into two types: backward and forward scattering. The backward scattering dose is approximately 20-fold as strong as the forward scattering dose [32]. Shielding against scattered radiation is usually accomplished by wearing protective clothing. The standard lead protection protocol requires the use of 0.35-mm lead aprons, thyroid shields, and eyeglasses with lead lining for the operating surgeon and 0.25-mm lead aprons for other personnel [33]. However, protection from scattered radiation by wearing protective clothes is incomplete, especially for the arms, eyes, feet, and brain.

The radiation exposure dose to the surgeon performing PCNL with a mean ED of 12.7 mSV per procedure is higher than that with 11.6 μSV during URS because of the longer FT and less distance between the source of radiation and the surgeon [8, 34]. Some investigators reported the mean fluoroscopy screening time during PCNL was 4.5–6.04 min (range 1.0–12.16 min) [35]. Furthermore, the mean radiation exposures to the finger and eye of the surgeon were 0.28 mSv and 0.125 mSV, respectively, due to the nonuniform radiation exposure to the scattered radiation [36, 37]. Therefore, operators should also protect the hands and eyes from scattered radiation exposure using gloves and glasses with lead lining. Most endourologists perform the needle puncture under fluoroscopy for renal access. The operator who carries out the needle puncture under fluoroscopy often is exposed to direct irradiation. The operator must be aware of this behavior and that it presents a critical risk. The surgeon must take care not to come into the direct fluoroscopic radiation field. The US approach is more beneficial than the fluoroscopic approach for protecting surgeons from radiation exposure during PCNL. Yang et al. reported that using a radiation shield constructed from 0.5-mm lead sheeting effectively reduces the surgeon's radiation exposure [38].

The radiation exposure dose to the surgeon in almost cases is less during URS than during PCNL because of the shorter FT and greater distance between the radiation source and the surgeon. Pulsed fluoroscopy was introduced to reduce the radiation dose by limiting the time of exposure to X-rays and the number of exposures per second. The original application of this technology during URS was decreased from 4.7 to 0.62 min [25]. Current reports have shown that the mean fluoroscopy screening time during URS was 44.1 s (range 36.5–51.6 s) [39]. In addition, incorporating several measures—using a laser-guided C-arm, last image holding, a preoperative fluoroscopy checklist—has been shown to reduce the FT by as much as 82% (from 86.1 to 15.5 s) without altering patient outcomes [40]. Currently, the RADPAD shielding device, composed of a tungsten antimony lead-free material, has been used to protect against radiation exposure during interventional radiography. This use resulted in a 23–52% reduction of the total radiation dose exposure [41]. Additionally, Zöller et al. reported that a face-protection shield was effective in reducing eye lens radiation exposure during URS [42]. Inoue and associates also reported that using protective lead curtains on both sides and at the end of the operating table and under the image intensifier was useful for reducing radiation exposure for surgeons during URS. They studied the spatial scattered radiation dose in the operating room for management of urolithiasis using an anthropomorphic phantom and ionization chamber and measured the scattered radiation dose with and without protective lead curtains under the patient's table and image intensifier. Consequently, protective lead curtains led to a 75–80% reduction in the scattered radiation dose compared to that without the lead curtains (Fig. 4.2). Additionally, Inoue et al. found these lead curtains useful for protecting against radiation exposure to surgeons during URS in the clinical setting [43] (Fig. 4.3).

Time, distance, and shielding are generally critical factors for determining the level of radiation exposure. Shielding is usually performed with protective clothing, although its protection from scattered radiation is incomplete. Inoue et al. found that the operator during URS was exposed to radiation (0.10 ± 0.47 μSv) inside the lead apron, even when wearing protective clothes. Performing procedures wearing these clothes under fluoroscopy causes fatigue because of the heavy weight of the clothes and the difficulty of movement, resulting in uncomfortable circumstances during the URS procedure. Söylemez et al. studied urologists and found that wearing

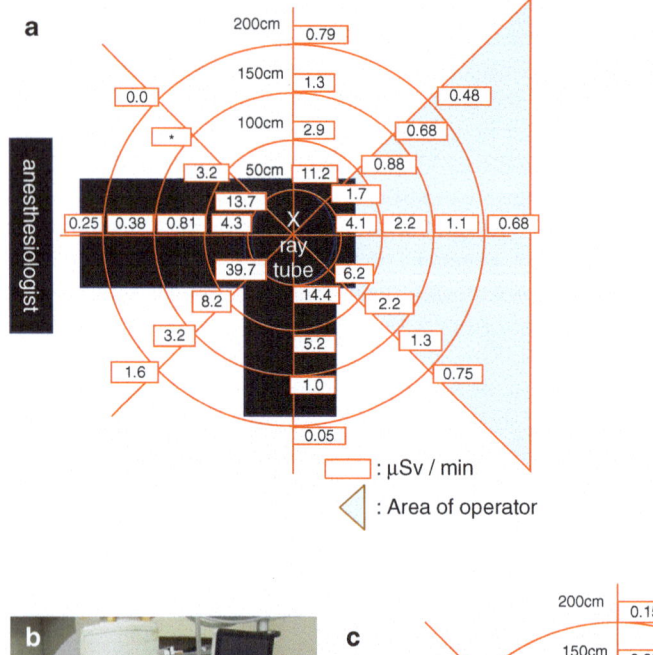

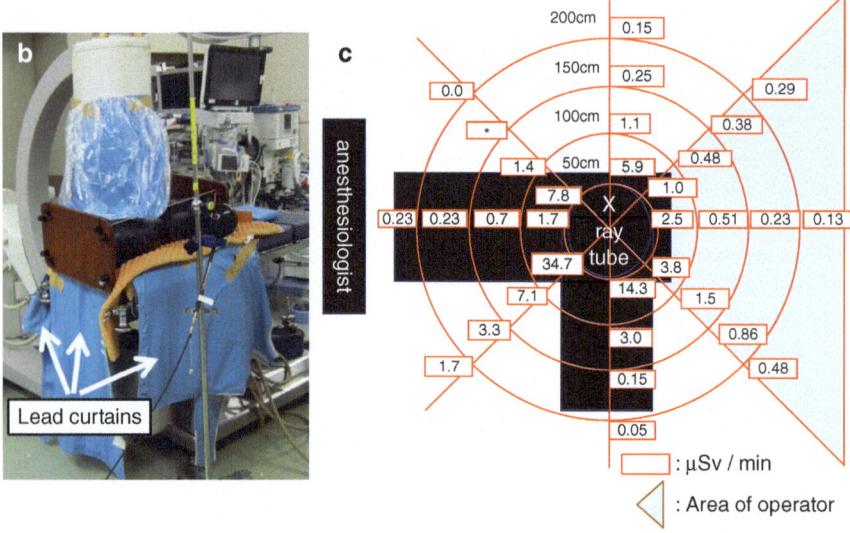

Fig. 4.2 Anthropomorphic phantom study to measure the scattered radiation dose. (**a**) Without protective lead curtains. (**b**) With lead protective curtains under the patient's table. (**c**) Image intensifier with protective lead curtains. (**b** From Inoue et al. [48], with permission of Elsevier)

protective clothing is not practical and causes deterioration of the surgeon's ergonomics [44]. Therefore, shielding from scattered radiation using protective lead devices on the operative table and circumstances may be of greater interest and potential hope.

In modern irradiation practice, active personal dosimeters are essential operational tools to satisfy the ALARA principle [45]. Most urologists have an

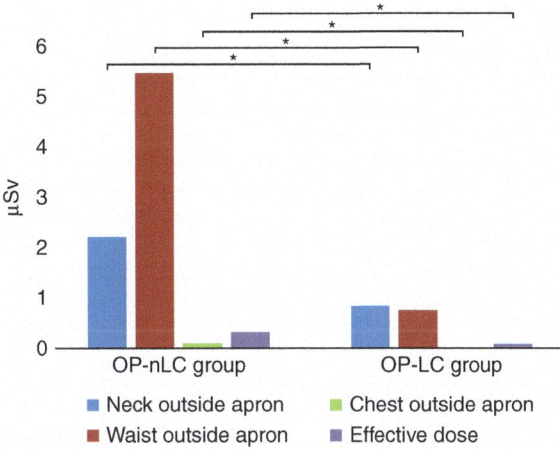

Fig. 4.3 Outcome of surgeon's radiation exposure during ureteroscopy for urolithiasis with and without lead protective curtains in a clinical study. OP-nLC group o-lead-curtain group, OP-LC group lead curtain group. $*p < 0.01$. (From Inoue et al. [48], with permission of Elsevier)

insufficient perception of radiation protection for themselves. A few previous studies showed that although 84.4% of urologists who were chronically exposed to ionizing radiation wore lead aprons, only 53.9% wore a thyroid shield, and 27.9% wore eye glasses with a lead lining. Moreover, only 23.6% of urologists put on a dosimeter [46]. Söylemez and colleagues found that urologists with lead aprons, a thyroid shield, eye glasses, or a dosimeter accounted for 75.2%, 46.6%, 23.1%, and 26.1%, respectively [44]. Awareness of physicians for occupational radiation exposure in the urological field remains low. Although the risks of harmful effects of occupational radiation exposure may be relatively small, they should not be ignored.

Furthermore as current technology has developed novel, robot-assisted, flexible ureteroscopes for management of urolithiasis, described by Rassweiler et al. in 2014. Although surgical outcomes—including the stone-free rate, complications, and operation time—need improvement, robotic surgery may contribute to reducing radiation exposure for surgeons and their assistants [47]. Additionally, it is potentially possible for surgeons to improve their ergonomics without wearing heavy radiation protectors.

In summary, long-term low-dose radiation exposure for patients with urolithiasis and medical professionals should not be ignored. Urologists must therefore acquire knowledge about, and the methods for, preventing radiation exposure. Other simple methods for minimizing occupational and patient radiation doses include minimizing the FT and the number of acquired images; collimating them; avoiding high-scatter areas; using the pulsed fluoroscopic mode; maximizing the distance between the X-ray tube and the patient; minimizing the distance between the patient and the image intensifier; using US instead of fluoroscopy whenever possible; using protective shielding; and wearing a personal dosimeter that provides feedback regarding the radiation dose to which one is already exposed per year (Table 4.1). Effective use of these methods requires both appropriate education and dedicated training in radiation exposure for all endourologists and their medical staff, as well as the availability of appropriate tools and equipment.

Table 4.1 Reduction technique from radiation exposure or patients and operators during surgery

Subjects	Methods ①	②	③	④
C-arm, image intensifier	Maximizing the distance between the X-ray tube and the patient	Minimizing the distance between patients and the image intensifier	Collimating	Pulsed fluoroscopic mode
Operator	Minimizing fluoroscopy time	Protective shielding for operator	Protective shielding for patient table	
Instrument	Using ultrasound instead of fluoroscopy	Laser guided C-arm	Last image hold	
Others	Dedicated educational training (including preoperative checklist)			

References

1. Pukkala E, Kesminiene A, Poliakov S, Ryzhov A, Drozdovitch V, Kovgan L, Kyyrönen P, Malakhova IV, Gulak L, Cardis E. Breast cancer in Belarus and Ukraine after the Chernobyl accident. Int J Cancer. 2006;119(3):651–8.
2. ICRP Publication 103 (ICRP-103) [3] 3. ICRP. The 2007 Recommendations of the International Commission on Radiological Protection. ICRP Publication 103. Ann ICRP. 2007;37(2–4):1–332.
3. Occupational dose limits for adults. Part 20-Standards for protection against radiation, Nuclear Regulatory Commission Regulations Title 10, Code of federal Regulation. Washington, D. C.: United States Nuclear Regulatory Commission; 1991.
4. Eken A, Aydin A, Erdem O, Akay C, Sanal HT, Soykut B, Sayal A, Somuncu I. Cytogenetic analysis of peripheral blood lymphocytes of hospital staff occupationally exposed to low doses of ionizing radiation. Toxicol Ind Health. 2010;26:273–80.
5. Dewey P, Incoll I. Evaluation of thyroid shield for reduction of radiation exposure to orthopaedic surgeons. Aust NZ J Surg. 1998;68:635–6.
6. Richardson DB, Cardis E, Daniels RD, Gillies M, O'Hagan JA, Hamra GB, Haylock R, Laurier D, Leuraud K, Moissonnier M, Schubauer-Berigan MK, Thierry-Chef I, Kesminiene A. Risk of cancer from occupational exposure to ionising radiation: retrospective cohort study of workers in France, the United Kingdom, and the United States (INWORKS). BMJ. 2015;20(351):h5359. https://doi.org/10.1136/bmj.h5359.
7. Preston DL, Kitahara CM, Freedman DM, Sigurdson AJ, Simon SL, Little MP, Cahoon EK, Rajaraman P, Miller JS, Alexander BH, Doody MM, Linet MS. Breast cancer risk and protracted low-to-moderate dose occupational radiation exposure in the US radiologic technologists cohort, 1983–2008. Br J Cancer. 2016;115(9):1105–12.
8. Hellawell GO, Mutch SJ, Thevendran G, Wells E, Morgan RJ. Radiation exposure and the urologist: what are the risks? J Urol. 2005;174:948–52.
9. Durán A, Hian SK, Miller DL, Le Heron J, Padovani R, Vano E. Recommendations for occupational radiation protection in interventional cardiology. Catheter Cardiovasc Interv. 2013;82:29–42.
10. Turk C, Knoll T, Petrik A, Sarica K, Skolarikos A, Straub M, Seitz C. Guidelines on urolithiasis of European Association of Urology; 2015. p. 12.
11. Niemann T, Kollmann T, Bongartz G. Diagnostic performance of low-dose CT for the detection of urolithiasis: a meta-analysis. AJR Am J Roentgenol. 2008;191:396–401.

12. Poletti PA, Platon A, Rutschmann OT, Schmidlin FR, Iselin CE, Becker CD. Low-dose versus standard-dose CT protocol in patients with clinically suspected renal colic. AJR Am J Roentgenol. 2007;188:927–33.
13. Fulgham PF, Assimos DG, Pearle MS, Preminger GM. Clinical effectiveness protocols for imaging in the management of ureteral calculous disease: AUA technology assessment. J Urol. 2013;189:1203–13.
14. Pooler BD, Lubner MG, Kim DH, Ryckman EM, Sivalingam S, Tang J, Nakada SY, Chen GH, Pickhardt PJ. Prospective trial of the detection of urolithiasis on ultralow dose (sub mSv) noncontrast computerized tomography: direct comparison against routine low dose reference standard. J Urol. 2014;192:1433–9.
15. Chen TT, Wang C, Ferrandino MN, Scales CD, Yoshizumi TT, Preminger GM, Lipkin ME. Radiation exposure during the evaluation and management of nephrolithiasis. J Urol. 2015;194:878–85.
16. Astroza GM, Neisius A, Wang AJ, Nguyen G, Toncheva G, Wang C, Januzis N, Lowry C, Ferrandino MN, Neville AN, Yoshizumi TT, Preminger GM, Lipkin ME. Radiation exposure in the follow-up of patients with urolithiasis comparing digital tomosynthesis, non-contrast CT, standard KUB, and IVU. J Endourol. 2013;27:1187–91.
17. Türk C (Chair), Neisius A, Petrik A, et al. European Association Urology, urolithiasis guideline 3.3.3.2. 2018. https://uroweb.org/wpcontent/uploads/EAU-Guidelines-on-Urolithiasis_2017_10-05V2.pdf.
18. Rizvi SAH, Hussain M, Askari SH, Hashmi A, Lal M, Zafar MN. Surgical outcomes of percutaneous nephrolithotomy in 3402 patients and results of stone analysis in 1559 patients. BJU Int. 2017;120:702–5.
19. Mancini JG, Raymundo EM, Lipkin M, Zilberman D, Yong D, Bañez LL, Miller MJ, Preminger GM, Ferrandino MN. Factors affecting patient radiation exposure during percutaneous nephrolithotomy. J Urol. 2010;184:2373–7.
20. Lipkin ME, Mancini JG, Zilberman DE, Raymundo ME, Yong D, Ferrandino MN, Miller MJ, Yoshizumi TT, Preminger GM. Reduced radiation exposure with the use of an air retrograde pyelogram during fluoroscopic access for percutaneous nephrolithotomy. J Endourol. 2011;25:563–7.
21. Usawachintachit M, Masic S, Chang HC, Allen IE, Chi T. Ultrasound guidance to assist percutaneous nephrolithotomy reduces radiation exposure in obese patients. Urology. 2016;98:32–8.
22. Alsyouf M, Arenas JL, Smith JC, Myklak K, Faaborg D, Jang M, Olgin G, Lehrman E, Baldwin DD. Direct endoscopic visualization combined with ultrasound guided access during percutaneous nephrolithotomy: a feasibility study and comparison to a conventional cohort. J Urol. 2016;196:227–33.
23. Lipkin ME, Wang AJ, Toncheva G, Ferrandino MN, Yoshizumi TT, Preminger GM. Determination of patient radiation dose during ureteroscopic treatment of urolithiasis using a validated model. J Urol. 2012;187:920–4.
24. Shin RH, Cabrera FJ, Nguyen G, Wang C, Youssef RF, Scales CD, Ferrandino MN, Preminger GM, Yoshizumi TT, Lipkin ME. Radiation dosimetry for ureteroscopy patients: a phantom study comparing the standard and obese patient models. J Endourol. 2015;30:57–62.
25. Bagley DH, Cubler-Goodman A. Radiation exposure during ureteroscopy. J Urol. 1990;144:1356–8.
26. Weld LR, Nwoye UO, Knight RB, Baumgartner TS, Ebertowski JS, Stringer MT, Kasprenski MC, Weld KJ. Safety, minimization, and awareness radiation training reduces fluoroscopy time during unilateral ureteroscopy. Urology. 2014;84:520–5.
27. Olgin G, Smith D, Alsyouf M, Arenas JL, Engebretsen S, Huang G, Arnold DC 2nd, Baldwin DD. Ureteroscopy without fluoroscopy: a feasibility study and comparison with conventional ureteroscopy. J Endourol. 2015;29:625–9.
28. Canales BK, Sinclair L, Kang D, Mench AM, Arreola M, Bird VG. Changing default fluoroscopy equipment setting decreases entrance skin dose in patients. J Urol. 2016;195:992–7.

29. Park S, Pearle MS. Imaging for percutaneous renal access and management of renal calculi. Urol Clin North Am. 2006;33:353–64.
30. Yecies TS, Fombona A, Semins MJ. Single pulse-per-second setting reduces fluoroscopy time during ureteroscopy. Urology. 2017;103:63–7.
31. Smith DL, Heldt JP, Richards GD, Agarwal G, Brisbane WG, Chen CJ, Chamberlin JD, Baldwin DD. Radiation exposure during continuous and pulsed fluoroscopy. J Endourol. 2013;27:384–8.
32. Lee K, Lee KM, Park MS, Lee B, Kwon DG, Chung CY. Measurements of surgeons' exposure to ionizing radiation dose during intraoperative use of C-arm fluoroscopy. Spine. 2012;37:1240–4.
33. Medical and dental guidance notes: a good practice guide on all aspects of ionising radiation protection in the clinical environment. York: Institute of Physics and Engineering in Medicine; 2002.
34. Safak M, Olgar T, Bor D, Berkmen G, Gogus C. Radiation doses of patients and urologists during percutaneous nephrolithotomy. J Radiol Prot. 2009;29:409–15.
35. Kumari G, Kumar P, Wadhwa P, Aron M, Gupta NP, Dogra PN. Radiation exposure to the patient and operating room personnel during percutaneous nephrolithotomy. Int Urol Nephrol. 2006;38:207–10.
36. Majidpour HS. Risk of radiation exposure during PCNL. Urol J. 2010;7:87–9.
37. Taylor ER, Kramer B, Frye TP, Wang S, Schwartz BF, Köhler TS. Ocular radiation exposure in modern urological practice. J Urol. 2013;190:139–43.
38. Yang RM, Morgan T, Bellman GC. Radiation protection during percutaneous nephrolithotomy: a new urologic surgery radiation shield. J Endourol. 2002;16:727–31.
39. Elkoushy MA, Shahrour W, Andonian S. Pulsed fluoroscopy in ureteroscopy and percutaneous nephrolithotomy. Urology. 2012;79:1230–5.
40. Leschied JR, Glazer DI, Bailey JE, Maturen KE. Improving our PRODUCT: a quality and safety improvement project demonstrating the value of a preprocedural checklist for fluoroscopy. Acad Radiol. 2015;22:400–7.
41. Gilligan P, Lynch J, Eder H, Maguire S, Fox E, Doyle B, Casserly I, McCann H, Foley D. Assessment of clinical occupational dose reduction effect of a new interventional cardiology shield for radial access combined with a scatter reducing drape. Cather Cardiovas Interv. 2015;86:935–40.
42. Zöller G, Figel M, Denk J, Schulz K, Sabo A. Eye lens radiation exposure during ureteroscopy with and without a face protection shield: investigations on a phantom model. Urologe A. 2016;55:364–9.
43. Inoue T, Komemushi A, Murota T, Yoshida T, Taguchi M, Kinoshita H, Matsuda T. Effect of protective lead curtains on scattered radiation exposure to the operator during ureteroscopy for stone disease: a controlled trial. Urology. 2017;109:60–6.
44. Söylemez H, Altunoluk B, Bozkurt Y, Sancaktutar AA, Penbegül N, Atar M. Radiation exposure – do urologists take it seriously in Turkey? J Urol. 2012 Apr;187(4):1301–5.
45. Bolognese-Milsztajn T, Ginjaume M, Luszik-Bhadra M. Active personal dosimeters for individual monitoring and other new development. Radiat Prot Dosim. 2004;112:141–68.
46. Borges CF, Reggio E, Vicentini FC, Reis LO, Carnelli GR, Fregonesi A. How are we protecting ourselves from radiation exposure? A nationwide survey. Int Urol Nephrol. 2015;47:271–4.
47. Saglam R, Muslumanoglu AY, Tokatlı Z, Caşkurlu T, Sarica K, Taşçi Aİ, Erkurt B, Süer E, Kabakci AS, Preminger G, Traxer O, Rassweiler JJ. A new robot for flexible ureteroscopy: development and early clinical results (IDEAL stage 1-2b). Eur Urol. 2014;66:1092–100.
48. Inoue T, Komemushi A, Murota T, Takashi Y, Taguchi M, Kinoshita H, Matsuda T. Effect of protective lead curtains on scattered radiation exposure to the operator during ureteroscopy for stone disease: a controlled trial. Urology. 2017;9:60–6.

Chapter 5
Safety and Care of Ureteroscopic Instruments

Panagiotis Kallidonis, Mohammed Alfozan, and Evangelos Liatsikos

Abbreviations

fURS   Flexible ureteroscopy

Introduction

Before the development of ureteroscopy, upper urinary tract diseases were managed through open procedures which led to a significant morbidity rate [1]. The constant interaction of engineering and medicine leads to the development of less invasive treatment modalities and improvement in the quality of clinical care; thus, the creation of digital sensor ureteroscopes, improvement of working elements, and the advent of the holmium laser had a great impact and allowed more complex procedures to be performed endoscopically [2].

The complex and fragile nature of flexible ureteroscopes leads to issues with reliability and cost of maintenance. The introduction of digital ureteroscopes was based on the image-to-digital data conversion and light-emitting diode, which resulted in great improvement and durability of these instruments, enabled significant design improvements, and reduced the use of fiber-optic scopes [3]. Despite the improvements in durability, the fragile nature of flexible ureteroscopes still poses a major financial burden for their clinical use [3]. Most failures are attributed to iatrogenic causes such as use of accessory equipment, sterilization, or improper handling at the time of sterilization [4].

P. Kallidonis (✉) · E. Liatsikos
Department of Urology, University Hospital of Patras, Patras, Greece

M. Alfozan
Department of Urology, University Hospital of Patras, Patras, Greece

College of Medicine, Prince Sattam Bin Abdulaziz University, Al Kharj, Saudi Arabia

© Springer Nature Switzerland AG 2020   63
B. F. Schwartz, J. D. Denstedt (eds.), *Ureteroscopy*,
https://doi.org/10.1007/978-3-030-26649-3_5

The introduction of digital ureteroscopes not only improved durability but also allowed for larger working channels, which permit superior rate of irrigation flow, the use of larger instruments, and removal of biopsy specimen through the channel [5]. Adequate irrigation flow is crucial for optimal visualization of the endoscopic field and for access to the urinary tract.

Durability of Flexible Ureteroscopes

Initial reports highlighted the excellent optical characteristics, design, and improved functions of these newly introduced digital instruments [6, 7]. However, studies evaluating and comparing the durability of new generations of ureteroscopes are limited. The durability of the ureteroscopes is related not only to the design but also to the technique of use and operator experience. Training in digital ureteroscope technique is a key component of subspecialty training in urology, mandatory for patient safety and the optimal care of instruments.

A study conducted by Sung et al. analyzed data on the characteristics of ureteroscope damage [8]. Data was obtained from the four major manufacturers (ACMI, Karl Storz, Richard Wolf, and Olympus). The frequency of repair increased with decreasing ureteroscope diameter and increasing scope length. Working channel laser burn and extreme scope deflection were major causes of damage to flexible ureteroscopes.

Afani et al. compared early generation flexible ureteroscopes and concluded that although luminosity and irrigation flow remained unchanged, there was significant deterioration (2–28%) in active deflection after the ureteroscopes were used for 6–15 uses (3–13 h) [9]. Information gained in this early study is useful because it serves as a reference point for subsequent studies. Another study did not observe any statistical significance between the durability of six flexible ureteroscopes originating from different manufacturers. Between 10 and 34 procedures were carried out with the flexible ureteroscopes before they needed major repair [10]. Carey et al. concluded that among the most important risk factors for predicting the number of uses of a ureteroscope was the age of the device and history of prior repair [4].

Traxer et al. reported on specific damage that occurred to Storz Flex X ureteroscope after 50 ureteroscopies. Maximal ventral deflection deteriorated from 270° to 208°, and maximal dorsal deflection deteriorated from 270° to 133°. There were six broken image fibers. The authors concluded that the new generation of flexible ureteroscopes needed less frequent repair, although no direct comparison was made with the previous generation of scopes [5]. Several other investigators have marked the improved durability of the recent generations of flexible ureteroscopes [11–14].

Perioperative Care of Flexible Ureteroscopes

General Considerations of Handling the Scopes

The longevity of ureteroscopes depends largely on operator skills; therefore, training in ureteroscopy is necessary to ensure the safety of both patients and equipment [15]. Care of the small-diameter flexible ureteroscopes begins with meticulous handling. Insertion of the flexible ureteroscope should be a smooth process. The scope should be straight during insertion, and the insertion should be done over a guide wire [22]. Fluoroscopy could be very useful under a variety of circumstances: determining the nature of the obstruction, ruling out any buckling of the ureteroscope in the bladder secondary to pathology, or determining if there is enough support by the guide wire [22]. A retrograde pyelogram or inspection of the distal ureter with ureteroscope could aid in identifying the cause of obstruction. Once inserted, the ureteroscope should be straight from the urethral meatus to the lens [23]. No instruments should be passed when the tip is deflected beyond 30° [23]. The ureteroscope shaft should not be twisted, as this may damage the fiber-optic bundles [22]. The instrument should be in its own trolley and other instruments should not be placed on it [24]. Support staff should be well trained since most scope damage occurs outside of the patient, during cleaning and storage [24]. Appropriate training of the supporting staff for optimal outpatient handling of the flexible scopes could be considered equally important as intraoperative handling of the instruments by the urologists [25]. The most common damage caused by support staff is overcurling of the scope or crushing of the scope by closing the storage case on the scope shaft [8]. Training the staff extends the life of the scopes and is cheaper than repairing or replacing the ureteroscope. Moreover, regular maintenance and service contract costs are also reduced [24].

Intraoperative Care of Flexible Ureteroscopes

The active deflection unit is the most fragile part of the flexible ureteroscope. Several studies showed that the leading cause of scope damage was working with a deflected tip, occurring either by direct damage to the deflection mechanism or by the introduction of instruments during deflection [15]. The active deflection mechanism eventually wears out with repeated use, necessitating repair or replacement of the ureteroscope [9]. Several techniques for preventing damage to the scope during intraoperative care have been proposed in the literature. Ghani et al. described a technique where they evacuated the collecting system with a syringe to draw the stone closer to the scope. Moreover, they proposed the use of a nitinol basket to reposition the lower pole stones into the middle or upper calyx, which allows working with a lesser degree of deflection and enables the passage of larger laser fibers [16].

The introduction of lasers for contact lithotripsy, tissue destruction, incision, and fulguration has significantly increased the use of the flexible ureteroscope. Small diameter laser fibers allow scope deflection, while bigger diameters deliver more power. Care must be taken during the insertion of the fiber against a deflected tip as this may cause perforations or scraping of the inner lining of the working channel. Also, the laser must not be activated if the fiber tip is not advanced outside the channel. Working with maximum deflection can cause microfractures and laser firing within the channel [2].

Ureteral access sheaths are used to facilitate ureteroscopy by decreasing the intrarenal pressure, providing better irrigation flow and visibility, as well as increasing the longevity of the ureteroscopy by providing support. Moreover, the sheaths decrease the resistance and buckling of the scope in the bladder [12, 17]. Nonetheless, the scope deflection mechanism should always be out of the sheath to avoid interfering with scope flexibility and to prevent damage to the deflection mechanism (Fig. 5.1a, b). Many studies demonstrated that the use of ureteral access sheaths decreased the operative time and cost, minimized the patient morbidity, and optimized the overall success of the ureteroscopy [18]. Ureteral access sheaths should be considered if multiple passes of a ureteroscope are necessary or if the ureteroscope cannot be negotiated easily into the upper urinary tract. Injuries and long-term complications of ureteral access sheath insertion are mainly related to maneuvers of insertion and largely can be decreased by preoperative ureteric stent insertion and by avoiding forceful insertion [19, 20].

Most modern accessories are made of nitinol, which resists kinking and causes minimal loss of deflection. Crucial factors to avoid complications and damage to the scope include carefully selecting extraction devices, using a safety guide wire, maintaining good visualization all the time, avoiding forceful or blind manipulation, and introducing the device while the scope is straight [21].

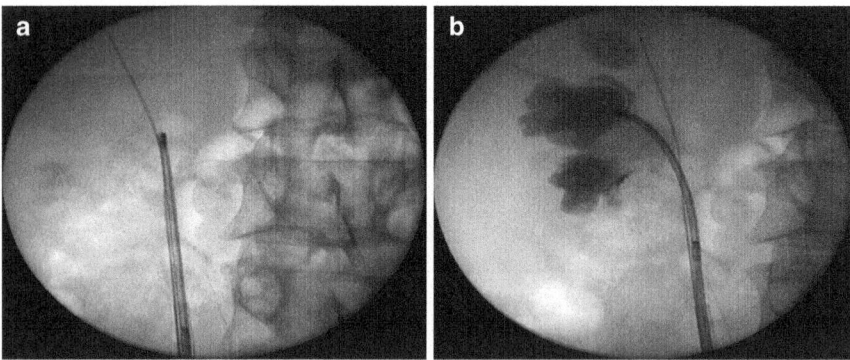

Fig. 5.1 (**a**) The flexible ureteroscope has been inserted in the sheath, but its deflection mechanism remains inside it. The deflection is significantly limited, and the mechanism of deflection is under tension and could be easily damaged. (**b**) The deflection mechanism is out of the access sheath. The scope can deflect efficiently. Notice the radiopaque ring at the site that the deflecting distal part of the flexible ureteroscope scope is connected to the shaft of the scope. This site should always be outside the sheath in order to prevent damage to the deflection mechanism

Processing, Cleaning, and Sterilization of Flexible Ureteroscopes

A main cause of damage outside the patient is the cleaning technique. Some available cleaning techniques do not ensure instrument viability and appropriate sterilization. Thus, the method of cleaning should be based on the manufacturer's guidelines [26]. Patient safety and optimal clearing of the instrument should be ensured by documenting and monitoring the cleaning process and sterilization. A study by McDougall et al. investigated if cleaning techniques and personal errors could affect ureteroscope failure, showing that when the processing and handling of the scopes was done by the surgeons and endourology support staff, the durability of the scopes was not affected [11]. Another study compared handling of the scope by endourology staff with handling by the central processing unit. Results showed that when the endourology staff handled the ureteroscopes, the average number of uses was 28.1 before any repair. The number of uses before repair was only 10.8 when the scopes were handled by the central unit [27]. Thus, the staff should be aware of the fragility of the ureteroscope and make every effort to prevent the onset of corrosion, pitting, and rusting [28].

Prior to each use, every new, repaired, and refurbished ureteroscope should be checked, cleaned, and sterilized by following the methods recommended by the manufacturer [29]. Precleaning is necessary to remove any debris and to make the scope safe for handling. Flushing of working channels with enzymatic detergent or water and removing all visible soil from the interior and exterior of the scope are also recommended [30].

After every use, the scope should immediately be immersed in warm water. Prior to manual cleaning, a leak test should be done. To ensure that internal channels are intact and to avoid any damage to the scope, the instrument should be sent back to the manufacturer for repair if a leak is detected [30, 31]. If no leak is found, the scope should be disassembled and cleaned of all protein material using the recommended enzymatic detergent to facilitate a biocidal process [30–32]. After visual inspection and cleaning, a high-level disinfection or sterilization should be performed according to the manufacturer instructions and healthcare organization regulations [31]. Care must be taken to rinse the ureteroscope and flush the channels to remove any traces of disinfectant solution [30]. Adherence to strict protocols and documentation and monitoring of the process are crucial to avoid any infectious outbreaks, damage to the scope, and compromise of staff safety.

The quality of water used for the processing has a great influence on the proper function and durability of the ureteroscope. A hard layer (lime deposits, scale) might form on the ureteroscope depending on water hardness and temperature and can sometimes be very difficult to dissolve. Cleaning solutions relying on tap water—even when using deionized water—will leave mineral residues on ureteroscopes that will not wash off completely. These factors can negatively affect the instrument's proper function. The quality of the rinsing water for final disinfection and cleaning should be free of pathogenic microorganisms. When an instrument is rinsed in tap water, recontamination can occur [28].

Routine sterilization is recommended for initial and subsequent sterilization of all instruments. Before sterilization, the ureteroscope must be fully cleaned, with all visible organic material, blood, and cleaning solution completely removed [31]. Instruments may be sterilized in ethylene oxide (EtO), steam, STERRAD® sterilization systems, or STERIS® Amsco V-PRO® sterilization systems. Sterilization is highly recommended for "critical" instruments to be used for hysteroscopy, neuroendoscopy, laparoscopy, or arthroscopy. High-level disinfection is recommended for "semi-critical" instruments which come into contact only with intact mucous membranes or non-intact skin [31].

Single-Use Ureteroscopes

Flexible ureteroscopy (fURS) has evolved to be the most used modality for surgical treatment of renal stones over the past 15 years [33]. Despite technological advances, the durability of flexible ureteroscopes is still a major concern. Due to limited durability and the relatively high cost of repair, the multiuse (reusable) ureteroscope continues to be a significant financial obstacle to initiating flexible ureteroscopy programs worldwide. Moreover, the maintenance, processing, and sterilization of flexible ureteroscopes lead to significant costs.

Flexible ureteroscope repair has been clearly stated in the literature as a significant cost parameter in several studies [37, 38]. Knudsen et al. showed that 46–59% of the cost of a flexible ureteroscopy program results from ureteroscope repairs [34]. Landman et al. evaluated flexible ureteroscopes from different manufacturers and calculated the overall costs associated with the use of each of the ureteroscopes for 25, 50, 75, and 100 cases during the 1st year (while under warranty) and with subsequent use. They concluded that 70% of the major ureteroscope repairs may result from operator-induced damage [35]. When the newer digital scopes were evaluated, the investigators observed an average of 12 uses before the need to repair the digital scopes [36]. In an attempt to address costly issues with durability and need for repairs, the single-use disposable ureteroscope was introduced; these scopes have to withstand only one case and do not require any repair or maintenance.

The LithoVue (Boston Scientific, Marlborough, MA) was the first disposable ureteroscope introduced on the market. The scope was shown to be comparable to conventional scopes in terms of visibility and manipulation in a cadaveric study [39]. Usawachintachit et al. reported the clinical outcomes between two randomized groups of patients undergoing flexible ureteroscopy for upper urinary tract pathology. The first group underwent surgery utilizing LithoVue, and the second group used reusable fiber-optic flexible ureteroscopes. LithoVue was related to an average 15.5-min reduction in operating room time and a 12.6% reduction in complications. Instrument failures were similar between LithoVue and the reusable flexible ureteroscopes [40]. Similar results showing the efficacy of single-use flexible ureteroscopes, including scopes other than LithoVue, have been published and suggest that the single-use flexible ureteroscopes could be a promising alternative to reusable flexible ureteroscopes without compromising the clinical outcome of fURS [41]. Nonetheless, the purchase cost of these scopes remains high and represents a limiting factor for their acceptance. However, recent economic studies calculating the cost of purchase, repair, maintenance, and sterilization showed that the single-use scopes could be considered more cost-effective in specific clinical settings [42, 43].

Conclusion

The clinical use of flexible ureteroscopes requires training of and care by surgeons as well as support personnel related to the maintenance, cleaning, storage, and sterilization of these instruments. The repair costs of these instruments are high and may represent a significant financial burden. The use of single-use flexible ureteroscopes may be cost-effective in some clinical settings by avoiding the need for maintenance and repair.

References

1. Wickham JE. Treatment of urinary tract stones. BMJ (Clin Res Ed). 1993;307(6916):1414–7.
2. Beiko DT, Denstedt JD. Advances in ureterorenoscopy. Urol Clin North Am. 2007;34(3):397–408.
3. Papatsoris AG, Kachrilas S, Howairis ME, Masood J, Buchholz N. Novel technologies in flexible ureterorenoscopy. Arab J Urol. 2011;9(1):41–6.
4. Carey RI, Gomez CS, Maurici G, Lynne CM, Leveillee RJ, Bird VG. Frequency of ureteroscope damage seen at a tertiary care center. J Urol. 2006;176(2):607–10; discussion 10.
5. Traxer O, Dubosq F, Jamali K, Gattegno B, Thibault P. New-generation flexible ureterorenoscopes are more durable than previous ones. Urology. 2006;68(2):276–9. discussion 80
6. Al-Qahtani SM, Geavlete B, Geavlette BP, de Medina SG-D, Traxer OP. The new Olympus digital flexible ureteroscope (URF-V): initial experience. Urology annals. 2011;3(3):133–7.
7. Binbay M, Yuruk E, Akman T, Ozgor F, Seyrek M, Ozkuvanci U, et al. Is there a difference in outcomes between digital and fiberoptic flexible ureterorenoscopy procedures? J Endourol. 2010;24(12):1929–34.
8. Sung JC, Springhart WP, Marguet CG, L'Esperance JO, Tan YH, Albala DM, et al. Location and etiology of flexible and semirigid ureteroscope damage. Urology. 2005;66(5):958–63.
9. Afane JS, Olweny EO, Bercowsky E, Sundaram CP, Dunn MD, Shalhav AL, et al. Flexible ureteroscopes: a single center evaluation of the durability and function of the new endoscopes smaller than 9Fr. J Urol. 2000;164(4):1164–8.
10. User HM, Hua V, Blunt LW, Wambi C, Gonzalez CM, Nadler RB. Performance and durability of leading flexible ureteroscopes. J Endourol. 2004;18(8):735–8.
11. McDougall EM, Afane JS, Dunn MD, Shalhav AL, Clayman RV. Laparoscopic management of retrovesical cystic disease: Washington University experience and review of the literature. J Endourol. 2001;15(8):815–9.

12. Pietrow PK, Auge BK, Delvecchio FC, Silverstein AD, Weizer AZ, Albala DM, et al. Techniques to maximize flexible ureteroscope longevity. Urology. 2002;60(5):784–8.
13. Wendth-Nordahl G, Mut T, Krombach P, et al. Do new generation ureterorenoscopes offer a higher treatment success than their predecessors? Urol Res. 2011;39. SRC – BaiduScholar:185–8.
14. Zilberman DE, Tsivian M, Yong D, Albala DM. Surgical steps that elongate operative time in robot-assisted radical prostatectomy among the obese population. J Endourol. 2011;25(5):793–6.
15. Karaolides T, Bach C, Kachrilas S, Goyal A, Masood J, Buchholz N. Improving the durability of digital flexible ureteroscopes. Urology. 2013;81(4):717–22.
16. Ghani KR, Bultitude M, Hegarty N, Thomas K, Glass J. Flexible ureterorenoscopy (URS) for lower pole calculi. BJU Int. 2012;110(2):294–8.
17. Ng YH, Somani BK, Dennison A, Kata SG, Nabi G, Brown S. Irrigant flow and intrarenal pressure during flexible ureteroscopy: the effect of different access sheaths, working channel instruments, and hydrostatic pressure. J Endourol. 2010;24(12):1915–20.
18. Kourambas J, Byrne RR, Preminger GM. Does a ureteral access sheath facilitate ureteroscopy? J Urol. 2001;165(3):789–93.
19. Breda A, Territo A, López-Martínez JM. Benefits and risks of ureteral access sheaths for retrograde renal access. Curr Opin Urol. 2016;26(1):70–5.
20. Traxer O, Thomas A. Prospective evaluation and classification of ureteral wall injuries resulting from insertion of a ureteral access sheath during retrograde intrarenal surgery. J Urol. 2013;189(2):580–4.
21. Somani BK, Aboumarzouk O, Srivastava A, Traxer O. Flexible ureterorenoscopy: tips and tricks. Urology Ann. 2013;5(1):1–6.
22. Sprunger JK, Herrell SD. Techniques of ureteroscopy. Urol Clin North Am. 2004;31(1):61–9.
23. Monga M, Dretler SP, Landman J, Slaton JW, Conradie MC, Clayman RV. Maximizing ureteroscope deflection: "play it straight". Urology. 2002;60(5):902–5.
24. Sooriakumaran P, Kaba R, Andrews HO, Buchholz NPN. Evaluation of the mechanisms of damage to flexible ureteroscopes and suggestions for ureteroscope preservation. Asian J Androl. 2005;7(4):433–8.
25. Sooriakumaran P, Buchholz NPN. Who broke the ureteroscope? BJU Int. 2004;94(1):4–5.
26. Aiello AE, Larson EL, Sedlak R. Hidden heroes of the health revolution. Sanitation and personal hygiene. Am J Infect Control. 2008;36(10 Suppl):S128–51.
27. Semins MJ, George S, Allaf ME, Matlaga BR. Ureteroscope cleaning and sterilization by the urology operating room team: the effect on repair costs. J Endourol. 2009;23(6):903–5.
28. Recommended practices for cleaning and caring for surgical instruments and powered equipment. AORN J. 2002;75:627–41.
29. Vrancich A. Instrumental care. Creating longevity through proper maintenance. Mater Manag Health Care. 2003;12(3):22–5.
30. Clemens JQ. Afferent neurourology: an epidemiological perspective. J Urol. 2010;184(2):432–9.
31. Association for the Advancement of Medical Instrumentation. ST91 Flexible and semirigid endoscope processing in health care facilities. 2015.
32. Rutala WA, Weber DJ. Reprocessing semicritical items: current issues and new technologies. Am J Infect Control. 2016;44(5 Suppl):e53–62.
33. Ordon M, Urbach D, Mamdani M, Saskin R, Honey RJDA, Pace KT. A population based study of the changing demographics of patients undergoing definitive treatment for kidney stone disease. J Urol. 2015;193(3):869–74.
34. Knudsen B, Miyaoka R, Shah K, Holden T, Turk TMT, Pedro RN, et al. Durability of the next-generation flexible fiberoptic ureteroscopes: a randomized prospective multi-institutional clinical trial. Urology. 2010;75(3):534–8.
35. Landman J, Lee DI, Lee C, Monga M. Evaluation of overall costs of currently available small flexible ureteroscopes. Urology. 2003;62(2):218–22.
36. Shah K, Monga M, Knudsen B. Prospective randomized trial comparing 2 flexible digital ureteroscopes: ACMI/Olympus Invisio DUR-D and Olympus URF-V. Urology. 2015;85(6):1267–71.

37. Kramolowsky E, McDowell Z, Moore B, Booth B, Wood N. Cost analysis of flexible ureteroscope repairs: evaluation of 655 procedures in a community-based practice. J Endourol. 2016;30(3):254–6.
38. Taguchi K, Harper JD, Stoller ML, Duty BD, Sorensen MD, Sur RL, et al. Identifying factors associated with need for flexible ureteroscope repair: a Western Endourology STone (WEST) research consortium prospective cohort study. Urolithiasis. 2018;46(6):559–66. https://doi.org/10.1007/s00240-017-1013-y.
39. Proietti S, Dragos L, Molina W, Doizi S, Giusti G, Traxer O. Comparison of new single-use digital flexible ureteroscope versus nondisposable fiber optic and digital ureteroscope in a cadaveric model. J Endourol. 2016;30(6):655–9.
40. Usawachintachit M, Isaacson DS, Taguchi K, Tzou DT, Hsi RS, Sherer BA, et al. A prospective case-control study comparing LithoVue, a single-use, flexible disposable ureteroscope, with flexible, reusable fiber-optic ureteroscopes. J Endourol. 2017;31(5):468–75.
41. Davis NF, Quinlan MR, Browne C, Bhatt NR, Manecksha RP, D'Arcy FT, et al. Single-use flexible ureteropyeloscopy: a systematic review. World J Urol. 2018;36(4):529–36.
42. Taguchi K, Usawachintachit M, Tzou DT, Sherer BA, Metzler I, Isaacson D, et al. Microcosting analysis demonstrates comparable costs for LithoVue compared to reusable flexible fiberoptic ureteroscopes. J Endourol. 2018;32(4):267–73.
43. Martin CJ, McAdams SB, Abdul-Muhsin H, Lim VM, Nunez-Nateras R, Tyson MD, et al. The economic implications of a reusable flexible digital ureteroscope: a cost-benefit analysis. J Urol. 2017;197(3 Pt 1):730–5.

Chapter 6
Single-Use Flexible Ureteroscopes

Brenton Winship and Michael Lipkin

Introduction

The development of the flexible ureteroscope revolutionized the treatment of urinary tract stone disease. Modern scopes allow for the treatment of all but the largest stones in nearly any location within the ureter or kidney. The flexible scope's greatest asset, its narrow and flexible shaft, however, is also its greatest weakness. The delicate components are not only expensive, they are prone to frequent breakage, difficult and expensive to repair, and challenging to sterilize. Accordingly, single-use or partially single-use flexible ureteroscopes appeared shortly after the first reusable flexible ureteroscopes [1]. Recently, single-use scopes have improved in optics and handling such that they are nearly equivalent to their reusable counterparts. By virtue of their disposability, single-use scopes remove concerns regarding repairs and sterilization. The cost/benefit analysis of single-use versus reusable flexible scope is highly dependent on a number of factors that are institution specific including case volume, repair frequency, and negotiated supply and service contracts.

Acquisition and Repair Costs of Reusable Flexible Ureteroscopes

Since their introduction into clinical use, flexible ureteroscopes have felt an evolutionary-like pressure to become as small and flexible as possible to allow near universal upper urinary tract access and decrease surgical morbidity. Most available

B. Winship · M. Lipkin (✉)
Department of Urology, Duke University Medical Center, Durham, NC, USA
e-mail: Michael.lipkin@duke.edu

© Springer Nature Switzerland AG 2020   73
B. F. Schwartz, J. D. Denstedt (eds.), *Ureteroscopy*,
https://doi.org/10.1007/978-3-030-26649-3_6

flexible scopes today range in shaft size from 7 to 10fr. Unfortunately, as demonstrated by Sung et al. [2], there is an inverse relationship between scope shaft size and frequency of damage requiring repair.

Reusable flexible ureteroscopes are extremely expensive instruments. New instruments range greatly in price and have been reported to cost as much as $52,000 and $70,000 USD [3]. The prices of different reusable flexible ureteroscopes may vary based on contracts between institutions and scope companies, as well as geographic location. However, it is not the purchase price of the instruments that drive costs for their use. Repairs of flexible scopes are responsible for about 50% of the costs associated with performing flexible ureteroscopy [4]. The average repair ranges from $2480 to $4535 USD [5]. The number of cases each scope can complete before requiring repair is widely variable and has been reported as low as 7.5 [3] and as high as 79 [6] procedures. A number of authors from academic centers involved in training urology residents have published reports with flexible scope durability averaging around 12 cases per repair [7, 8]. Conversely, a report from a specialized surgical center with no urology trainees reported a higher average durability of 21 cases [9]. Additionally, scope durability worsens with each subsequent repair. Multiple authors have reported that a single repair can decrease the number of cases performed before the next repair is required by up to 25% [8, 10, 11]. Given these considerations, the cost per case allotted to ureteroscope repairs varies by institution but has been reported to range between $358 and $957 USD [3–5, 8, 12].

Reprocessing and Sterilization Issues

Reprocessing flexible ureteroscopes between cases can cause damage and further elevate associated repair costs. The personnel performing this task can make a significant impact on repair frequency and therefore costs. Semins et al. [13] reported their experience in transitioning scope reprocessing from a central sterile processing unit to the urology OR nursing staff. This change nearly tripled the average number of cases their scopes could perform before requiring repair from 10.8 to 28.1 cases. This subsequently dropped their per case repair cost from $418 to $120 USD. Kramolowsky et al. [9] reported a similar finding at a specialized surgical center with reprocessing staff trained to specially handle ureteroscopes.

A single reprocessing has the potential to cause significant scope damage, but many ureteroscopes are subjected to multiple reprocessing cycles between cases. The average ureteroscope is reprocessed 1.8 times per case [6], and 12% of scopes must be rejected during case setup due to newly discovered damage or visible contamination [14]. Similarly, but of potentially much greater clinical and financial concern, contaminated scopes may be a vehicle for transmission of bacteria or viruses between patients. Ofstead et al. [15] examined the sterile processing of ureteroscopes at 2 centers and discovered protein in all examined scopes, hemoglobin in over half, and bacterial culture swabs from 2 of 16 patient-ready scopes grew organisms after the scopes had undergone sterilization. The clinical implications of such findings are unclear; however, examples of contaminated ureteroscopes acting as disease vectors have been published. For example, Chang et al. [16] published a report of ertapenem-resistant *Enterobacter cloacae* transmission linked to contaminated ureteroscopes in 2013. The potential expenses related to litigation of such cases could easily surpass any scope maintenance costs by many times.

Evolution of Single-Use Flexible Ureteroscopes

A single-use, disposable ureteroscope offers many potential advantages, obviating concerns regarding repairs and sterilization and allowing flexible ureteroscopy to expand its reach to areas without reprocessing and repair facilities. While flexible ureteroscopy was still in its relative infancy, Bagley reported his experience with a flexible ureteroscope with a reusable handle and disposable flexible tips [1]. However, it was not until 2009 and later that such devices became widely available for use [17]. The SemiFlex scope was the first such device. It was a fiberoptic ureteroscope with a reusable handle and eyepiece with a disposable semiflexible shaft. The published evaluation of this scope demonstrated acceptable benchtop performance relative to a reusable ureteroscope, but the scope failed to gain popularity and was eventually discontinued [17, 18]. The PolyScope was the next semi-reusable scope to enter the market. It offered a flexible, single-use shaft with reusable optical components in the form of fiberoptic bundles. The scope had a unique syringe-like handle that only allowed unidirectional deflection of 180° (Fig. 6.1). Despite reports that documented its performance relative to reusable scopes as adequate, it too failed to establish a foothold in the market [17]. In 2013, the Flexor Vue was released by Cook Medical. This scope had a 15fr single-use sheath designed to act as its own access sheath with a flexible tip and a hand piece that can be used up to ten times [19]. The scope's relatively large diameter and associated change in procedural steps required to use this hybrid access sheath/scope likely played a role in its

Fig. 6.1 The PolyDiagnost PolyScope

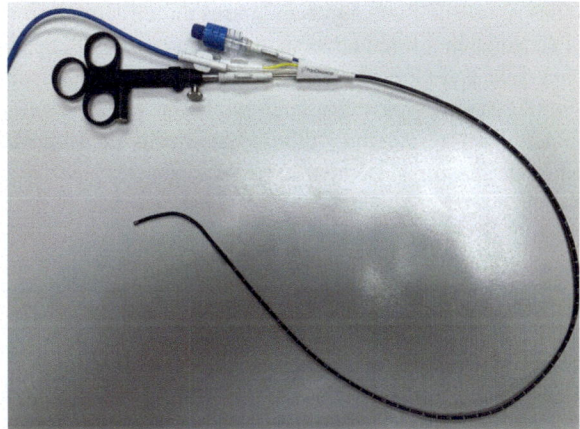

Fig. 6.2 The Boston
Scientific LithoVue

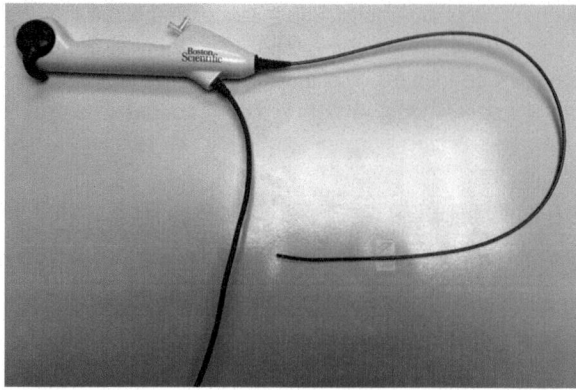

Fig. 6.3 The Pusen
PU3022a

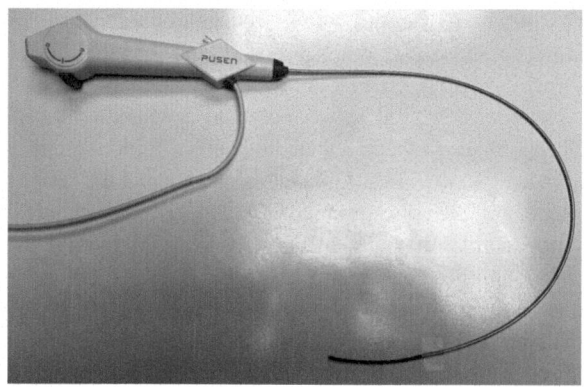

eventual discontinuation. In 2015, Boston Scientific (Marlborough, MA) released the LithoVue, a single-use digital scope designed to be a disposable mimic of reusable ureteroscopes. The LithoVue has 7.7fr flexible tip, 9.5fr shaft, and 3.6fr working channel and allows at least 270′ of tip deflection in two directions (Fig. 6.2). It has a built-in light source and plugs directly into its own monitor via a single cable [17]. Since that time, other manufacturers (i.e., PUSEN (Zhuhai, China) (Fig. 6.3)) have released single-use scopes which appear and function similarly to reusable scopes. Such scopes have been well received by urologists worldwide and for the remainder of this chapter, unless specifically mentioned, will be the scopes intended when discussing single-use ureteroscopes.

Comparing Single-Use and Reusable Flexible Scopes

The LithoVue and other similar scopes offer a nearly 1:1 exchange for a reusable scope in the domains of optics, flexibility, and other performance characteristics. Dale et al. [20] performed a series of benchtop comparisons of the LithoVue to fiberoptic and digital reusable scopes. They demonstrated that the LithoVue offers superior deflection of up to 276' with an empty working channel and maintains superior maximal deflection with a 200 nm laser fiber or 1.9fr basket in the channel relative to the reusable scopes. Optical resolution was on par with the digital scope, the Storz Flex-Xc (Karl Storz, Germany), and superior to the fiberoptic scope, the Wolf Cobra (Richard Wolf, Germany). Additionally, LithoVue maintained higher irrigant flow via the working channel with instruments in place. Similar benchtop studies comparing the LithoVue to other single-use scopes as well as both fiberoptic and digital reusable scopes have confirmed parity between devices with a few exceptions [21, 22]. Dragos et al. [23] examined the tip deflection characteristics of a number of fiberoptic and digital reusable scopes as well as the LithoVue. They demonstrated that the relatively longer inflexible tip housing the camera chip found on all digital scopes, LithoVue included, limits the ability to enter an acutely angled calyx when compared to a fiberoptic scope. Additionally, in another report, Dragos et al. [24] demonstrated that stiff instruments such as PTFE wires or biopsy forceps have a greater impact on loss of maximal deflection in single-use scopes relative to reusable scopes.

Clinically, the LithoVue has been evaluated relative to reusable uretereoscopes in many reports. Usawachintachit et al. [25] performed a case-control study to compare the LithoVue to the Olympus URF-P6 fiberoptic reusable scope. They demonstrate that in clinical use, the single-use scope had a 4.4% failure rate versus 7% for the reusable scope. Interestingly, they also found that the single-use scope saved about 10 min of OR time and was associated with fewer perioperative complications. They postulated the time difference observed may be due to simplified setup of the single-use scope (LithoVue requires plugging in a single cable versus the individual light cord and camera for the fiberoptic reusable scope). The reduced complications are not as easily explained; however, none of the differences in complications were secondary to infectious etiology, nor were they serious complications (all Clavien grade 1 or 2 regardless of scope used). Such significant differences in OR time and postoperative complications have not been reproduced in subsequent studies comparing single-use to reusable ureteroscopes.

Mager et al. [3] performed a prospective cohort study to compare the LithoVue to both a fiberoptic reusable scope and digital reusable scope. They report no difference between any of the scopes in terms of case success (ability to reach the target anatomy), perioperative complications, OR time, or radiography exposure time.

Given the disposable nature of single-use scopes, there have been concerns raised by urologists regarding sufficient durability to complete a prolonged or difficult case. In the above-referenced study [3], of the 68 cases completed with LithoVue, only one scope failure was reported. This failure occurred early in the case and was deemed to be due to a faulty scope which was replaced at no cost. Additionally, Doizi et al. [17] examined the maximal deflection of LithoVue at the start and completion of 40 consecutive cases with no significant difference found between the time points.

Some concerns about single-use scope durability may arise from the feel of these scopes in the surgeon's hands. Single-use scopes are far lighter than reusable scopes, which may create the feel of a poorly made device. However, rather than be a detriment, this may actually be an advantage. Proietti et al. [26] assessed the weight of a number of clinically available flexible ureteroscopes including digital and fiberoptic as well as single-use (LithoVue). The single-use scope was by far the lightest of the scopes at 277.5 g. On the other end of the spectrum, the Olympus URF-V2 digital reusable scope weighs in at 942 g. The relative weight of the ureteroscope may not seem important, but as demonstrated by Ludwig et al. [27], significantly more muscle work is required to complete a standard flexible ureteroscopy training task when using a heavier scope. Single-use scopes may thus allow less surgeon fatigue during longer cases or after multiple cases, which may improve efficiency in the OR. Such claims have been studied with other fatigue reducing surgical equipment, most notably the surgical robot [28, 29]. Although they used time as a measure of surgeon fatigue, Seklehner et al. [30] demonstrated a correlation between time in the OR and worsened stone-free rates. Such studies suggest the economic implications of using single-use scopes may go well beyond device acquisition and maintenance cost.

At the time of this writing, single-use scopes similar to the LithoVue such as the Pusen PU3022 have undergone limited published trials. Marchini et al. [31] performed in vitro comparison of the LithoVue and Pusen scopes and noted differences in resolution, irrigation flow rates, deflection loss with an instrument in the working channel, etc. Many of these differences were statistically significant, but relatively subtle as they were similar to the variation seen between different manufacturers of reusable scopes and their clinical significance is unclear. Clinically, Salvadó [32] reported on the Pusen scope in 11 cases and found no performance deficits.

Environmental Impact

The modern operating room creates an enormous amount of waste. This translates not only into cost to the healthcare system but potentially cost to the environment. One concern with single-use scopes is the exacerbation of this problem by adding yet another item to the waste bin at the completion of a case. At the time of writing, only one study has attempted to illuminate this issue with regard to single-use scopes. Davis et al. [33] examined the carbon footprint of a single-use scope (LithoVue) and a digital reusable scope (Olympus URF-V2). The solid waste produced and energy consumption required for the manufacture, repair, sterilization, and ultimate disposal of each scope was estimated and this converted to the equivalent mass of CO_2 produced. The authors used data from their own institution, including an average of 16 cases before the reusable scope required repair and 180 total cases before final disposal. They reported an average of 4.43 kg of CO_2 produced per case for a single-use scope and 4.47 kg of CO_2 produced for the reusable scope. Thus, it appears the potential environmental impact of single-use scopes is comparable to reusable scopes when measured by carbon footprint.

Cost Analysis

Performance issues aside, the logic of a single-use ureteroscope hinges upon its cost. Single-use ureteroscopes are a fraction of the price of a new reusable scope, but they remain relatively expensive as a line item for every case as a disposable instrument. Nonetheless, they eliminate the significant and uncertain repair costs associated with reusable scopes, offer the urologist a scope with consistency, like new performance in nearly every case, and remove the possibility of delayed or canceled cases due to sterilization or breakage issues.

Unfortunately, determining the economic impact of using a single-use ureteroscope is not a simple task. Negotiated prices for all ureteroscope-related services from initial scope acquisition to repair costs are variable and often confidential. At the time of this writing, the most commonly published price for the LithoVue is $1500 USD [34], and this is the price point upon which nearly all cost analysis studies have been based.

Note that the majority of centers that have performed cost analyses are academic training centers. As previously discussed, the number of cases a reusable flexible scope can be used before needing repair may be dependent on who is using the scope. Thus, cost analysis of single-use scopes differ significantly at centers not involved in training residents.

Martin et al. [7] performed a cost-benefit analysis comparing the LithoVue to a digital flexible ureteroscope (Storz Flex-XC, Karl Storz, Germany). They examined 160 cases completed with the reusable scope and compared the actual cost of these procedures to the projected costs of using a single-use scope for every case assuming a fixed cost for the LithoVue of $1500 USD per scope. They did not include the purchase price of the reusable scopes in their analysis, so this analysis may not be applicable to centers looking to establish or upgrade an existing fleet of ureteroscopes. They report the cases completed with reusable scopes cost on average $848 USD. At that price point, the authors concluded that if a center is performing 99 or more ureteroscopies per year, the reusable scopes were the more economical option.

A similar analysis by Mager et al. [3] reported the "breakpoint" for single-use scopes to be between 61 and 118 cases per year.

Taguchi et al. [12] performed a micro-costing analysis of cases completed with a fiberoptic reusable ureteoscope (Olympus URV-P6) and cases completed with the LithoVue. Their analysis assigned a price to every step of every procedure including steps such as disposal of the single-use scopes. One week of consecutive cases performed with each scope were analyzed. They report the average cost for the reusable scope cases was $2799 USD and for the single-use scope cases was $2852 USD. Note this study reported relatively high reusable scope repair cost at $957 USD per case and despite being performed at the same center as the Usawachintachit et al. study [25], found no significant OR time advantage to using the single-use scope.

Providing a slightly different angle, Tosoian et al. [5] reported that at their high volume academic center, they would remain profitable so long as average repair costs for their reusable scopes remained under $1199 USD per case.

Selective Use of Single-Use Scopes

Ozimek et al. [35] performed a cost analysis comparing a mix of cases completed with fiberoptic and digital reusable scopes to projected costs with a LithoVue. Similar to Martin et al. [7], they report that scope-related costs would have nearly doubled if they switched to single-use scopes for all cases. However, in examining their cases, they noted the majority of scope repairs were required following cases in which access to a lower pole calyx with an infundibulo-pelvic angle of <50° was required. The authors point out that if a single-use scope were used in these cases, the cost savings to their institution would have been enormous. They postulated that not only would repair costs have been decreased but total case number would have increased as case delays and cancelations would have been avoided, increasing overall revenue.

This report suggests that for high and potentially even moderate volume centers, selective use of single-use scopes may offer a major economic advantage. In addition to lower pole stones, other high-risk cases for scope damage have been identified including antegrade ureteroscopy and attempted ureteroscopic treatment of stones over 2 cm [6]. Additionally, Keller et al. [36] suggested that certain maneuvers to improve ureteroscope deflection can create enormous stress on the instrument and should only be employed with a single-use scope. For example, forced tip deflection, which is performed by forcing the scope to flex prior to the flexible tip fully exiting the access sheath, will decrease the deflection diameter of the scope by 66%. This allows entry into very steeply angled calyces but creates 4x more torque on the scope than regular full flexion.

Molina et al. [37] reported their results of selective use of the LithoVue at their center. They used a single-use scope in any case where the greatest stone diameter was over 15 mm or the stone was of any size requiring lithotripsy for treatment but located in a lower pole calyx and could not be easily relocated to an upper or middle calyx for lithotripsy. Over 15 months, they performed 228 ureteroscopies, 17 with a single-use scope per their selection criteria. They report a cost savings of over $52,000 USD relative to the prior 228 cases performed at their center. This translates to about $229 USD of savings per case.

Scope damage during difficult cases is not only a problem from an economic standpoint. Huynh et al. [38] reported on two cases of reusable ureteroscopes becoming entrapped in patients during surgery. One was able to be removed with endoscopic maneuvers, the other required open surgical extraction. Analysis of scope use in the second case revealed the scope had been used over 80 times for more than 2000 h of service. Accordioning of the distal bending rubber on the ureteroscopes was felt to be the initiating event in each case. Similar findings are echoed in a report examining the most common indications for repair of reusable scopes [39] as well as a review of mechanisms related to intraoperative ureteral avulsion injuries [40]. Certainly single-use scopes are not immune to structural failure; however, these data suggest the most dangerous failures are likely unique to reusable scopes used during multiple prior cases.

Conclusions

Despite much evidence suggesting single-use scopes are nearly equal to reusable flexible ureteroscopes in benchtop and clinical testing and recent work demonstrating there may be an economic advantage to using a single-use scope in selected cases, there persists a sentiment among urologists that reusable scopes are superior. Certainly, what differences exist between the two categories of scopes are subtle and difficult to objectively measure. For example, the authors have noted the LithoVue has a tendency to "white out" the center of the image, especially during laser activation. This phenomenon is not as pronounced in reusable digital scopes and will likely improve with advancing technology. In fact, the authors have noted improvement in this area with interval software improvements to the monitor's image processing software. Additionally, the currently clinically available single-use ureteroscopes all have larger tip and shaft diameters than most fiberoptic reusable scopes [20, 23, 24], potentially limiting their ability to gain access via a narrow ureter. Nonetheless, the most difficult cases that put ureteroscopes under the greatest strain and thus have the most potential for single-use scopes to assert an economic advantage are often the cases most urologists would choose to use their most high-performing scope.

As flexible ureteroscopes continue to evolve, single-use scopes may overcome this performance barrier. Digital imaging technology will continue to improve and become smaller and cheaper, allowing more maneuverable, higher definition scopes. New single-use scopes from multiple suppliers will enter the market, drive down proves, and/or improve on scope performance. It is likely that current reusable scope manufacturers will either join the single-use market or innovate ways to decrease repair costs. Fortunately, these changes will likely increase the availability of flexible ureteroscopy around the world by reducing the costs to low volume centers without access to repair or reprocessing facilities. If we look to the evolution of laser fibers, baskets, and many other endoscopic tools as examples, a near future with a completely disposable endourologic tool chest is not hard to imagine.

References

1. Bagley DH. Flexible ureteropyeloscopy with modular, "disposable" endoscope. Urology. 1987;29(3):296–300.
2. Sung JC, Springhart WP, Marguet CG, L'Esperance JO, Tan YH, Albala DM, et al. Location and etiology of flexible and semirigid ureteroscope damage. Urology. 2005;66(5):958–63.

3. Mager R, Kurosch M, Hofner T, Frees S, Haferkamp A, Neisius A. Clinical outcomes and costs of reusable and single-use flexible ureterorenoscopes: a prospective cohort study. Urolithiasis. 2018;46:587.
4. Landman J, Lee DI, Lee C, Monga M. Evaluation of overall costs of currently available small flexible ureteroscopes. Urology. 2003;62(2):218–22.
5. Tosoian JJ, Ludwig W, Sopko N, Mullins JK, Matlaga BR. The effect of repair costs on the profitability of a ureteroscopy program. J Endourol. 2015;29(4):406–9.
6. Legemate JD, Kamphuis GM, Freund JE, Baard J, Zanetti SP, Catellani M, et al. Durability of flexible Ureteroscopes: a prospective evaluation of longevity, the factors that affect it, and damage mechanisms. Eur Urol Focus. 2018. https://doi.org/10.1016/j.euf.2018.03.001.
7. Martin CJ, McAdams SB, Abdul-Muhsin H, Lim VM, Nunez-Nateras R, Tyson MD, et al. The economic implications of a reusable flexible digital Ureteroscope: a cost-benefit analysis. J Urol. 2017;197(3 Pt 1):730–5.
8. Hennessey DB, Fojecki GL, Papa NP, Lawrentschuk N, Bolton D. Single-use disposable digital flexible ureteroscopes: an ex vivo assessment and cost analysis. BJU Int. 2018;121 Suppl 3:55–61.
9. Kramolowsky E, McDowell Z, Moore B, Booth B, Wood N. Cost analysis of flexible Ureteroscope repairs: evaluation of 655 procedures in a community-based practice. J Endourol. 2016;30(3):254–6.
10. Canales BK, Gleason JM, Hicks N, Monga M. Independent analysis of Olympus flexible ureteroscope repairs. Urology. 2007;70(1):11–5.
11. Carey RI, Gomez CS, Maurici G, Lynne CM, Leveillee RJ, Bird VG. Frequency of ureteroscope damage seen at a tertiary care center. J Urol. 2006;176(2):607–10. discussion 10
12. Taguchi K, Usawachintachit M, Tzou DT, Sherer BA, Metzler I, Isaacson D, et al. Microcosting analysis demonstrates comparable costs for LithoVue compared to reusable flexible fiberoptic ureteroscopes. J Endourol. 2018;32(4):267–73.
13. Semins MJ, George S, Allaf ME, Matlaga BR. Ureteroscope cleaning and sterilization by the urology operating room team: the effect on repair costs. J Endourol. 2009;23(6):903–5.
14. Calio B, Hubosky S, Healy KA, Bagley D. MP89-17 bad out of the box: a report on preoperative failure rates of reusable flexible ureteroscopes at a single institution. J Urol. 2018;199(4):e1212.
15. Ofstead CL, Heymann OL, Quick MR, Johnson EA, Eiland JE, Wetzler HP. The effectiveness of sterilization for flexible ureteroscopes: a real-world study. Am J Infect Control. 2017;45(8):888–95.
16. Chang CL, Su LH, Lu CM, Tai FT, Huang YC, Chang KK. Outbreak of ertapenem-resistant Enterobacter cloacae urinary tract infections due to a contaminated ureteroscope. J Hosp Infect. 2013;85(2):118–24.
17. Doizi S, Kamphuis G, Giusti G, Andreassen KH, Knoll T, Osther PJ, et al. First clinical evaluation of a new single-use flexible ureteroscope (LithoVue): a European prospective multicentric feasibility study. World J Urol. 2017;35(5):809–18.
18. Boylu U, Oommen M, Thomas R, Lee BR. In vitro comparison of a disposable flexible ureteroscope and conventional flexible ureteroscopes. J Urol. 2009;182(5):2347–51.
19. Schlager D, Hein S, Obaid MA, Wilhelm K, Miernik A, Schoenthaler M. Performance of single-use flexorVue vs reusable boaVision ureteroscope for visualization of calices and stone extraction in an artificial kidney model. J Endourol. 2017;31(11):1139–44.
20. Dale J, Kaplan AG, Radvak D, Shin R, Ackerman A, Chen T, et al. Evaluation of a novel single-use flexible Ureteroscope. J Endourol. epub 2017.
21. Talso M, Proietti S, Emiliani E, Gallioli A, Dragos L, Orosa A, et al. Comparison of flexible Ureterorenoscope quality of vision: an in vitro study. J Endourol. 2018;32(6):523–8.
22. Tom WR, Wollin DA, Jiang R, Radvak D, Simmons WN, Preminger GM, et al. Next-generation single-use Ureteroscopes: an in vitro comparison. J Endourol. 2017;31(12):1301–6.
23. Dragos LB, Somani BK, Sener ET, Buttice S, Proietti S, Ploumidis A, et al. Which flexible Ureteroscopes (digital vs. fiber-optic) can easily reach the difficult lower pole calices and have better end-tip deflection: in vitro study on K-box. A PETRA evaluation. J Endourol. 2017;31(7):630–7.

24. Dragos L, Martis SM, Somani BK, Rodriguez-Monsalve Herrero M, Keller EX, De Coninck VMJ, et al. MP68-03 comparison of eight digital (reusable and disposable) flexible ureteroscopes deflection properties: in-vitro study in 10 different scope settings. J Urol. 2018;199(4):e917.
25. Usawachintachit M, Isaacson DS, Taguchi K, Tzou DT, Hsi RS, Sherer BA, et al. A prospective case-control study comparing LithoVue, a single-use, flexible disposable Ureteroscope, with flexible, Reusable Fiber-Optic Ureteroscopes. J Endourol. 2017;31(5):468–75.
26. Proietti S, Somani B, Sofer M, Pietropaolo A, Rosso M, Saitta G, et al. The "body mass index" of flexible ureteroscopes. J Endourol. 2017;31(10):1090–5.
27. Ludwig WW, Lee G, Ziemba JB, Ko JS, Matlaga BR. Evaluating the ergonomics of flexible ureteroscopy. J Endourol. 2017;31(10):1062–6.
28. Heemskerk J, Zandbergen HR, Keet SW, Martijnse I, van Montfort G, Peters RJ, et al. Relax, it's just laparoscopy! A prospective randomized trial on heart rate variability of the surgeon in robot-assisted versus conventional laparoscopic cholecystectomy. Dig Surg. 2014;31(3):225–32.
29. Hubert N, Gilles M, Desbrosses K, Meyer JP, Felblinger J, Hubert J. Ergonomic assessment of the surgeon's physical workload during standard and robotic assisted laparoscopic procedures. Int J Med Robot. 2013;9(2):142–7.
30. Seklehner S, Heissler O, Engelhardt PF, Hruby S, Riedl C. Impact of hours worked by a urologist prior to performing ureteroscopy on its safety and efficacy. Scand J Urol. 2016;50(1):56–60.
31. Marchini GS, Batagello CA, Monga M, Torricelli FCM, Vicentini FC, Danilovic A, et al. In vitro evaluation of single-use digital flexible ureteroscopes: a practical comparison for a patient-centered approach. J Endourol. 2018;32(3):184–91.
32. Salvadó JA, Velasco A, Olivares R, Cabello JM, Díaz M, Moreno S. PD35-11 new digital single-use flexible ureteroscope (pusen ^{TM}): first clinical experience. J Urol. 2017;197(4):e667.
33. Davis NF, McGrath S, Quinlan M, Jack G, Lawrentschuk N, Bolton DM. Carbon footprint in flexible ureteroscopy: a comparative study on the environmental impact of reusable and single-use ureteroscopes. J Endourol. 2018;32(3):214–7.
34. Davis NF, Quinlan MR, Browne C, Bhatt NR, Manecksha RP, D'Arcy FT, et al. Single-use flexible ureteropyeloscopy: a systematic review. World J Urol. 2018;36(4):529–36.
35. Ozimek T, Schneider MH, Hupe MC, Wiessmeyer JR, Cordes J, Chlosta PL, et al. Retrospective cost analysis of a single-center reusable flexible ureterorenoscopy program: a comparative cost simulation of disposable fURS as an alternative. J Endourol. 2017;31(12):1226–30.
36. Keller EX, De Coninck V, Rodriguez-Monsalve M, Dragos L, Doizi S, Traxer O. MP68-05 taking advantage of single-use flexible ureteroscopes: techniques of forced tip deflection and forced torque. J Urol. 2018;199(4):e918.
37. Molina W, Warncke J, Donalisio da Silva R, Gustafson D, Nogueira L, Kim F. PD53-03 cost analysis of utilization of disposable flexible ureteroscopes in high risk for breakage cases. J Urol. 2018;199(4):e1047.
38. Huynh M, Telfer S, Pautler S, Denstedt J, Razvi H. Retained digital flexible Ureteroscopes. J Endourol Caser Rep. 2017;3(1):24–7.
39. Canales BK, Gleason JM, Hicks N, Monga M. Independent analysis of Olympus flexible Ureteroscope repairs. Urology. 2007;70(1):11–5.
40. Tanimoto R, Cleary RC, Bagley DH, Hubosky SG. Ureteral avulsion associated with ureteroscopy: insights from the MAUDE database. J Endourol. 2016;30(3):257–61.

Chapter 7
Devices for Stone Management

Robert C. Calvert

Stone Retrieval Devices

History

Hugh Hampton Young performed the first recorded ureteroscopy in 1912 [1], but the first specifically designed ureteroscope was not produced until 1979 [2, 3], and ureteroscopic stone treatment did not start to become commonplace until the 1980s. Endoscopic extraction of smaller ureteral stones which had not passed spontaneously was frequently used as an alternative to open ureterolithotomy. Various extraction devices were in use from an early time: including the Council extractor (1926 [4]), the Johnson extractor (1936 [5]) and the improved Dormia extractor (1958 [6]). These extractors looked like large versions of modern day baskets and were inserted cystoscopically into the ureter (see Fig. 7.1). X-ray guidance was normally utilised to help engage the stone and extract it. Ureteral dilation was often required, and although this technique provided a welcome alternative to open surgery, there was no fragmentation, so engaging too large a stone was problematic and risked serious ureteral injury including avulsion. It was readily apparent that there was a lot of variability in the tightness of the lower ureter in different patients, so predicting which stones would be suitable for endoscopic management was haphazard, and basket impaction was not uncommon [7, 8]. This was normally dealt with by incising the vesico-ureteral junction endoscopically or by converting to open ureterolithotomy. There were some reports of serious ureteric injuries in the literature, and although they were not common, it is likely that there was under-reporting.

R. C. Calvert (✉)
Gow Gibbon Department of Urology, Royal Liverpool and Broadgreen University Hospitals NHS Trust, Kent, Lodge, Broadgreen Hospital, Thomas Drive, UK
e-mail: robert.calvert@rlbuht.nhs.uk

© Springer Nature Switzerland AG 2020   85
B. F. Schwartz, J. D. Denstedt (eds.), *Ureteroscopy*,
https://doi.org/10.1007/978-3-030-26649-3_7

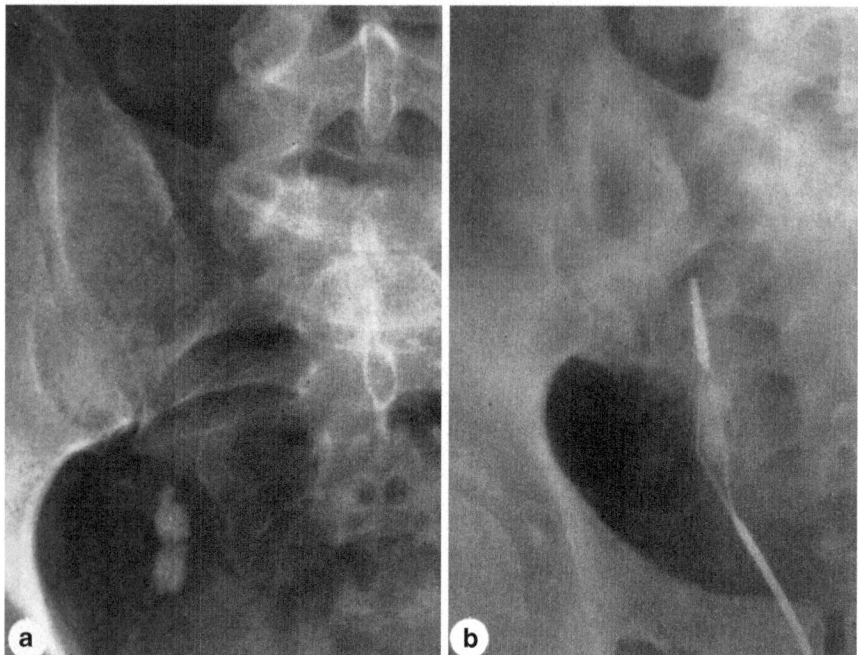

Fig. 7.1 A historic example of improper case selection for endoscopic manipulation (blind basketing) with a Johnson extractor. Open ureterotomy needed to release extractor and recover stone. (From Butt [8])

Modern Usage

The advent of rigid and semirigid ureteroscopes allowed the direct visualisation of the stone to allow more accurate assessment of the stone size in relation to the ureter and more precise engagement of retrieval instruments. Furthermore, ureteroscopy afforded the opportunity to apply stone fragmentation energies such as electrohydraulic lithotripsy, pneumatic lithotripsy and, latterly and most successfully, laser energy.

Miniaturisation and improvement in optics revolutionised the success and safety of ureteral stone retrieval, and blind basketing and open ureterolithotomy are no longer performed, having been replaced by ureteroscopy, shockwave lithotripsy and medical expulsive therapies. The advent of flexible ureteroscopes allowed retrograde fragmentation of stones within the renal pelvis or calyces, and its improvement with miniaturisation and exaggerated-deflection scopes in the years immediately following the millennium led to a dramatic growth in retrograde intrarenal surgery [9, 10].

Techniques of endoscopic stone management are discussed in Chapter 8. Small stones can sometimes be removed without fragmentation with a basket or forceps, but such stones have often passed spontaneously and not required ureteroscopy. The majority of ureteral or kidney stone treated will require at least some fragmentation. The holmium:YAG laser offers the possibility of disrupting the stone with a high-frequency energy so that it is partially vaporised and the residue becomes fine dust which can then be allowed to wash out (dusting). An alternative approach is to use the laser at a lower frequency but higher energy per pulse to cause the stone to fragment into a small number of intermediate-sized pieces that can be retrieved with a basket or forceps (fragmenting). The use of the fragmenting techniques in the kidney normally requires the surgeon to place a ureteral access sheath, as normally a number of passes of the scope and basket are required. The surgeon should be aware that the number of scope passes is proportionate to the stone volume and that the stone volume is proportionate to the third power of the stone's maximum diameter (assuming a spherical stone shape). Stone volume is the best predictor of operative time [11].

The surgeon will need to judge how small a fragment needs to be before it is appropriate to attempt to retrieve it. When treating a ureteral stone, it is not uncommon to push the stone back a little from its initial resting position which might be associated with mucosal oedema. It is not uncommon to attempt to remove too large a fragment which might not pass the tighter lower ureter or vesico-ureteral junction, so the surgeon should withdraw with care and under full vision. The use of a ureteral forceps allows easier release of stone fragments, but the surgeon might be more likely to inadvertently drop smaller fragments compared to using a basket. The surgeon needs to be particularly careful when using a basket in the upper ureter given the greater distance of ureter needed to be traversed.

When treating kidney stones, careful consideration also must be given to the fragment size and access sheath choice. Larger access sheaths have improved flow and allow the surgeon to remove larger fragments, but their deployment in tight and unstented ureters can be associated with risk to the ureter (see chapters 9 and 12). Fragmenting a kidney stone too much will increase the number of scope passes required for retrieval, or it may force you to change from a fragmenting strategy to a dusting strategy. It is probable that most cases of fragmenting involve at least some element of dusting.

Repositioning Stones

Baskets or forceps may also be used to reposition stones before laser treatment. The placing of a device through a flexible ureteroscope inevitably causes some loss of deflection. The first generation of flexible ureteroscopes could deflect to about 100–150° with an empty instrument channel. When a laser fibre was placed through the working channel, the scopes could barely deflect 90°, so that it was not possible to treat lower-pole stones. Importantly, about half of kidney stones sit in the lower pole. The disposable baskets tend to be less rigid than even a 200 μm laser fibre, and it was often possible to reposition the lower-pole stone into an upper-pole calyx to allow the laser to be used there [12, 13].

With currently available exaggerated-deflection flexible ureteroscopes, it is normally possible to target lower-pole stones in situ, but there are other reasons why the surgeon might still choose to reposition the stone. Firstly, it might simply be easier to treat the stone in an upper-pole calyx, and you might choose a calyx where the stone resulting fragments might be less likely to shoot off but be encouraged to bounce back and forth in front of your firing laser fibre improving fragmentation efficiency (popcorning). Secondly, if you have chosen a dusting approach to a stone, the small residue might be more likely to complete wash out if it is sitting in an upper-pole calyx. This consideration might be important if the lower-pole calyx has a long, narrow infundibulum and a tight pelvi-calyceal angle. Finally, using a laser at high energy setting with a high degree of deflection risks melting the laser fibre at the point of maximum deflection which is likely to destroy your flexible ureteroscope. There is quite a lot of variability in laser energy ratings of the differently available fine laser fibres, and the surgeon should consider this when choosing the most appropriate stone treatment strategy.

Types of Retrieval Devices

An ideal stone retrieval device needs to be strong and durable enough to last a long procedure but narrow enough to not obstruct the flow of irrigation through the working channel and flexible enough to not reduce the deflection of the flexible ureteroscope. The retrieval device should be able to efficiently pick up a range of stone fragment sizes but must also be able to release them easily.

Early ureteroscopists tend to use baskets that had been designed for cystoscopic manipulation such as the Dormia basket which was a helical device of stainless steel wires [14]. The stone was picked up by a rotational movement and later iterations of the basket and similar baskets such as the Bagley basket, and the double-helical Gemini baskets (see Fig. 7.2) are still in use. Such baskets tend to be fairly sturdy but large and are for use through a semirigid ureteroscope. Some variants have a filiform tip which might be of use in guiding the point tip of the basket safely past the stone reducing the risk of ureteral damage. The filiform tips can also help the surgeon re-enter the ureteric orifice after depositing stone fragments in the bladder. The size of these baskets does tend to cause a significant reduction in irrigation flow in most modern small diameter semirigid ureteroscopes.

The Segura™ basket (Boston Scientific Corp, MA, USA) was introduced in the early 1980s and consisted of four flat wires (Fig. 7.3). This basket had the advantage of being able to be opened wide in quite a small space, but the sharp edges of the wires could traumatise the mucosa. It became quite popular, but the stiffness of the basket limited its use with flexible scopes. The development of baskets made from the extraordinary nickel titanium alloy, Nitinol, has revolutionised stone retrieval devices, and nowadays most baskets are made from this. Nitinol is strong, is light, has a shape memory effect and is superelastic, allowing the wires to be folded into a narrow sheath to be passed through the scope and then to jump quickly to its

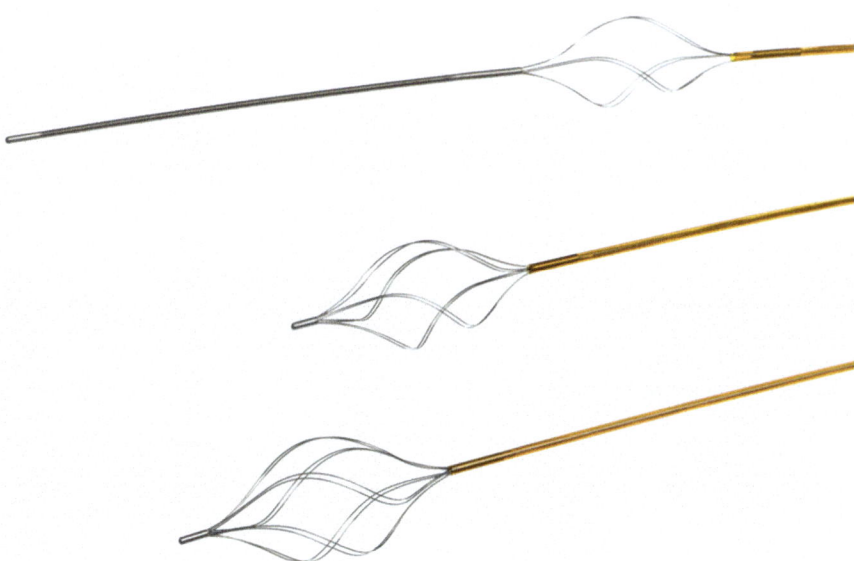

Fig. 7.2 Gemini baskets (Boston Scientific Corp, MA, USA). (Image courtesy of Boston Scientific Corporation)

Fig. 7.3 A/3B The Segura™ flat-wire basket (Boston Scientific Corp, MA, USA). (Image courtesy of Boston Scientific Corporation)

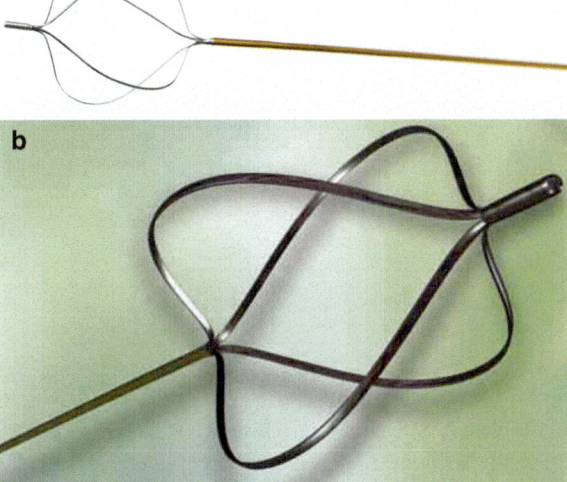

preformed shape as it is extended forward from its sheath. The spherical configuration without a tip is popular as typified by the Zero Tip™ Basket (Fig. 7.4, Boston Scientific Corp, MA, USA), the Halo™ (Fig. 7.5, Sacred Heart Medical Inc., MN, USA), the NCircle® (Fig. 7.6, Cook Medical LLC, IN USA) or the Dormia® No-Tip

Fig. 7.4 Zero Tip™
basket (Boston Scientific
Corp, MA, USA). (Image
courtesy of Boston
Scientific Corporation)

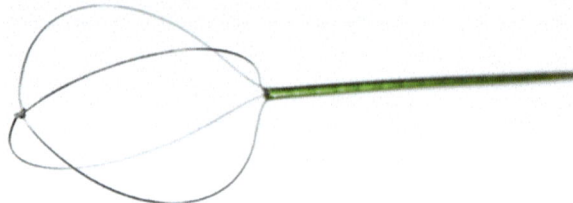

Fig. 7.5 Sacred Heart
Halo 1.5 Fr. Nitinol Tipless
Stone Basket (Sacred Heart
Medical Inc., MN, USA).
(Image courtesy of Sacred
Heart Medical)

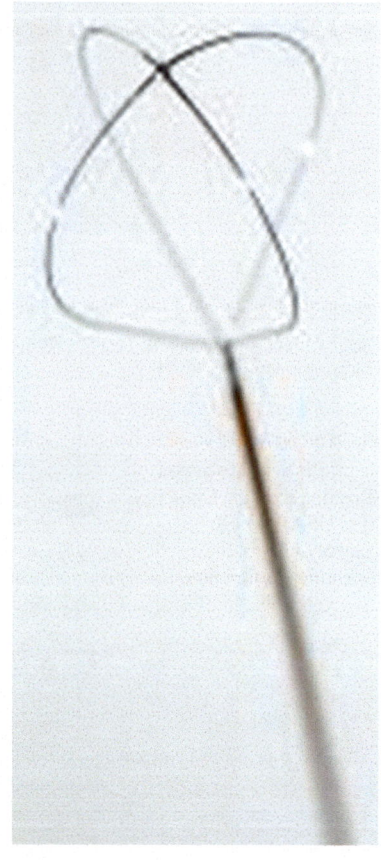

(Coloplast A/S, Denmark). This sort of basket allows stones in calyces to be picked up easily without traumatising the papillae.

Nitinol helical baskets have also been produced, e.g. NForce® (Fig. 7.6, Cook Medical LLC, IN USA) and Dormia® N.Stone® (Coloplast A/S, Denmark), and tend to be lighter in weight and more flexible than the stainless steel helical baskets.

Some manufacturers have produced baskets with a finer mesh designed to sweep smaller fragments from a calyx or ureter, e.g. the NCompass® (Fig. 7.6, Cook Medical LLC, IN USA) or the Leslie Parachute™ (Boston Scientific Corp, MA,

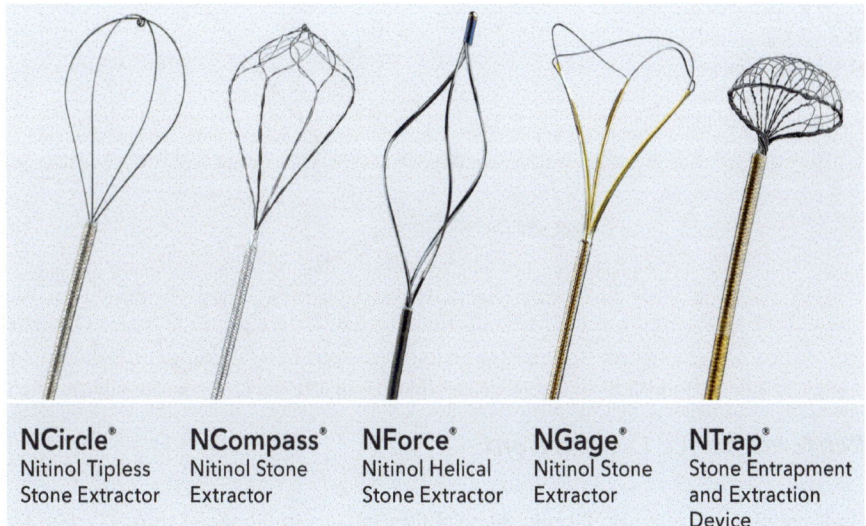

NCircle®	NCompass®	NForce®	NGage®	NTrap®
Nitinol Tipless Stone Extractor	Nitinol Stone Extractor	Nitinol Helical Stone Extractor	Nitinol Stone Extractor	Stone Entrapment and Extraction Device

Fig. 7.6 A range of different nitinol stone retrieving devices (Cook Medical LLC, IN, USA). (Permission for use granted by Cook Medical, Bloomington, Indiana)

Fig. 7.7 Rigid reusable stone graspers (Karl Storz-Endoskope, Germany). (©2019 KARL STORZ Endoscopy-America, Inc.)

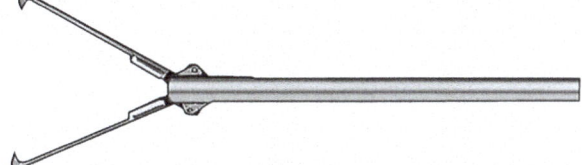

USA). These might be kept as part of the armamentarium of an endourologist for use in situations where it might be particularly important to clear all very small fragments.

Graspers can also be used to efficiently retrieve stone fragments. Various companies make reusable and single-use products, both rigid and flexible (see Fig. 7.7, KARL STORZ Endoscopy-America, Inc). The rigid graspers are mostly two-pronged, and they tend to be 3–4 FG in diameter which may preclude their use in some smaller semirigid ureteroscopes and will certainly substantially reduce irrigation flow. They are more robust than most of the baskets discussed and effective in removing larger fragments where the ureter will allow it. They are also the instrument of choice for removing retropulsed stents.

Three-pronged graspers such as the disposable Tricep™ grasper (Fig. 7.8, Boston Scientific Corp, MA, USA) are also available. Cook produce a product called NGage® (see Fig. 7.6) which is effectively a hybrid between triradiate forceps and a basket and might be useful to pick stones up which are adherent to urothelium of Randall's plaques.

Fig. 7.8 Tricep™ forceps
(Boston Scientific Corp,
MA, USA). (Image
courtesy of Boston
Scientific Corporation)

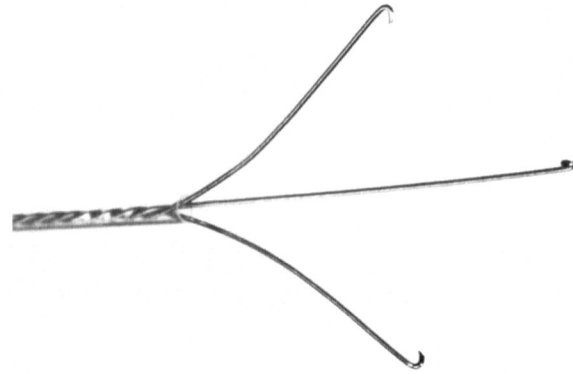

Retrieval Device Comparisons

Undoubtedly, personal preference plays a role in selecting a stone retrieval device, but several investigators have conducted comparative trials to help guide what device might be safest and most efficient in a range of circumstances. Hudson et al. [15] showed that the failure rate to pass a ureteroscope increased dramatically once the scope size reaches 9FG, and larger scopes will also have reduced irrigation outflow between the scope and inner ureteral wall. However, smaller scopes will inevitably have a small working channel also limiting irrigation flow. To optimise irrigation flow there will be a trade-off between external scope size and internal working channel size. Placing wires or baskets through the working channel has a dramatic effect on flow, and the relationship between basket diameter and flow is marked. Bedke et al. [16] demonstrated that using a 1.2FG basket resulted in a 13.6x increase in irrigation flow compared to a 2.2FG basket in the flexible ureteroscope they tested, albeit the 1.2FG was very much weaker on their breaking strength tests. There is a further trade-off between basket size and strength.

An in vitro model comparing five different basket types showed that the double-helical and parachute basket types performed best in retrieving different-sized beads from a simulated ureter. The flat-wire basket performed poorly. In a simulated calyx, the only basket to successfully remove beads was a tipless basket [17]. Monga et al. [18] evaluated the characteristics of 17 commercially available baskets in 2004. He found that tipless baskets opened more quickly to their target basket width than flat-wire or helical baskets and that the NCircle® basket exhibited linear opening allowing more precise control. A more recent comparison by Monga's group [19] found that the 1.5FG Halo™ basket performed better than the larger compared tipless baskets in the penetration force (safety metric), radial dilation force (functional metric for ureteral calculi), and limitation of deflection tests (functional metric).

Ptashnyk et al. [20] tested the efficiency and safety of a variety of stone retrieval devices in four ex vivo models including a single ureteral stone model, an impacted ureteral stone model, a steinstrasse model and a lower-pole kidney model. For the single ureteral stone and impacted ureteral stone models, the two-pronged grasper did best, and the helical basket also fared well. The three-pronged grasper and para-chute type basket caused most damage to the mucosa. For the steinstrasse model, the helical basket was more efficient than the two-pronged grasper, and the para-chute basket was found to risk significant ureteral damage. For the lower-pole stone model, no difference was found between the nitinol basket and graspers tested. Lukaswycz et al. [21] compared the efficiency of six tipless and four helical baskets in removing ureteral stones in a simulated model of the human ureter. Overall no significant difference was seen in the mean time of stone removal between the groups, and all devices removed the stone with a mean time of less than 16 s.

Complications Related to Retrieval Devices

A complete discussion of complications of ureteroscopy is in Chapter 12. Complications specifically related to retrieval devices may range from minor muco-sal abrasions to ureteral avulsion. Ureteral avulsion was reported in 0.5% of cases in a review from 1987 [22]. Thirty years later the Clinical Research Office of the Endourological Society (CROES) reported a rate of 0.1% ureteral avulsion in 8543 patients [23]. The risk was 0.3% in patients with impacted stones but 0.02% in unimpacted stones ($p < 0.001$). Avulsion often occurs while using a basket but can also occur by pushing a ureteroscope with excessive force into a tight ureter. Problems related to flexible ureteroscope deflection mechanism locking or bunch-ing of the distal bending rubber in a flexible ureteroscope [24] have also been reported to cause ureteral avulsion. This serious complication may be recognised immediately as the invaginated ureter is withdrawn into the bladder or out the ure-thra as the scope is withdrawn. It is likely that the risk is higher when using a basket in the upper ureter, and it is thought that the upper ureter has less muscular support than the lower ureter [25]. In benchtop and ex vivo porcine ureteroscopy models, Najafi et al. [26] found that only about 10 N of force was required to avulse a ureter. Ureteroscopists must be very aware of the risk of this complication and be ready to place a stent and return rather that exerting excessive force attempting to access a tight ureter. Care must be taken to not engage too large a stone in the basket, and impacted stones should be fragmented and disimpacted before extraction is attempted. Ureteral avulsion may be managed with early repair or nephrostomy and delayed repair, but complications following such reconstructions are high [27]. Lower ureteral avulsion injuries might be best managed with ureteral reimplanta-tion with or without a Boari flap.

Perforation of the ureter may be caused by basket or forceps tips or from tearing due to applying excessive force on a large stone fragment. They may be more likely with the more robust stainless steel retrieval devices and can normal be managed by ending the procedure promptly and placing a ureteral stent for a period of time [24].

Basket entrapment occurs when a surgeon engages a stone in the basket which is subsequently found to be too large to withdraw, but then the surgeon is unable to release the stone from the basket. Using excessive force in this situation risks serious injury including intussusception, tearing or avulsion of the ureter. Most baskets have a handle mechanism that can be disassembled. Doing so will allow the surgeon to withdraw the ureteroscope leaving the remaining basket and stone in situ. The surgeon can then reinsert the ureteroscope alongside the basket and fragment the stone sitting in the basket ultimately allowing retrieval of both [28]. Depending on the relative sizes of the basket and working channel, it may also be possible to place a laser fibre directly alongside the basket wire to fragment the stone without disassembling the basket handle. Entrapment is not a risk associated with the use of forceps for stone retrieval.

Repeated use during a long procedure can cause baskets to break, but laser energy, when applied directly, may also break a nitinol or stainless steel basket. Certain basket configurations, particularly tipped baskets, can spring open if broken, so care may be needed in withdrawing the basket to avoid lacerating the ureteral mucosa [29].

Antiretropulsion Devices

Semirigid ureteroscopes require saline irrigation to allow the surgeon to view the stone and safely perform stone fragmentation without damaging the ureteral mucosa. Ureteral stones often come to rest at a narrow point in the ureter, and gentle dislodging of the stone from the narrowed segment is into the more dilated proximal portion of ureter and allows the surgeon to get a clearer approach to the stone with the fragmentation device. Both the flow of irrigation and the actions of the fragmentation device (laser and, especially, the pneumatic lithotripter [30]) can cause further proximal migration of the stone into the kidney. This was a particular problem for upper ureteral stones in the earlier days of ureteroscopy when flexible ureteroscope and laser availability was poor. In such a situation, a ureteral stent was placed, and the patient needed to return for shockwave lithotripsy. Distal ureteral stones can also migrate into the proximal ureter during treatment, and this location can sometimes be more challenging to reach with a semirigid ureteroscope rendering the procedure more difficult [31]. A number of antiretropulsion devices have been developed to help avoid these problems. In modern practice some units will always have a flexible ureteroscope available so that if fragments of stone do wash back into the kidney, they can be dealt with at the same sitting. Other surgeons prefer to use antiretropulsion devices so that the stones can be completely extracted from the ureter to their satisfaction. A recent report from CROES database showed that 14.5% of 9877 ureteroscopies for ureteral stones were performed with an antiretropulsion device [32]. Moreover, the cases which employed such a device had marginally higher stone-free rates ($+2.8\%$; $p < 0.001$) and marginally shorter lengths of stay (-4.7%; $p = 0.001$).

Physical Techniques and Gels to Reduce Retropulsion of Stone Fragments

Control of irrigation pressure is likely to be the most important factor in reducing stone fragment retropulsion. Irrigation flow can determine the ureteroscopic view and may be increased by raising the height of the irrigation bottle or bag or by using pressure bags or pumps. A balance needs to be found between the perfection of the view and washing stones backwards. Placing the patient into a reverse Trendelenburg position might help but may compromise the surgeon's operating position.

Several authors have recommended injecting 1–2 ml of lidocaine jelly proximal to the stone through a 5 or 6FG ureteral catheter at the start of the procedure [33, 34]. The viscous jelly remains in the ureter long enough to slow down the fragment retropulsion before washing out, and Zehri et al. [35] found that retrograde stone migration was only 4% with this technique in a small randomised trial compared to the control procedure group where it was 28%. Stone clearance at 2 weeks was superior with the lidocaine jelly method (96% compared to 72%).

BackStop™ (Pluromed Inc., Woburn, MA, USA) is a reverse thermosensitive water-soluble polymer designed to be injected into the ureter proximal to the stone and used in the same way as lidocaine jelly. It later dissolves and washes out. Rane et al. [36] found that retropulsion occurred in 9% of cases using BackStop™ compared to 53% in a control group of ureteroscopic procedures, and it dissolved successfully in all cases.

The Range of Antiretropulsion Devices

The 12FG 4 cm Passport™ balloon (Boston Scientific Corp, Natick, MA, USA; see Fig. 7.9) was principally designed for ureteral dilation but has been used successfully to prevent stone retropulsion [37]. Ureteral baskets designed to collect small fragments such as the Lithocatch™ and Parachute™ (both Boston Scientific Corp., MA, USA) have also been deployed proximal to stone to prevent fragment migration [38].

Fig. 7.9 Passport™ balloon (Boston Scientific Corp., MA, USA). (Image courtesy of Boston Scientific Corporation)

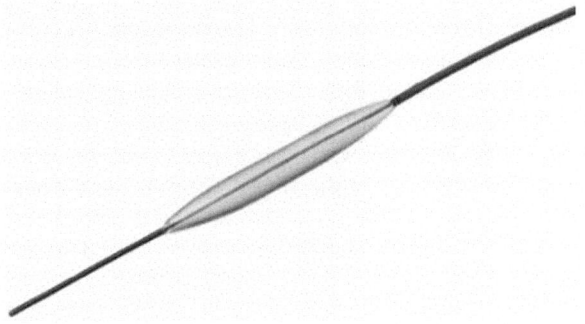

Fig. 7.10 Dretler Stone
Cone™ (Boston Scientific,
MA, USA). (Image
courtesy of Boston
Scientific Corporation)

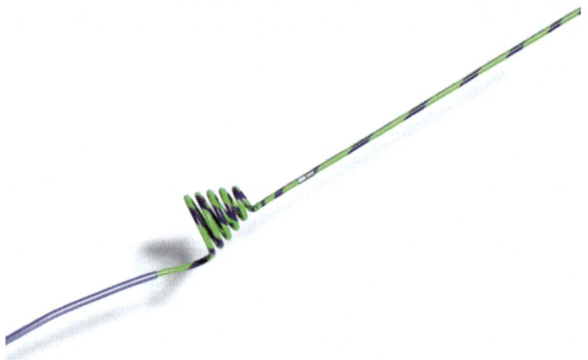

   The Dretler Stone Cone™ (Boston Scientific, MA, USA; see Fig. 7.10) consists
of a ureteral catheter with conical concentric coils which are deployed beyond the
stone to stop retropulsion of larger fragments [39]. The cone can also be used to
retrieve some fragments in its own right without risking fragment impaction. Desai
et al. found that using the Stone Cone™ during ureteroscopy resulted in fewer
residual fragments over 3 mm compared to a group of ureteroscopic procedures
where a flat-wire basket was used [40]. Twenty percent of the flat-wire basket group
needed an auxiliary procedure, but none of the Stone Cone™ group. In a randomised
clinical trial, Bastawisy et al. [41] found that proximal stone migration occurred in
15% of cases of ureteroscopic pneumatic lithotripsy using the lidocaine jelly
preventative technique, but not at all using a Stone Cone™. The Stone Cone™
comes in 7 mm and 10 mm outer diameter coil sizes and can be deployed
cystoscopically with screening although impacted stones often require it to be
deployed ureteroscopically. The Stone Cone™ is quite wide at 3FG which some
users have found this makes ureteroscopic access quite tight alongside within the
ureter [38].
   The NTrap® basket (Cook Urologic, IN, USA; see Fig. 7.6) is another type of
occlusive basket designed specifically to stop retropulsion of stone fragments during treatment. A meta-analysis of randomised trials [42] showed lower stone migration, a higher stone-free rate and less auxiliary shockwave lithotripsy in the patients
who had ureteroscopy using NTrap® compared to controls.
   Unlike the other devices mentioned above, the Escape™ nitinol retrieval basket
(Boston Scientific Corp., MA, USA; see Fig. 7.11) is 1.9FG and can be deployed
through the ureteroscope working channel with a laser fibre. An initial case series
has shown good stone clearance without complications [43].
   The Accordion™ (Percutaneous Systems, CA, USA) is a catheter-based mechanical occlusion device which has a hydrophilic flange that accordions together when
deployed proximal to the stone. This has been designed to reduce retropulsion,
allow increased irrigation flow to be used distally and to sweep out fragments without risking avulsion injuries. Wu et al. [44] found that its use improved the stone-free

Fig. 7.11 Escape™ basket
(Boston Scientific Corp.,
MA, USA). (Image
courtesy of Boston
Scientific Corporation)

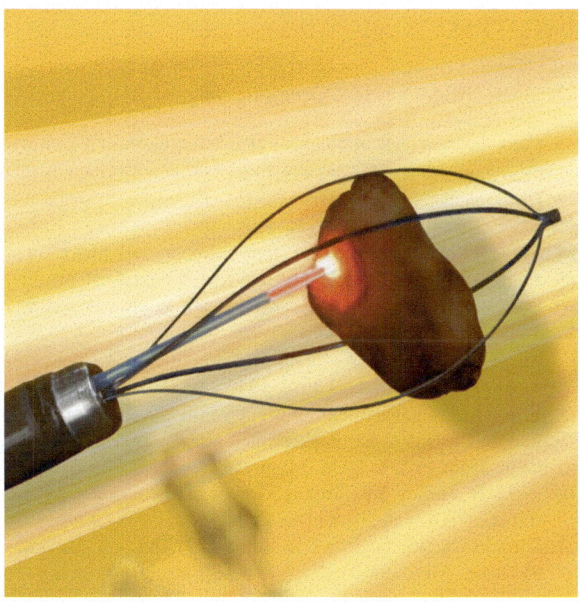

rate (84% vs 54%) compared to cases where it was not used in an institutional cohort comparison.

The Xenx™ (Rocamed, Monaco) is an antriretropulsion device which can function as an 0.038 inch guidewire when closed but opens to reveal a nitinol ureteral mesh. A comparative study of Xenx™ showed an improvement in the surgeons' assessment of intraoperative clearance of the stone, although lasering took longer in the XenX™ group compared to controls. There was no difference in stone-free rate at 4 weeks although 17% of the control group needed ancillary procedures to achieve this [45].

The cost of the aforementioned strategies varies significantly, but if the consequence of stone retropulsion is another procedure, then is this cost worth investing in? Ursiny and Eisner [46] constructed a decision analysis model to assess this. They calculated that it became cost-effective to use an antiretropulsion device with retropulsion rates above 6.3%. From their literature search, they determined that the weighted probability of retropulsion was 98% with an antiretropulsion device and 84% without one, so they calculated that these devices were cost-effective. Some, but not all of the studies on which these calculations and assumptions are based are for stone fragmentation using pneumatic lithotripsy where retropulsion rates are higher compared to laser stone fragmentation. Having a flexible ureteroscope available for all semirigid ureteroscopic procedures for ureteral stones might reduce the need, inconvenience and cost of ancillary procedures related to stone retropulsion, but sterilizing these flexible scopes frequently does itself have cost and may shorten their lifespans.

References

1. Young HH, McKay RW. Congenital valvular obstruction of the prostatic urethra. Surg Gynecol Obstet. 1929;24:25–42.
2. Lyon ES, Banno JJ, Shoenburg HW. Transurethral ureteroscopy in men using juvenile cystoscopy equipment. J Urol. 1979;122:152–3.
3. Huffman JL, Bagley DH, Lyon ES. Treatment of distal ureteric calculi using rigid ureteroscope. Urology. 1982;20:574–7.
4. Council WA. A new ureteral stone extractor and dilator. JAMA. 1926;86:1907–8.
5. Johnson FP. A new method of removing ureteral calculi. J Urol. 1937;37:84–9.
6. Dormia E. Due nuovi apparecchi per la rimozione dei calculi dall' uretere. Urologia. 1958;25:225–33.
7. Rusche CF, Bacon SK. Injury to the ureter due to cystoscopic intraureteral instrumentation: report of sixteen cases. J Urol. 1940;44:777–93.
8. Butt AJ, editor. Treatment of urinary lithiasis. Springfield: Charles C Thomas; 1960 Pub.
9. Leone NT, Garcia-Roig M, Bagley DH. Changing trends in the use of ureteroscopic instruments from 1996 to 2008. J Endourol. 2010;24:361–5.
10. Heers H, Turney BW. Trends in urological stone disease: a 5-year update of hospital episode statistics. BJU Int. 2016;118:785–9.
11. Sorokin I, Cardona-Grau DK, Rehfuss A, Birney A, Stavrakis C, Leinwand G, Herr A, Feustel PJ, White MD. Stone volume is best predictor of operative time required in retrograde intrarenal surgery for renal calculi: implications for surgical planning and quality improvement. Urolithiasis. 2016;44:545–50.
12. Auge BK, Dahm P, Wu NZ, Preminger GM. Ureteroscopic management of lower-pole renal calculi: technique of calculus displacement. J Endourol. 2001;15:835–8.
13. Bach T, Geavlete B, Herrmann TR, Gross AJ. Working tools in flexible ureterorenoscopy – influence on flow and deflection: what does matter? J Endourol. 2008;22:1639–43.
14. Dormia E. Dormia basket: standard technique, observations and general concepts. Urology. 1982;20:437.
15. Hudson RG, Conlin MJ, Bagley DH. Ureteric access with flexible ureteroscopes: effect of the size of the ureteroscope. BJU Int. 2005;95:1043–4.
16. Bedke J, Leichtle U, Lorenz A, Nagele U, Stenzl A, Kruck S. 1.2French stone retrieval baskets further enhance irrigation flow in flexible ureterorenoscopy. Urolithiasis. 2013;41:153–7.
17. El-Gabry EA, Bagley DH. Retrieval capabilities of different stone basket designs in vitro. J Endourol. 1999;13:305–7.
18. Monga M, Hendlin K, Lee C, Andersen JK. Systematic evaluation of stone basket dimensions. Urology. 2004;63:1042–4.
19. Patel N, Akhavein A, Hinck B, Jain R, Monga M. Tipless nitinol stone baskets: comparison of penetration force, radial dilation force, opening dynamics and deflection. Urology. 2017;103:256–60.
20. Ptashnyk T, Cueva-Martinez A, Michel MS, Alken P, Köhrmann KU. Comparative investigations of retrieval capabilities of various baskets and graspers in four ex vivo models. Eur Urol. 2002;41:406–10.
21. Lukaswycz S, Hoffman N, Botnaru A, Deka PM, Monga M. Comparison of tipless and helical baskets in an in vitro ureteral model. Urology. 2004;64:435–8.
22. Weinberg JJ, Ansong K, Smith AD. Complications of ureteroscopy in relation to experience: report of survey and authors experience. J Urol. 1987;137:384–5.
23. Legemate JD, Wijnstok NK, Matsuda T, Strijbos W, Erdogru T, Roth B, Kinoshita H, Palacios-Ramos J, Scarpa RM, de la Rosette JJ. Characteristics and outcomes of ureteroscopic treatment in 2650 patients with impacted ureteral stones. World J Urol. 2017;35:1497–506.
24. Tanimoto R, Cleary RC, Bagley DH, Hubosky SG. Ureteral avulsion associated with ureteroscopy: insights from the MAUDE database. J Endourol. 2016;30:257–61.

25. Huffman JL. Ureteroscopic injuries to the upper urinary tract. Urol Clin North Am. 1989;16:249–54.
26. Najafi Z, Tieu T, Mahajan AM, Schwartz BF. Significance of extraction forces in kidney stone basketing. J Endourol. 2015;29:1270–5.
27. De La Rosette JJ, Skreka T, Segura JW. Handling and prevention of complications in stone basketing. Eur Urol. 2006;50:991–9.
28. Motola JA, Smith AD. Complications of ureteoscopy: prevention and treatment. AUA Update Series, vol. 11, lesson 21, 1992.
29. Gallentine ML, Bishoff JT, Harmon WJ. The broken basket: configuration and technique for removal. J Endourol. 2001;15:911–4.
30. Knispel HH, Klan R, Heicappell R, Miller K. Pneumatic lithotripsy applied through deflected working channel of miniureterscope: results in 143 patients. J Endourol. 1998;12:513–5.
31. Robert M, Bennani A, Guiter J, Avérous M, Grasset D. Treatment of 150 ureteric calculi with the lithoclast. Eur Urol. 1994;26:212–5.
32. Saussine C, Andonian S, Pacik D, Popioloek M, Celia A, Buchholz N, Sountoulides P, Petrut B, de la Rosette JJMCH. Worldwide use of antiretropulsion techniques: observations from the clinical research office of the endourological society ureteroscopy global study. J Endourol. 2018;32:297–303.
33. Ali AA, Ali ZA, Halstead JC, Yousaf MW, Wah P. A novel method to prevent retrograde displacement of ureteric calculi during intracorporeal lithotripsy. BJU Int. 2004;94:441–2.
34. Mohseni MG, Arasteh S, Alizadeh F. Preventing retrograde stone displacement during pneumatic lithotripsy for ureteral calculi using lidocaine jelly. Urology. 2006;68:505–7.
35. Zehri AA, Ather MH, Siddiqui KM, Sulaiman MN. A randomized clinical trial of lignocaine jelly for prevention of inadvertent retrograde stone migration during pneumatic lithotripsy of ureteral stone. J Urol. 2008;180:966–8.
36. Rane A, Bradoo A, Rao P, Shivde S, Elhilali M, Anidjar M, Pace K, D'A Honey JR. The use of a novel reverse thermosensitive polymer to prevent ureteral stone retropulsion during intracorporeal lithotripsy: a randomized, controlled trial. J Urol. 2010;183:1417–21.
37. Dretler SP. Ureteroscopy for proximal ureteral calculi: prevention of stone migration. J Endourol. 2000;14:565–7.
38. Rane A, Sur R, Chew B. Retropulsion during intracorporal lithotripsy: what's out there to help? BJU Int. 2010;106:591–2.
39. Dretler SP. The stone cone: a new generation of basketry. J Urol. 2001;165:1593–6.
40. Desai MR, Patel SB, Desai MM, Kukreja R, Sabnis RB, Desai RM, Patel SH. The Dretler stone cone: a device to prevent ureteral stone migration-the initial clinical experience. J Urol. 2002;167:1985–8.
41. Bastawisy M, Gameel T, Radwan M, Ramadan A, Alkathiri M, Omar A. A comparison of stone cone versus lidocaine jelly in the prevention of ureteral stone migration during ureteroscopic lithotripsy. Ther Adv Urol. 2011;3:203–10.
42. Ding H, Wang Z, Du W, Zhang H. NTrap in prevention of stone migration during ureteroscopic lithotripsy for proximal ureteral stone: a meta-analysis. J Endourol. 2012;26:130–4.
43. Kesler SS, Pierre SA, Brison DI, Preminger GM, Munver R. Use of the escape nitinol stone retrieval basket facilitates fragmentation and extraction or ureteral and renal calculi: a pilot study. J Endourol. 2008;22:1213–7.
44. Wu JA, Ngo TC, Hagedorn JC, Macloed LC, Chung BI, Singal R. The accordion antiretropulsive device improves stone-free rates during laser lithotripsy. J Endourol. 2013;27:438–41.
45. Sanguedolce F, Montanari E, Alavrez-Maestro M, Macchione N, Hruby S, Papatsoris A, Kallidonis P, Villa L, Honeck P, Traxer O, Greco F, EAU Young Academic Urologists-Endourology and Urolithiasis Working Group. Use of XenX™, the latest ureteric occlusion device with guide wire-utility: results from a prospective multicentric comparative study. World J Urol. 2016;34:1583–9.
46. Ursiny M, Eisner BH. Cost-effectiveness of anti-retropulsion devices for ureteroscopic lithotripsy. J Urol. 2013;189:1762–6.

Chapter 8
Ho:YAG Laser Lithotripsy

Michael W. Sourial and Bodo E. Knudsen

Introduction

There have been numerous advances in holmium:YAG (Ho:YAG) laser lithotripsy since the preliminary reports of its use in urology were first published [1–3]. The Ho:YAG laser has become the gold standard for intracorporeal lithotripsy over the past few decades. This is based on two key features of the Ho:YAG laser: (1) its effectiveness in fragmenting stones of all compositions, a critically important property that limited the adoption of others types of laser for lithotripsy, and (2) its wide margin of safety.

Basic Physics

The word "laser" is derived from an acronym for "*l*ight *a*mplification by *s*timulated *e*mission of electromagnetic *r*adiation." Laser is a beam of energy (light) that is derived from a source of electromagnetic radiation. The properties of this light create the therapeutic effects used in surgical procedures. Laser consoles consist of an energy source (electric current) which is used to energize the atoms and generate light in the active medium. A resonant cavity is created using mirrors to reflect light, allowing it to have many passes through the medium. A small portion of the amplified light escapes out of the resonant cavity and forms the beam of laser light. The light exits the console in electromagnetic waves, with the light traveling in a highly ordered array, at the same wavelength and in the same direction, a term called "coherence."

M. W. Sourial · B. E. Knudsen (✉)
Department of Urology, The Ohio State University Wexner Medical Center, Columbus, OH, USA
e-mail: bodo.knudsen@osumc.edu

© Springer Nature Switzerland AG 2020
B. F. Schwartz, J. D. Denstedt (eds.), *Ureteroscopy*,
https://doi.org/10.1007/978-3-030-26649-3_8

Wavelength

The Ho:YAG laser operates at a wavelength of approximately 2140 nm in the near-infrared spectrum. This results in the laser energy being absorbed in water and thereby is ideal for the aqueous environment in which laser lithotripsy is performed [4].

Mechanism of Stone Fragmentation

The process of fragmenting calculi by the Ho:YAG laser will depend on pulse duration [5, 6]. At shorter pulse durations (less than a few microseconds), stones are fragmented by means of shockwaves that follow the breakdown and plasma expansion of ionized water or calculus compositions or by cavitation collapse, thus manifesting a *photoacoustical* effect. At longer pulse durations (>100 μs), the acoustic waves that accompany the collapse of vapor bubbles are of insufficient pressure magnitude to mechanically damage or fragment calculi. The mechanism of fragmentation with longer pulse duration is primarily *photothermal*, with increasing thermal collateral damage as pulse duration increased (>20 ms) [5]. The Ho:YAG lasers used clinically in urology operate with a dominant photothermal effect and typically have a pulse duration of 300 μs or longer depending on the model of laser used. Some weak photoacoustic effects can be seen, and this can result in movement and retropulsion of the stones when treated.

Laser Generators

Two components are required to deliver the laser energy to the stone: (1) a Ho:YAG laser console and (2) a fiber delivery system. A wide range of laser console options are available that start with low power systems capable of delivering 10–20 W of power up to newer high powered 120–140 W systems capable of delivering both high pulse energy and frequency.

The lower powered laser consoles will operate on a standard 110 volt outlet thus allowing operation in almost any type of procedure room – an advantage if the surgeon expects to use it in various locations with existing electrical infrastructure. The disadvantage of the lower powered systems is they are generally not capable of reaching the high pulse energy settings (2.0–3.5 J) and the high pulse frequency settings (50–80 Hz) of the high-power systems. This high pulse energy settings are important for soft tissue applications such as holmium laser enucleation of the prostate (HoLEP). The high pulse frequency settings have become increasingly used as surgeons employ "dusting" strategies to treat renal stones where low pulse energy and high pulse frequency are used. While Lumenis (Lumenis Ltd., Yokneam, Israel) have historically been the dominant purveyor of high-powered systems, more

Fig. 8.1 Example of
high-powered laser

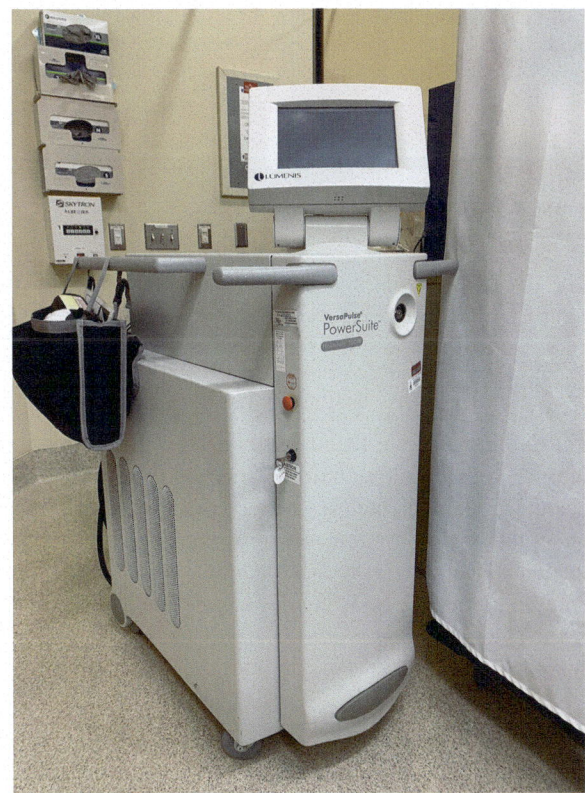

recently other manufacturers have released high-powered variants. The disadvantage
of the high-power systems is that they are large and bulky due to the extensive
cooling systems needed. Further, they require special electrical service. The
Lumenis Pulse™ 100H (*see* Fig. 8.1) and the Olympus EMPOWER 65 (Olympus
Surgical Technologies America, Southborough, MA), capable of pulse frequencies
of 50 and 60 Hz respectively, both require 20 amp electrical service. The Lumenis
MOSES Pulse™ 120H, which can operate at up to 80 Hz at some settings, requires
50 amp electrical service which can be a limiting factor when planning installation.
Some operating and procedure rooms do not have the infrastructure to support this
type of power, or it may require a costly upgrade to retrofit.

Lumenis (Yokneam, Israel) has developed a new technology for their Lumenis
Pulse™ 120H laser dubbed the "Moses effect." The laser pulse is modulated to
create a vapor channel between the tip of the fiber and the target stone or tissue. The
Olympus EMPOWER H65 system employs a "stabilization mode" to provide a
similar vapor channel effect. Pulse modulation is designed to improve energy
transmission to the target stone or tissue and thereby improve fragmentation, reduce
retropulsion, and ideally shorten procedural times [7]. Future Ho:YAG laser designs
will likely further work to optimize pulse modulation.

Fig. 8.2 Components
of fiber

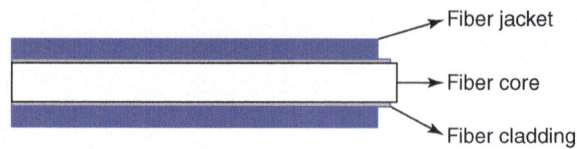

Fiber jacket

Fiber core

Fiber cladding

Laser Fibers

The Ho:YAG laser allows for the use of low hydroxyl silica optical fibers which are robust but relatively inexpensive fibers and are available in a variety of diameters and core sizes. The laser fiber is constructed of three key components: a core, a cladding, and a jacket (see Fig. 8.2).

The (1) silica glass core of the fibers used with the Ho:YAG laser is the laser light transmitting portion. Ideally laser energy should travel efficiently through the core through a process termed total internal reflection. The core is surrounded by the cladding. The (2) cladding may be made of similar material to the core but has a lower index of refraction, which is important for total internal reflection to occur at the boundary of the core and cladding. The (3) jacket, or outer coating, encases the core and cladding and functions to protect the delicate glass components of the fiber. The jackets are often colored which aids in visualizing the fiber both endoscopically and outside the patient.

Laser Fiber Size

The diameter of a laser fiber affects how that fiber might perform. For example, larger fibers may be less flexible and limit irrigation flow. Often urologists will request a "200 μm" laser fiber to use for their procedures not necessarily understanding that the fibers are not 200 μm in overall diameter. In fact, there are few commercially available fibers that can be used for laser lithotripsy that are 200 μm in diameter. The true diameter of most fibers is significantly greater as the diameter must take into account the combination of the fiber's core, cladding, and jacket. For example, the Cook (Spencer, IN) HLF-S200 fiber is marketed as having a 200 μm diameter, but it is the fiber core that measures 200 μm and the true diameter of the fiber, when taking the core, cladding, and jacket into account, is approximately 374 μm. Another even more confusing example is the Boston Scientific (Marlborough, MA) Flexiva 200 fiber. While the name of the fiber implies it is 200 μm, the core is about 240 μm and the true diameter of the fiber is 443 μm, so in fact no part of the fiber is 200 μm [8].

A range of fiber core sizes are used for Ho:YAG laser lithotripsy with a range of approximately 150–1000 μm. The choice of fiber core size should depend on the application and instrument through which it is used (Table 8.1). Smaller core sizes (150–300 μm) are typically used in flexible ureteroscopes, while larger core sizes

Table 8.1 Preferred laser fiber core diameter

Location/ureteroscope	Core size	Notes
Kidney/flexible ureteroscope	240–272 μm	Ball-tip fiber preferred to preserve inner lining of flexible ureteroscope
Ureter/flexible ureteroscope	240–272 μm	Ball-tip fiber preferred to preserve inner lining of flexible ureteroscope
Semirigid ureteroscopes (4.5–6F)	240–272 μm	Flat-tipped fiber
Semirigid ureteroscopes (>6F)	365 μm	Flat-tipped fiber

(200–365 μm) can be used in semirigid ureteroscopes or mini-PCNL nephroscopes which have larger working channels and can still provide adequate irrigant flow. The 550–1000 μm core fibers are usually reserved for use through large rigid instruments such as standard 24F nephroscopes and cystoscopes, as they lack flexibility and can be too large to fit through the working channel of endoscopes used for ureteroscopy. These large fibers can be used for holmium laser enucleation of the prostate, PCNL, or cystolitholapaxy.

The beam profile of the Ho:YAG lasers couples best with core sizes of greater than 200 μm and ideally larger than about 240 μm. Smaller core sizes risk launching the laser energy into the cladding which can damage or destroy the fiber. Prior bench testing of fibers has demonstrated that fibers with core sizes <240 μm were more prone to failure [9]. For flexible ureteroscopy with intracorporeal lithotripsy, choosing a fiber with a core size of 240–270 μm offers a fair trade-off between durability and size.

Fiber Performance: Flexibility

The flexibility of a laser fiber is an important performance component for fibers used during ureteroscopy, especially for stones located in the lower pole. The flexibility of a fiber is affected by both the diameter of the fiber and the components used to construct the fiber. The deflection of a ureteroscope can be limited if a stiffer laser fiber is used, potentially limiting access to lower pole stones in certain situations. When a selection of fibers with 240–270 μm core diameters were evaluated for flexibility, approximately 30–60° of baseline deflection was lost when inserted into a Stryker (Kalamazoo, MI) U-500 flexible ureteroscope that has 275° of baseline deflection. Fibers with a slightly smaller core size of 200 μm had slightly less deflection loss, averaging 20–30° of deflection loss in the U-500 [8]. Therefore if maximal deflection is needed to reach a stone, then a 200 μm core fiber may be the best option to reach the target. Stiffer, less flexible fibers have the potential to put added strain on the deflection mechanism of a delicate flexible ureteroscope which could lead to premature failure of the device.

Fiber Performance: Durability

Durability refers to the resistance of the fiber to fracture with bending. Typically the fibers do not fail with bending alone but rather fail when the laser is activated with the fiber in a deflected position. The concept is that with bending, there can be a loss of total internal reflection of the laser energy within the fiber core, and when the energy leaks into the cladding and especially the jacket, the fiber will fail due to thermal damage [4]. Increasing both the pulse energy setting of the laser and the tightness of the fiber bend increases the risk of fiber failure [10]. Should this occur during a clinical case, it could result in catastrophic damage to the flexible uretero-scope secondary to damage from the laser energy. The broken piece of the fiber could fall into the kidney and require extraction, which may be technically difficult. Moving and displacing stones from the lower pole to an easier to access location such as the renal pelvis or upper pole is also a prudent strategy to reduce the risk of fiber failure. This decreases the strain on the deflection mechanism of the flexible ureteroscope and may increase the stone-free rates after the procedure [11, 12].

Fiber Tip

Historically the tips of the laser fibers used in urology have been primarily flat. More recently manufacturers have introduced modifications to the fiber tip. The most common of these is a round or "ball tip" (see Fig. 8.3). By placing a ball tip on the end of the fiber, it allows for the fiber to be passed with less resistance through a flexible ureteroscope. The concept is that the ball-tip slides more freely in the working channel of the ureteroscope and is less likely to dig in or gouge the delicate inner lining. During a procedure, a ball tip allows a fiber to be advanced through the channel with the ureteroscope in a deflected position, something that would not be recommended with a flat tip fiber. This may be helpful when there is a difficult-to-reach lower pole stone and the surgeon does not want to pull the ureteroscope out of

Fig. 8.3 Ball-tip fiber

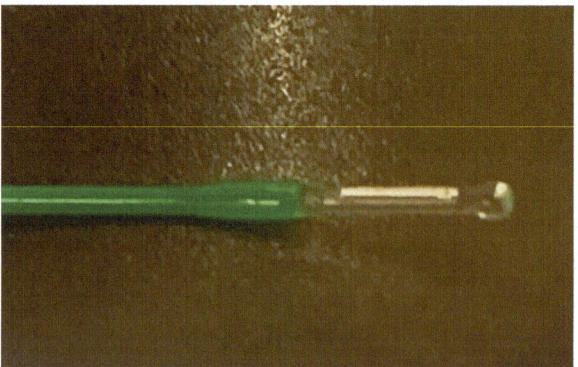

the lower pole to advance the fiber once he or she has identified the target. Studies have determined that the ablative properties were not changed whether the tip configuration of a fiber is flat or ball tip [13, 14].

The fiber tip is often degraded with burnback. Preparation of the fiber tip consists of stripping the terminal portion of the jacket and then cleaving several mm off the end of the core. Specialized tools such as laser fiber strippers and ceramic scissors exist for that purpose. In one in vitro study, the coated fibers (compared to stripped) regardless of how they were cut (metal or ceramic scissors) yielded better lithotripsy performance. The authors hypothesized that stripping the fibers may damage the cladding layer [15].

Single-Use Versus Reusable Fibers

There is currently a wide range of commercially available laser fibers, with both single use and reusable variants available. Historically, reusable fibers were more costly to purchase, but with repeated use the cost is amortized over the life of the fiber and reusable fibers can be more cost-effective than single-use variants [16]. In general terms, performance between single-use and reusable fibers has been similar, although there have been examples where the reusable version from a manufacturer outperformed their single-use version [9, 10]. In recent years, a shift has begun to occur with some laser fiber manufacturers focusing on high-cost, single-use fibers. An example of this is the Boston Scientific Flexiva and Flexiva TracTip 200 fiber line. The fibers are single use only and reusable variants are not available. These fibers sit at the high end of the price spectrum for Ho:YAG fibers but have been shown to have excellent performance characteristics [17].

Use of Laser Fibers in Ureteroscopy

The primary advantage of the Ho:YAG laser in ureteroscopy is that it can be used to fragment stones of any composition. The procedure is performed by carefully advancing the laser fiber in through the working channel of the ureteroscope. The tip of the fiber should always be visualized. The tip of the fiber should be in contact with the stone for efficient fragmentation. Failure to see the tip of the fiber may indicate that the fiber is inside the working channel of the ureteroscope and, if activated, can cause catastrophic damage to the ureteroscope. Furthermore, the cavitation bubble collapse created by the individual pulses may be of sufficient magnitude to damage the ureteroscope. In one study, when the laser fiber was advanced out to a point that it occupied a quarter of the video screen, the bubble generated by laser activation never touched the flexible ureteroscope tip, thus preserving the scope from damage. The authors dubbed this the "safety-distance concept" [18].

Outcomes of Ho:YAG Laser Lithotripsy

Preliminary experience using the Ho:YAG laser to fragment stones highlighted a few important points [2]. First, the laser proved *effective* at treating stones, with a stone-free rate of 92% in 21 patients. Second, the laser was *versatile* in treating stones located throughout the entire urinary tract and proved particularly helpful in treating calyceal stones away from the nephrostomy tract in percutaneous nephrolithotomy when used in flexible nephroscopy. Third, the laser had the ability to treat stones of *all* compositions, including cystine stones and calcium oxalate monohydrate stones, which had failed previously attempted treatment modalities. In addition, the laser proved to be safe, with one case of ureteral perforation when the device was used under fluoroscopic control rather than direct visualization.

Larger series with over 500 patients validated the initial findings and had similar conclusions highlighting the Ho:YAG laser's efficacy at treating stones, with stone-free rates >90% and very low rates of complications including ureteral perforation and stricture formation (<1%) [19, 20].

As experience with Ho:YAG laser lithotripsy grew, studies began to investigate its use with more challenging patient populations. Excellent outcomes were reported in various clinical situations, including patients with morbid obesity [21], bleeding diatheses [22, 23], anomalous kidneys [24], and the gravid [25] and pediatric [26] patient population. The combination of small caliber highly deflectable ureteroscopes coupled with Ho:YAG laser allowed surgeons to perform procedures that may have historically required more invasive means such as percutaneous or even open approaches [27, 28].

One caveat is that most series use plain abdominal radiograph and renal ultrasound to report stone-free rates, which may overestimate the true stone-free rates. When evaluating stone-free rates using computed tomography, the true stone-free rates appear to be much lower (~50%) [29] (Table 8.2). In one retrospective multicenter trial, the natural history of stone fragments in 232 patients after ureteroscopy at a mean follow-up of 16.8 months was evaluated. In this cohort, 44% of patients experienced a stone-related event, defined as stone growth, stone passage, and need for re-intervention or complication (e.g., symptoms, emergency department (ED) visit, hospital admission, or worsening renal function). Among this group, 29% of patients required surgical re-intervention, and 15% experienced a complication that did not culminate in re-intervention. Furthermore, patients with residual fragments larger than 4 mm were significantly more likely to experience complications or

Table 8.2 URS outcomes – KUB/RUS versus CT follow-ups

Study	N	Follow-up	Imaging modality	SFR
Sofer et al. (2002)	598	6–12 weeks	KUB/RUS	97%
Jiang et al. (2007)	697	2–4 weeks	KUB/RUS	92%
Rippel et al. (2012)	265	30–90 days	CT	62%
Portis et al. (2006)	58	30 days	CT	54%
Macejko et al. (2009)	92	1 day–16.9 months (mean 3 months)	CT	50%

stone growth or to require re-intervention than patients with fragments smaller than 4 mm [30].

Ureteroscopy remains one of the most efficacious, safe, and versatile treatment modalities to treat urolithiasis; however the procedure should be optimized to reduce residual fragments to ultimately reduce potential postoperative morbidity.

Dusting vs Fragmenting

Traditional fragmentation of stones utilized higher energy settings (0.6–1 J) and lower-frequency settings (6–15 Hz). The stone would fragment into pieces that were then amenable to basket removal. Recently there has been an interest in the "dusting" technique where lower energy settings (0.2–0.4 J) and higher-frequency settings (50–80 Hz) are utilized to pulverize the stone into "dust." The goal in dusting is to leave no large fragments behind, avoiding the need to basket stones. A ureteral access sheath may also be omitted in these cases since multiple in/out passages to the kidney are no longer required.

More recently, many consoles have the additional option of varying the pulse duration or modulating the pulse generated that can impact the performance of the system. In an in vitro dusting model, a longer laser pulse duration provided effective stone comminution with the advantage of reducing laser fiber tip degradation and stone retropulsion [31]. Lumenis (Yokneam, Israel) has developed a modulated pulse for their Lumenis Pulse™ 120H laser dubbed the "Moses effect." Although the exact details of the mechanism have not been fully reported, it appears to work by employing a double pulse of the laser. The first pulse is delivered to create a vapor channel to the stone, and then the second pulse contacts the target stone and provides the lithotripsy effect. Reports demonstrate the potential for reduced retropulsion and greater ablation efficiency as compared to standard short pulse modes [7].

A prospective, multicenter trial [32] from the EDGE (Endourology Disease Group for Excellence) Research Consortium aimed to determine which modality (dusting or fragmenting) produced a higher stone-free rate with the fewest complications. A total of 84 and 75 patients with 5–20 mm renal stone burden were enrolled in the basketing and dusting arms, respectively. The stone-free rate was significantly higher in the basketing group on univariate analysis (74.3% vs 58.2%, $p = 0.04$) but not on multivariate analysis (1.9 OR, 95% CI 0.9–4.3, $p = 0.11$). In patients who underwent a basketing procedure, operative time was 37.7 min longer than in those treated with a dusting procedure (95% CI 23.8–51.7, $p < 0.001$). There was no statistically significant difference in complication rates, hospital readmissions, or additional procedures between the groups.

Ultimately, both modalities should be readily available to the urologist, and one can oftentimes revert between the two depending on the specific clinical situation (Table 8.3).

Table 8.3 Recommended laser settings

Stone location	Fragmentation vs dusting	Settings	Pulse duration
Kidney	Fragmentation	Energy: 0.6–1.0 J	Short
		Frequency: 6–10 Hz	
	Dusting	Energy: 0.2–0.4 J	Long or pulse modulation mode
		Frequency: 40–80 Hz[a]	
Ureter	Fragmentation	Energy: 0.6–0.8 J	Short
		Frequency: 6–8 Hz	
	Dusting	Energy: 0.2–0.4 J	Long or pulse modulation mode
		Frequency: 40–80 Hz[a]	
Bladder	Mixed (residual pieces cleared with Elik evacuator)	Energy: 1.5–2.0 J	Long or pulse modulation mode
		Frequency: 50 Hz[a]	

[a]If laser console is not capable of high-frequency setting, a lower setting may be used, but this will increase the duration of the procedure

Safety

The Ho:YAG laser is a safe and efficient technology for the treatment of urolithiasis in all groups of patient. Its safety has been confirmed in the young and elderly, in pregnant patients, in renal transplants, and in patients on anticoagulation [23]. A few precautions specific to the Ho:YAG laser are worth mentioning. The risk of ureteral perforation is extremely low; however at least three deaths were reported as a result of ureteral perforation with the Ho:YAG laser (specific procedure performed was not specified) [33]. Ho:YAG lithotripsy of pure uric acid stone produces cyanide by a photothermal mechanism; however the amount produced is clinically insignificant [34]. In an ex vivo study, Ho:YAG laser induced corneal lesions in unprotected eyes, ranging from superficial burning lesions to full-thickness necrotic areas, and was directly related to pulse energy and time of exposure and inversely related to the distance from the eye. However, when the laser was placed 5 cm or more, no corneal damage was observed regardless of the laser setting and the time of exposure. Eyeglasses were equally as effective in preventing laser damage as laser safety glasses.

More recently, given the advent of new higher powered laser, attention has been given to local temperature rapidly rising at the site of laser lithotripsy, particularly without irrigation [35, 36]. This could potentially cause structural damage to the surrounding urothelium and renal parenchyma with protein denaturation occurring at temperatures as low as 43 °C. In one study, Ho:YAG fiber activation at 1 J and 10 Hz can cause the temperature to rise 60 degrees Celsius in under 60 seconds. This rapid rise in temperature seems to be mitigated with irrigant flow, and thus care should be given to ensure adequate irrigation, or intermittent laser stoppage to avoid thermal damage, particularly in cases of obstructed calyces where flow is limited [35–37].

Conclusion

The Ho:YAG laser is currently the gold standard for ureteroscopic intracorporeal lithotripsy, based on its effectiveness and wide margin of safety. Laser fibers vary greatly in their performance characteristics including their flexibility and durability. New higher-powered laser consoles can provide higher energy and frequency settings, allowing for more efficient stone fragmentation. Newer technologies such as varying the pulse duration or the "Moses" pulse modulation can also potentially performance characteristics of the lasers.

References

1. Erhard MJ, Bagley DH. Urologic applications of the holmium laser: preliminary experience. J Endourol. 1995;9(5):383–6.
2. Denstedt JD, Razvi HA, Sales JL, Eberwein PM. Preliminary experience with holmium: YAG laser lithotripsy. J Endourol. 1995;9(3):255–8.
3. Matsuoka K, Iida S, Nakanami M, Koga H, Shimada A, Mihara T, et al. Holmium: yttrium-aluminum-garnet laser for endoscopic lithotripsy. Urology. 1995;45(6):947–52.
4. Marks AJ, Teichman JM. Lasers in clinical urology: state of the art and new horizons. World J Urol. 2007;25(3):227–33.
5. Chan KF, Pfefer TJ, Teichman JM, Welch AJ. A perspective on laser lithotripsy: the fragmentation processes. J Endourol. 2001;15(3):257–73.
6. Vassar GJ, Chan KF, Teichman JM, Glickman RD, Weintraub ST, Pfefer TJ, et al. Holmium: YAG lithotripsy: photothermal mechanism. J Endourol. 1999;13(3):181–90.
7. Elhilali MM, Badaan S, Ibrahim A, Andonian S. Use of the moses technology to improve holmium laser lithotripsy outcomes: a preclinical study. J Endourol. 2017;31(6):598–604.
8. Akar EC, Knudsen BE. Evaluation of 16 new holmium:yttrium-aluminum-garnet laser optical fibers for ureteroscopy. Urology. 2015;86(2):230–5.
9. Mues AC, Teichman JM, Knudsen BE. Evaluation of 24 holmium:YAG laser optical fibers for flexible ureteroscopy. J Urol. 2009;182(1):348–54.
10. Knudsen BE, Glickman RD, Stallman KJ, Maswadi S, Chew BH, Beiko DT, et al. Performance and safety of holmium: YAG laser optical fibers. J Endourol. 2005;19(9):1092–7.
11. Auge BK, Dahm P, Wu NZ, Preminger GM. Ureteroscopic management of lower-pole renal calculi: technique of calculus displacement. J Endourol. 2001;15(8):835–8.
12. Wolf JS Jr. Ureteroscopic treatment of lower pole calculi: comparison of lithotripsy in situ and after displacement. Int Braz J Urol. 2002;28(4):367–8.
13. Kronenberg P, Traxer O. Lithotripsy performance of specially designed laser fiber tips. J Urol. 2016;195(5):1606–12.
14. Shin RH, Lautz JM, Cabrera FJ, Shami CJ, Goldsmith ZG, Kuntz NJ, et al. Evaluation of novel ball-tip holmium laser fiber: impact on ureteroscope performance and fragmentation efficiency. J Endourol. 2016;30(2):189–94.
15. Kronenberg P, Traxer O. Are we all doing it wrong? Influence of stripping and cleaving methods of laser fibers on laser lithotripsy performance. J Urol. 2015;193(3):1030–5.
16. Knudsen BE, Pedro R, Hinck B, Monga M. Durability of reusable holmium:YAG laser fibers: a multicenter study. J Urol. 2011;185(1):160–3.
17. Khemees TA, Shore DM, Antiporda M, Teichman JM, Knudsen BE. Evaluation of a new 240-mum single-use holmium:YAG optical fiber for flexible ureteroscopy. J Endourol. 2013;27(4):475–9.

18. Talso M, Emiliani E, Haddad M, Berthe L, Baghdadi M, Montanari E, et al. Laser Fiber and flexible Ureterorenoscopy: the safety distance concept. J Endourol. 2016;30(12):1269–74.
19. Sofer M, Watterson JD, Wollin TA, Nott L, Razvi H, Denstedt JD. Holmium:YAG laser lithotripsy for upper urinary tract calculi in 598 patients. J Urol. 2002;167(1):31–4.
20. Jiang H, Wu Z, Ding Q, Zhang Y. Ureteroscopic treatment of ureteral calculi with holmium: YAG laser lithotripsy. J Endourol. 2007;21(2):151–4.
21. Doizi S, Letendre J, Bonneau C, Gil Diez de Medina S, Traxer O. Comparative study of the treatment of renal stones with flexible ureterorenoscopy in normal weight, obese, and morbidly obese patients. Urology. 2015;85(1):38–44.
22. Watterson JD, Girvan AR, Cook AJ, Beiko DT, Nott L, Auge BK, et al. Safety and efficacy of holmium:YAG laser lithotripsy in patients with bleeding diatheses. J Urol. 2002;168(2):442–5.
23. Sharaf A, Amer T, Somani BK, Aboumarzouk OM. Ureteroscopy in patients with bleeding diatheses, anticoagulated, and on anti-platelet agents: a systematic review and meta-analysis of the literature. J Endourol. 2017;31(12):1217–25.
24. Weizer AZ, Springhart WP, Ekeruo WO, Matlaga BR, Tan YH, Assimos DG, et al. Ureteroscopic management of renal calculi in anomalous kidneys. Urology. 2005;65(2):265–9.
25. Bozkurt Y, Soylemez H, Atar M, Sancaktutar AA, Penbegul N, Hatipoglu NK, et al. Effectiveness and safety of ureteroscopy in pregnant women: a comparative study. Urolithiasis. 2013;41(1):37–42.
26. Xiao J, Wang X, Li J, Wang M, Han T, Zhang C, et al. Treatment of upper urinary tract stones with flexible ureteroscopy in children. Can Urol Assoc J. 2019;13:E78.
27. Aboumarzouk OM, Monga M, Kata SG, Traxer O, Somani BK. Flexible ureteroscopy and laser lithotripsy for stones >2 cm: a systematic review and meta-analysis. J Endourol. 2012;26(10):1257–63.
28. Pevzner M, Stisser BC, Luskin J, Yeamans JC, Cheng-Lucey M, Pahira JJ. Alternative management of complex renal stones. Int Urol Nephrol. 2011;43(3):631–8.
29. Pearle MS. Is ureteroscopy as good as we think? J Urol. 2016;195(4 Pt 1):823–4.
30. Chew BH, Brotherhood HL, Sur RL, Wang AQ, Knudsen BE, Yong C, et al. Natural history, complications and re-intervention rates of asymptomatic residual stone fragments after ureteroscopy: a report from the EDGE Research Consortium. J Urol. 2016;195(4 Pt 1):982–6.
31. Wollin DA, Ackerman A, Yang C, Chen T, Simmons WN, Preminger GM, et al. Variable pulse duration from a new holmium:YAG laser: the effect on stone comminution, fiber tip degradation, and retropulsion in a dusting model. Urology. 2017;103:47–51.
32. Humphreys MR, Shah OD, Monga M, Chang YH, Krambeck AE, Sur RL, et al. Dusting versus basketing during ureteroscopy-which technique is more efficacious? A prospective multicenter trial from the EDGE Research Consortium. J Urol. 2018;199(5):1272–6.
33. Althunayan AM, Elkoushy MA, Elhilali MM, Andonian S. Adverse events resulting from lasers used in urology. J Endourol. 2014;28(2):256–60.
34. Zagone RL, Waldmann TM, Conlin MJ. Fragmentation of uric acid calculi with the holmium: YAG laser produces cyanide. Lasers Surg Med. 2002;31(4):230–2.
35. Sourial MW, Ebel J, Francois N, Box GN, Knudsen BE. Holmium-YAG laser: impact of pulse energy and frequency on local fluid temperature in an in-vitro obstructed kidney calyx model. J Biomed Opt. 2018;23(10):1–4.
36. Aldoukhi AH, Ghani KR, Hall TL, Roberts WW. Thermal response to high-power holmium laser lithotripsy. J Endourol. 2017;31(12):1308–12.
37. Wollin DA, Carlos EC, Tom WR, Simmons WN, Preminger GM, Lipkin ME. Effect of laser settings and irrigation rates on ureteral temperature during holmium laser lithotripsy, an in vitro model. J Endourol. 2018;32(1):59–63.

Chapter 9
Ureteral Access Sheaths and Irrigation Devices

Karen L. Stern and Manoj Monga

Ureteral Access Sheaths

Ureteral access sheaths have become an increasingly popular tool for urologists in the endoscopic management of ureteral and renal calculi. Advantages include ease of multiple reentries to the upper tract with the ureteroscope, increased irrigation, and decreased intrarenal pressures [1]. First described in 1974 by Takayasu and Aso, the "guide tube" was developed to aid in access to the proximal ureter with the rigid scope [2]. In the 1980s, a reported high ureteral perforation rate of 19% limited the use of access sheaths [3]. However, with multiple improvements, including a hydrophilic coating, a locking mechanism to aid in passing the dilator and sheath together, kink-resistant designs, and a variety of available diameters and lengths, sheaths have again regained popularity [1, 3, 4].

The normal diameter of a human non-stented ureter is 9–10 Fr [5], but that diameter can stretch to accommodate ureteral access sheaths up to 18 Fr in outer diameter [4]. In general, the access sheath has a tapered inner dilator and hydrophilic outer sheath, allowing for atraumatic advancement through the lumen of the ureter up to the level of the stone or proximal ureter for renal stones. Once in place, the sheath allows for multiple passes of the ureteroscope without needing to backload over a wire and leads to a significant reduction of intrarenal pressures, up to 57–75% [3, 6]. High intrarenal pressures are associated with postoperative urinary sepsis, and the decreased pressure can help to avoid bacterial backflow [7]. Although the sheath is an added direct cost to the procedure, its use can actually be cost efficient [1]. Ureteral access sheaths are cheaper than a balloon dilation kit, and a more

K. L. Stern
Department of Urology, Cleveland Clinic Foundation, Cleveland, OH, USA

M. Monga (✉)
Glickman Urologic and Kidney Institute, The Cleveland Clinic, Cleveland, OH, USA
e-mail: mongam@ccf.org

© Springer Nature Switzerland AG 2020
B. F. Schwartz, J. D. Denstedt (eds.), *Ureteroscopy*,
https://doi.org/10.1007/978-3-030-26649-3_9

efficient stone removal can lead to a decreased operative time and therefore significant cost savings [1, 3]. In addition, the use of a sheath has been shown to aid in
ureteroscope longevity by reducing the stress on the tip of the scope during advancement through the ureter [3]. Pietrow et al. found that a ureteral access sheath may
increase the scope average life from an average of 6–15 cases up to 27.5 separate
operative procedures [8].

Testing has been done to evaluate various makes and models of ureteral access
sheaths. Monga et al. looked at the insertion forces necessary to buckle a sheath and
tested several different sheaths. First, they reported that urology residents apply a
significantly lower maximum force than staff urologists, 4.84 N versus 6.55 N,
respectively [9]. A force of approximately 4.7–7.6 N is necessary to result in perforation, but commercially available sheaths generally buckle at 3–6 N [9]. Looking
at various sheaths, the Cook Flexor sheath required the most force to buckle, and the
ACMI UroPass was the most resistant to kinking [10]. A more recent study of newer
sheath models, including the Glideway, Pathway, and Navigator HD, revealed the
Boston Scientific Navigator HD (Fig. 9.1) to have a higher safety and performance
profile [11]. Specifically, the Navigator has a blunter inner dilator and a milder taper
of the other sheath. The Navigator also required more force for tip perforation

Fig. 9.1 Boston scientific Navigator™ HD ureteral access sheath

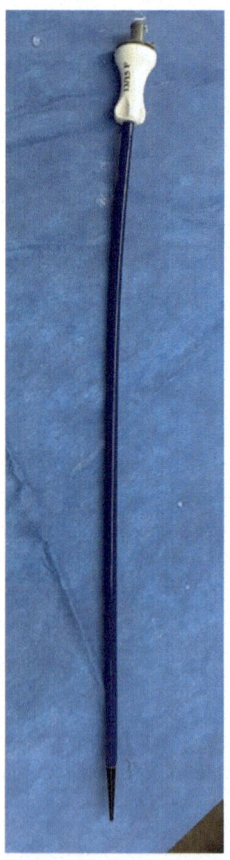

compared to the other two sheaths and required the least force for advancement through the biological model. In addition, it was more radiopaque, theoretically making it easier to place using fluoroscopic guidance [11].

Data on stone-free rates with the use of ureteral access sheaths is conflicting. L'Esperance et al. compared 173 cases with an access sheath to 83 without and found a significantly higher stone-free rate in the access sheath group, 79% versus 67% [12]. Contrary to the prior study, Berquet et al. retrospectively reviewed 280 ureteroscopy cases, 157 with an access sheath and 123 without. They found no significant difference in postoperative stone-free rate [13]. On multivariate analysis, the only factor predictive of a higher stone-free rate was stone size [13]. A recent meta-analysis including 3099 patients and 3127 procedures found there was no significant difference in stone-free rates between patients in whom an access sheath had been used and patients in whom a sheath had not been used, $p = 0.45$ [14]. However, as with studies on multiple other topics without endourology, weakness lies in absence of CT scans to determine postoperative stone-free rates.

Some of the main criticisms of ureteral access sheaths, including decreased blood flow to the ureter and tissue inflammation and necrosis, come from studies done in the porcine model. Lallas et al. studied blood flow to the ureter with the use of access sheaths [15]. Blood flow to the porcine ureter was measured with a Doppler ultrasound after the placement of a 10/12 Fr, 12/14 Fr, or 14/16 Fr sheath in the ureter for 70 min. He found there was an initial decrease in ureteral blood flow; however it was followed by a gradual rise toward baseline. Blood flow in the ureters with the 10/12 Fr sheath changed the least with an average nadir blood flow of 75% before compensation to 88.4% of baseline blood flow by the end of the procedure. The 12/14 Fr and 14/16 Fr had nearly identical blood flow nadirs, 34.6% and 34.4%, respectively, but the larger sheath reached the nadir more rapidly and rose toward compensation more slowly [15]. Lallas also looked at the histopathology of the ureters at 3 time points – directly after the procedure, at 48 h, and at 72 h. Overall there were inflammatory changes but no evidence of ischemic necrosis to the deeper muscularis propria layer [15]. Another study looked at the more long-term histopathologic changes in the ureter after the use of a 9.5/11.5 Fr access sheath inserted in the ureter for 30 min and 60 min [16]. Again there were findings of inflammatory changes, more pronounced in the distal than proximal ureter, but by 2 weeks, the changes were minimal. The ureters that had the sheaths inserted for 30 min showed no inflammation at 2 weeks, and the ureters that had the sheaths for 60 min showed minimal inflammation with intact epithelium [16]. Lildal et al. confirmed that COX-2 and TNF-α mRNA are increased in ureteral tissue after the use of a 13/15 Fr access sheath, more so in the distal ureter than proximal ureter [17]. While the expression of these markers is associated with inflammation and is found in urinary obstruction, the clinical significance is unknown. In addition, the study was done without a comparison arm looking to see if just inserting a ureteroscope would have a similar effect.

Another criticism of ureteral access sheaths is the prevalence of ureteral wall injuries. While the overall rate of intraoperative complications with an access sheath has not been shown to be different than that of ureteroscopy without a sheath, the rate of patients with a visible ureteral injury after a sheath is 46.5% [5, 14]. The

Table 9.1 Endoscopic grading system for ureteral injuries

Grade	Ureteral wall
0	No ureteral lesion or only mucosal petechiae
1	Mucosal erosion or mucosal flap without smooth muscle injury
2	Injury involves mucosa and smooth muscle, but not adventitia
3	Full-thickness ureteral perforation
4	Ureteral avulsion with loss of ureteral continuity

Traxer ureteral injury scale determines the grade of injury on the depth of ureteral damage (Table 9.1), with a low-grade injury classified as a grade 0 or 1 injury and high-grade as grade 2, 3, or 4 [5]. Traxer studied 359 consecutive patients who had ureteroscopy with a 12/14 Fr access sheath. Of the 46.5% with a visible injury, 86.6% of them were low-grade. Higher grade injuries were more common in male patients and older patients. Pre-stenting decreased the risk of severe injury sevenfold. Although ureteral injury is not uncommon, the long-term clinical impact of such an injury does not appear to be significant [18, 19]. The stricture rate after ureteroscopy with an access sheath is reported to be around 1–2%, which is similar to the overall stricture rate without an access sheath [18]. Other postoperative complications appear to be similar between patients with a sheath and without; however there is some data that indicates the postoperative infectious complication rate is lower with a ureteral access sheath [20, 21].

As mentioned above, patients who are pre-stented have a lower rate of ureteral injury with the use of an access sheath. Pre-stenting has been found to be predictive of an effective ureteral access sheath insertion [22], and a preoperative stent is associated with an increased stone-free rate and decreased procedure-related events such as patient phone calls and emergency department visits [21]. When looking at the necessity of leaving a postoperative ureteral stent, the literature is more conflicting. Torricelli et al. compared 51 patients who had a stent placed after ureteroscopy with a ureteral access sheath to 51 patients without a postoperative stent [23]. He found that patients in whom a ureteral stent was not left had a significantly increased amount of postoperative pain and more unplanned encounters than stented patients. However, there was no difference in the number of admissions, overall complication rate, UTI, or hematuria between the two groups. There was also no notable effect of pre-stenting or sheath size [23]. Astroza et al. specifically studied pre-stented patients to see if a postoperative stent is necessary after using a ureteral access sheath [24]. They found no difference in operative time, emergency department visits, UTIs, or reported renal colic, therefore indicating that patients who are pre-stented do not need a postoperative stent, saving the cost of a secondary procedure to remove the stent [24].

The advantages versus disadvantages to using a larger diameter access sheath are often debated. A larger access sheath allows for larger scopes, increased irrigation, as well as the removal of larger stone fragments. Ureteroscopes are oval, while the access sheaths are circular. Therefore, just because a ureteroscope has a smaller diameter than the diameter of the access sheath, it may not be useable. Overall, access sheaths with a diameter of at least 12 Fr can accommodate most flexible ureteroscopes [25]. While an 11/13 Fr sheath can accept all ureteroscopes, the Olympus digital scope has high resistance and low maneuverability [25]. But is bigger better? Tracy et al. found a 30% more efficient rate of stone treatment and removal when using a 14/16 Fr sheath versus a 12/14 Fr sheath, although the overall stone-free rate did not differ [21]. In addition, the complication rate was not different between the two sheath sizes [21].

Literature on the use of ureteral access sheaths in the pediatric population is limited, with reported risks of the development of vesicoureteral reflux and ureteral injury. Wang et al. retrospectively reviewed 40 patients under the age of 21 who had ureteroscopy with a ureteral access sheath used [26]. They found an increased rate of intraoperative complications and postoperative stent placement. Patients in whom the sheath was used tended to have a higher stone burden and a history of other stone procedures. Only seven patients (10%) had postoperative imaging, but of those four had notable hydronephrosis. Three out of the four had spontaneous resolution, and none of the patients had a clinically confirmed postoperative ureteral stricture. There was a trend toward a higher stone-free rate with patients without a ureteral access sheath, but again, very few patients had postoperative imaging [26]. Another study looked specifically at pre-stented preschool aged children less than 20 kg and found that the ureteral access sheath was inserted without complication in 93.8% of patients, and none had long-term complications [27]. Therefore, while there is no clear advantage to using an access sheath in the pediatric population, it does appear to be relatively safe with no long-term complications.

The use of ureteral access sheaths is not just limited to the surgical management of stones. Endourologists often diagnose and manage upper tract urothelial carcinoma, when nephroureterectomy is not indicated or desired. One of the limitations in the diagnosis of upper tract urothelial carcinoma is the difficulty of obtaining an adequate biopsy specimen. Theoretically, an access sheath would aid in the diagnosis by allowing a larger lumen to atraumatically remove tissue and easily facilitate multiple passes of the ureteroscope. No clinical trials exist between the endoscopic management of upper tract disease with and without the use of ureteral access sheaths, given the low prevalence of the disease, but Gorin et al. published a study looking at 88 patients with UTUC diagnosed or treated with a ureteral access sheath [28]. He found a high diagnostic yield with concordance between tumor grade of the biopsy and tumor grade of the final specimen after nephroureterectomy in 88.6% of patients [28].

In our practice we often use a ureteral access sheath during both ureteroscopy and percutaneous nephrolithotomy and decide the diameter of the sheath to use after an estimate of ureteral capacity during semirigid ureteroscopy or retrograde pyelogram. If the patient was pre-stented for any reason, we feel more comfortable using a larger sheath. We feel the sheath aids in visualization of the upper tract and helps with stone removal efficiency. The ureter is inspected while withdrawing the sheath at the conclusion of the case, and any injuries are noted. It is our routine practice to place a postoperative stent and leave it in place for 7–10 days, even if a high-grade ureteral injury is noted. In our patient population, the long-term stricture rate is negligible, even in patients with a high-grade injury from an access sheath.

Irrigation Devices

During ureteroscopy, visualization is of utmost importance. Pressurized irrigation is necessary to maintain adequate distention of the urinary tract and visualization of the lumen [29]. There are multiple irrigation devices commercially available, from gravity pressure bags to foot pumps and various hand-operated devices to automated devices. Ultimately, the best device limits retropulsion but has enough pressure to clear debris and blood to keep visualization optimal. In addition, the optimal device is ergonomic and limits surgeon or assistant fatigue.

Multiple studies have compared the devices. In 2008, Hendlin et al. compared gravity-pressurized irrigation to the EMS Peditrol foot pump, the Cook Ureteroscopy Irrigation System, ACMI Irri-Flo System, the Boston Scientific Single-Action-Pump (SAP) hand pump (Fig. 9.2), and the Kosin Piggyback Irrigation System

Fig. 9.2 Boston scientific single-action pump (SAP) hand-pump

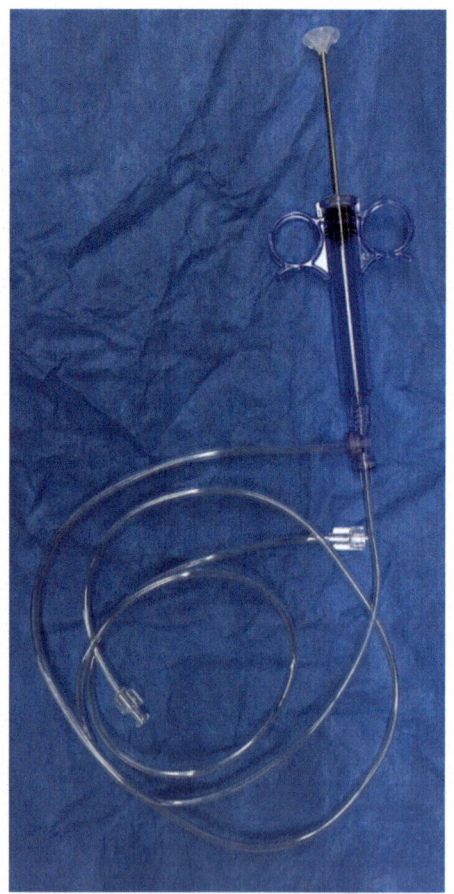

Fig. 9.3 Pathfinder Plus
bulb hand pump

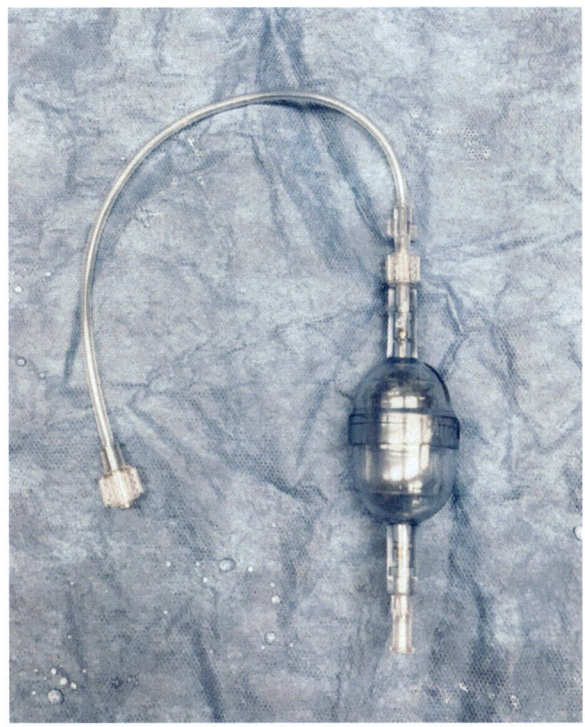

(UPIS). Of the manually operated systems, the SAP required the fewest number of pumps per second to maintain a clear field, versus the Peditrol which required the most. The gravity-based systems exerted a significantly less total maximum impulse than the hand or foot pump devices [30]. In 2012, Hedlin et al. compared the Boston Scientific SAP to the NuVista Medical Flo-Assist foot pump. They were comparable on the amount of pumps required to maintain a clear field; however the SAP device exerted less average maximum force on the stone, theoretically decreasing retropulsion [31]. More recently, Tarplin et al. compared the SAP to the Pathfinder Plus bulb hand pump (Fig. 9.3). The flow rate with the SAP was significantly larger than with the Pathfinder bulb with a maximum flow rate approximately threefold larger. However, the SAP was associated with a significant decrease of grip strength at 10 min, while the Pathfinder was not associated with a decrease in grip strength and, therefore, leads to less operator fatigue [29]. Although pressurized irrigation systems such as the Thermedx have been shown to be inaccurate in their pressure and flow estimates, they may contribute to decreased procedure times and increased stone-free rates [32, 33].

At our institution, multiple different devices are employed, all based on surgeon preference. The three main staff endourologists use three different irrigation devices – one uses the SAP, one uses an automated device, and the third uses the Pathfinder.

Conclusion

Every ureteroscopy case is unique, and the tools necessary for the best surgical outcome vary from case to case. Whether the urologist decides to utilize or forego a ureteral access sheath or use one irrigation device over another depends on surgeon preference and comfort with those devices. The most important tool is the knowledge of the various available devices as well as their and pros and cons. In this chapter we outlined the advantages and disadvantages to ureteral access sheaths and the fundamentals of the different irrigation devices currently available to urologists. Urologists should use this knowledge to improve the efficacy and efficiency of each ureteroscopy case as well as to encourage future research and development of superior instruments.

References

1. Yong C, Knudsen BE. Ureteroscopy: accessory devices. In: Humphreys M, editor. Ureteroscopy for stone disease. MUN. Roma, Italy: Minerva Medica; 2016. p. 55–70.
2. Takayasu H, Aso Y. Recent development for pyeloureteroscopy: guide tube method for its introduction into the ureter. J Urol. 1974;112:176–8.
3. Rizkala ER, Monga M. Controversies in ureteroscopy: wire, basket, and sheath. Indian J Urol. 2013;29:244–8.
4. Kaplan AG, Lipkin ME, Scales CD, Preminger GM. Use of ureteral access sheaths in ureteroscopy. Nat Rev Urol. 2016;13:135–40.
5. Traxer O, Thomas A. Prospective evaluation and classification of ureteral wall injuries resulting from insertion of a ureteral access sheath during retrograde intrarenal surgery. J Urol. 2013;189:580–4.
6. Auge BK, Pietrow PK, Lallas CD, Raj CV, Santa-Cruz RW, Preminger GM. Ureteral access sheath provides protection against elevated renal pressures during routine flexible ureteroscopic stone manipulation. J Endourol. 2004;18:33–6.
7. Breda A, Territo A, Lopez-Martinez JM. Benefits and risks of ureteral access sheaths for retrograde renal access. Curr Opin Urol. 2016;26:70–5.
8. Pietrow PK, Auge BK, Delvecchio FC, Silverstein AD, Weizer AZ, Albala DM, Preminger GM. Techniques to maximize flexible ureteroscope longevity. Urology. 2002;60:784–8.
9. Pedro RN, Weiland D, Reardon S, Monga M. Ureteral access sheath insertion forces: implications for design and training. Urol Res. 2007;35:107–9.
10. Pedro RN, Hendlin K, Durfee WK, Monga M. Physical characteristics of next-generation ureteral access sheaths: buckling and kinking. Urology. 2007;70:440–2.
11. Patel N, Monga M. Ureteral access sheaths: a comprehensive comparison of physical and mechanical properties. Int Braz J Urol. 2017;44:524–35.
12. L'esperance JO, Ekeruo WO, Scales CD, Marguet CG, Springhart WP, Maloney ME, et al. Effect of ureteral access sheath on stone-free rates in patients undergoing ureteroscopic management of renal calculi. Urology. 2005;66:252–5.
13. Berquet G, Prunel P, Verhoest G, Mathieu R, Bensalah K. The use of a ureteral access sheath does not improve stone-free rate after ureteroscopy for upper urinary tract stones. World J Urol. 2014;32:229–32.
14. Huang J, Zhao Z, Alsmadi JK, Liang X, Zhong F, Zeng T, et al. Use of the ureteral access sheath during ureteroscopy: a systematic review and meta-analysis. PLoS One. 2018;13:e0193600. eCollection.

15. Lallas CD, Auge BK, Raj GV, Santa-Cruz R, Madden JF, Preminger GM. Laser Doppler flow-metric determination of ureteral blood flow after ureteral access sheath placement. J Endourol. 2002;16:583–90.
16. Ozsoy M, Kyriazis I, Vrettos T, Kotsiris D, Ntasiotis P, Seitz C, et al. Histological changes caused by the prolonged placement of ureteral access sheaths: an experimental study in porcine model. Urolithiasis. 2018;46(4):397–404.
17. Lidal SK, Norregaard R, Andreassen KH, Christiansen FE, Jung H, Pedersen MR, Osther PJ. Ureteral access sheath influence on the ureteral wall evaluated by cyclooxygenase-2 and tumor necrosis factor-α in a porcine model. J Endourol. 2017;31:307–13.
18. Delvecchio FC, Auge BK, Brizuela RM, Weizer AZ, Silverstein AD, Lallas CD, et al. Assessment of stricture formation with the ureteral access sheath. Urology. 2003;61:518–22.
19. Patel RM, Okhunov Zhamshid O, Kaler K, Clayman RV. Aftermath of grade 3 ureteral injury from passage of a ureteral access sheath: disaster or deliverance? J Endourol Case Rep. 2016;21:169–71.
20. Traxer O, Wendt-Nordahl G, Sodha H, Rassweiler J, Meretyk S, Tefekli A, et al. Differences in renal stone treatment and outcomes for patients treated either with or without the support of a ureteral access sheath: the Clinical Research Office of the Endourological Society Ureteroscopy Global Study. World J Urol. 2015;33:2137–44.
21. Tracy CR, Ghareeb GM, Paul CJ, Brooks NA. Increasing the size of ureteral access sheath during retrograde intrarenal surgery improves surgical efficiency without increasing complications. World J Urol. 2018;36:971.
22. Mogilevkin Y, Sofer M, Margel D, Greensetin A, Lifshitz D. Predicting an effective ureteral access sheath insertion: a bicenter prospective study. J Endourol. 2014;28:1414–7.
23. Torricelli FC, De S, Hinck B, Noble M, Monga M. Flexible ureteroscopy with a ureteral access sheath: when to stent? Urology. 2014;83:278–81.
24. Astroza G, Catalan M, Consigliere L, Selman T, Salvado J, Rubilar F. Is a ureteral stent required after use of a ureteral access sheath in prestented patients who undergo flexible ureteroscopy? Cent Eur J Urol. 2017;70:88–92.
25. Al-Qahtani SM, Letendre J, Thomas A, Natalin R, Saussez T, Traxer O. Which ureteral access sheath is compatible with your flexible ureteroscope? J Endourol. 2014;28:286–90.
26. Wang HH, Huang L, Routh JC, Kokorowski P, Cilento BG, Nelson CP. Use of the ureteral access sheath during ureteroscopy in children. J Urol. 2011;186:1728–33.
27. Berrettin A, Boeri L, Montanari E, Mogiatti M, Acquati P, Lorenzis ED, et al. Retrograde intrarenal surgery using ureteral access sheaths is a safe and effective treatment for renal stones in children weight < 20 kg. J Pediatr Urol. 2018;14:59.e1–6.
28. Gorin M, Cortes JA, Kyle CC, Carey RI, Bird VG. Initial clinical experience with use of ureteral access sheaths in the diagnosis and treatment of upper tract urothelial carcinoma. Urology. 2011;78:523–7.
29. Tarplin S, Byrne M, Farrell N, Monga M, Sivalingam S. Endoscopic valves and irrigation devices for flexible ureteroscopy: is there a difference? J Endourol. 2015;29:983–92.
30. Hendlin K, Weiland D, Monga M. Impact of irrigation systems on stone migration. J Endourol. 2008;22:453–8.
31. Hendlin K, Sarkissian C, Duffey B, Monga M. Systematic evaluation of a novel foot-pump ureteroscopic irrigation system. J Endourol. 2012;26:126–9.
32. Lechevallier E, Luciani M, Nahon O, Lay F, Coulange C. Transurethral ureteronolithotripsy using new automated irrigation/suction system controlling pressure and flow compared to standard irrigation: a randomized pilot study. J Endourol. 2003;17:97–101.
33. De S, Miranda TF, Sarkissian C, Ganesh K, Monga M. Evaluating the automated Thermedx fluid management system in a ureteroscopy model. J Endourol. 2014;28:549–53.

Chapter 10
Quality of Life After Ureteroscopy

Blake Anderson, Joshua M. Heiman, and Amy Krambeck

Background

In addition to the clinical effectiveness of any procedure, such as stone-free rate for ureteroscopy (URS), at the forefront of the patient's mind is how their quality of life will be impacted. With endoscopic stone procedures, it is not uncommon for patients to question when they will return to work and how much pain they will endure with the procedure. Several tools exist to help urologists quantify their patients' quality of life after URS. Prior studies have demonstrated reported outcomes that help urologists guide patients on what they may experience postoperatively [1–4]. Patient questionnaires have been developed and validated for assessing the patient experience with the URS procedure, postoperative stents, and stone disease in general. For example, the USSQ (Ureteral Stent Symptom Questionnaire) is a validated questionnaire to assess stent-related symptoms [5]. The WISQOL (Wisconsin Stone Quality of Life Questionnaire) is another validated stone-related symptom questionnaire that was designed for understanding quality of life in patients with kidney stones (**see** Fig. 10.1) [6, 7]. Herein, this chapter provides the most current evidence to help urologist counsel patients on what they may experience from a quality of life standpoint following URS.

Analgesia and Narcotic Use After URS

Given the narcotic epidemic and the multitude of negative side effects associated with narcotic pain medication, urologists and patients alike are considering other treatment options of postoperative pain control (Table 10.1). Deaths due to

B. Anderson (✉) · J. M. Heiman · A. Krambeck
Department of Urology, Indiana University School of Medicine, IU Health Urology
Methodist Hospital, Indianapolis, IN, USA

© Springer Nature Switzerland AG 2020
B. F. Schwartz, J. D. Denstedt (eds.), *Ureteroscopy*,
https://doi.org/10.1007/978-3-030-26649-3_10

Wisconsin Stone-QOL

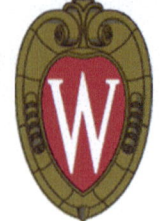

THE WISCONSIN "LIVING WITH KIDNEY STONES" QUESTIONNAIRE

This questionnaire is designed to understand the quality of life of patients with a history of kidney stones. The questions below ask about how problems with kidney stones have affected you **during the past month**.

Some questions may look very similar or have similar wording, but each one is different. Please answer the questions as honestly as possible. THE QUESTIONNAIRE IS 2-SIDED. Although you may have a number of physical or medical problems, **please do your best to think only about your problems related to kidney stones.** All information is confidential. Thank you for your input!

1. In the last 4 weeks, how true for you are the following statements?

	Very true	Mostly true	Somewhat true	A little true	Not at all true
A.) My energy level during the day is less than usual	1	2	3	4	5
B.) I feel very tired or fatigued	1	2	3	4	5
C.) My activity is limited	1	2	3	4	5

2. Because of kidney stones, how true have any of these problems been for you within the last 4 weeks?

	Very true	Mostly true	Somewhat true	A little true	Not at all true
A.) Trouble getting to sleep or with waking up while trying to sleep	1	2	3	4	5
B.) Needing to get up frequently while sleeping to urinate	1	2	3	4	5
C.) Poor quality sleep or not feeling rested after sleeping	1	2	3	4	5
D.) Difficulty returning to sleep	1	2	3	4	5

3. Because of kidney stones, how true for you over the last 4 weeks are the following?

	Very true	Mostly true	Somewhat true	A little true	Not at all true
A.) I don't feel the usual freedom to travel or to attend or participate in social events	1	2	3	4	5
B.) I force myself to go to work or school, to exercise, or to fulfill other responsibilities	1	2	3	4	5
C.) I have missed work or family time, or lost leisure or recreation time	1	2	3	4	5
D.) I make frequent adjustments or changes to my daily schedule	1	2	3	4	5
E.) I have less ability than usual to focus on my work, family, or other commitments or interests	1	2	3	4	5

Please answer questions on other side...

Copyright © 2017

Fig. 10.1 Wisconsin stone-QOL questionnaire. (With permission. Please visit www.urology.wisc.edu/wisqol for further information on using the WISQOL and to register for its use)

4. How often have you experienced or felt the following in the last 4 weeks because of kidney stones?

	Always or almost always	Very often	Somewhat often	Hardly at all	Not at all, never
A.) Problems or difficulties sticking to the diet recommendations	1	2	3	4	5
B.) Problems tolerating or taking prescription medications as directed	1	2	3	4	5
C.) Concern about my general health	1	2	3	4	5

5. Below are some physical symptoms that might be related to kidney stones. In the last 4 weeks, how often have you felt these symptoms?

	Always or almost always	Very often	Somewhat often	Hardly at all	Not at all, never
A.) Nausea, stomach upset or cramps	1	2	3	4	5
B.) Physical pain	1	2	3	4	5
C.) Urinary frequency (feeling like you have to go more than usual)	1	2	3	4	5
D.) Urinary urgency (sudden or unstoppable urge to urinate)	1	2	3	4	5

6. Because of kidney stones, in the last 4 weeks, how true are the following for you?

	Very true	Mostly true	Somewhat true	A little true	Not at all true
A.) I have less interest in sex or less sexual contact than usual	1	2	3	4	5
B.) I need to make special arrangements when traveling	1	2	3	4	5
C.) I have less interest than usual in socializing/ being around others	1	2	3	4	5

7. In the last 4 weeks, because of your kidney stones, how much have you felt the following?

	Very much	Quite a lot	Somewhat	A little bit	Not at all, never
A.) Frustrated with my situation	1	2	3	4	5
B.) Worried about what is wrong now	1	2	3	4	5
C.) Anxious or nervous about what might go wrong in the future	1	2	3	4	5
D.) Annoyed at the nuisances and inconveniences of my situation	1	2	3	4	5
E.) Reduced ability, compared to usual, to cope with everyday issues or responsibilities	1	2	3	4	5
F.) More irritable than usual	1	2	3	4	5

** A few questions about you... **WITHIN THE LAST 4 WEEKS** (PLEASE CIRCLE YOUR RESPONSE):*

1.) Did or do you **currently have stones** in your urinary system?	Yes	No	Not sure
2.) Did you currently have any **pain or symptoms related to kidney stones?**	Yes	No	Not sure
3.) Did you go to the Emergency Room or urgent care because of kidney stones?	Yes	No	Not sure
4.) Did you have a traumatic or very upsetting life event **in the last 4 weeks?**	Yes	No	Not sure
5.) Were you hospitalized or otherwise seriously affected by some health problem **NOT** related to kidney stones?	Yes	No	Not sure
6.) Your gender *(circle one):* Male Female	7.) Your age:		

Fig. 10.1 (continued)

Table 10.1 Recommended medications to prescribe post URS

Medication	Recommended use	Mechanism of action	Major side effects	Dosing
Diclofenac (Voltaren) [64]	Post URS and stent pain	NSAID: Inhibits cyclooxygenase, reducing prostaglandin and thromboxane synthesis	Stroke, myocardial infarction, GI ulcers and bleeding, gastric perforation	50 mg PO TID
Tramadol (Ultram) [65]	For patients with contraindications to NSAIDs	Central opioid agonist and weakly inhibits norepinephrine/serotonin reuptake	Nausea, dizziness, drowsiness, sweating, vomiting, dry mouth	50 mg PO q6
Tamsulosin (Flomax) [66]	Stent pain with concurrent NSAID use	Alpha-1a adrenergic receptor antagonist, relaxing smooth muscle, and improving urine flow	Orthostatic hypotension, floppy iris syndrome, syncope, dizziness, abnormal ejaculation	0.4 mg PO qd
Oxybutynin (Ditropan) [67]	Stent-related bladder spasms	Muscarinic receptor antagonist relaxes bladder smooth muscle, inhibits involuntary detrusor muscle contractions	Dry mouth, dry eyes, constipation	10 mg PO qd
Phenazopyridine (Pyridium) [28]	Post URS and stent dysuria	Produces topical analgesia of urinary tract	Orange hue to bodily fluids	1.5 PO TID
Hydrocodone-acetaminophen (Norco) [9]	Refractory pain and contraindications to other medications	Opioid agonist, producing analgesia and sedation	Addiction, respiratory depression, hepatotoxicity, constipation	2.5–10 mg PO q4-6h

prescription narcotic pain medication have tripled since 1999 with a staggering 16,235 reported fatalities in 2013 [8]. Common reported side effects of opioid pain medication include constipation, nausea, vomiting, physical dependence, tolerance, dizziness, sedation, and respiratory depression. Black box warnings for hydrocodone-acetaminophen include addiction, abuse, misuse, respiratory depression, accidental ingestion, neonatal opioid withdrawal syndrome, CYP450 3A4 interaction, risks with concomitant benzodiazepines or central nervous system depressants (sedation, respiratory depression, coma, death), and hepatotoxicity [9]. Fortunately, patients after URS may be managed with or without narcotics, and there is evidence to suggest that using other forms of pain control, such as nonsteroidal anti-inflammatory drugs (NSAIDs), are effective and do not pose risk for addiction. For renal colic, it has been shown that intramuscular diclofenac was superior to both intravenous (IV) paracetamol and IV morphine in a randomized controlled trial [10]. Data presented at AUA 2018 by Sobel et al. revealed that 73% (151/206) of patients could be discharged after ureteroscopy without narcotic pain medication [11]. The authors found that elevated BMI, chronic kidney disease, and fibromyalgia were associated with a postoperative narcotic requirement. Diclofenac was used as the narcotic-free alternative in this study, and patients who received it had a lower rate of phone calls and refill requests. It is still important to discuss with patients the risks of NSAIDs like diclofenac which include black box warnings for cardiovascular (e.g., stroke, myocardial infarction) and gastrointestinal risk (ulcers, bleeding, gastric perforation). However, diclofenac has been shown to have less adverse effects than aspirin, only 7% more than placebo, but similar to ibuprofen in a study on osteoarthritis using the same dose as has been our practice after ureteroscopy (50 mg TID) but for 4–6 weeks or more [12]. Intravenous acetaminophen has shown promise in some studies on renal colic, but data is conflicting and limited [13]. Additionally, IV acetaminophen is not available as a generic, which presents a cost challenge ($42.48/1 g vial) for wider use [14]. Patients with contraindications to NSAIDs may certainly benefit from a short course of an opioid pain medication, but urologists must prescribe the medication thoughtfully with care to avoid overprescribing practices. A recent study of 74 consecutive patients found that the median opioid pill use after URS was 10 but by day 6 postoperatively was down to 0 with patients only using half of the total number of prescribed pills [15]. One opioid option for patients in whom NSAIDs are contraindicated is tramadol. Tramadol, a centrally acting analgesic, has two separate mechanisms of action. While it is a weak μ opioid agonist, it also inhibits norepinephrine and serotonin reuptake which activates descending monoaminergic spinal inhibition of pain [16]. Both IV and oral tramadol are effective with minimal adverse effects in patients with moderate or severe postoperative pain which may be due to its dual mechanisms of action [17]. The most common reported side effects occurring in 1.6–6.1% of patients are nausea, dizziness, drowsiness, sweating, vomiting, and dry mouth. Most importantly, tramadol has no clinically significant cardiac or respiratory effects at recommended doses in adult or pediatric patients and is unlikely to lead to abuse or dependence. It is our practice to prescribe a limited number of tramadol pills after URS for patients who cannot take NSAIDS due to allergy, renal dysfunction, cardiac disease, or bleeding tendencies.

In addition to NSAID or narcotic pain medications, use of an alpha blocker for patients who have a ureteral stent placed at the time of URS does decrease bothersome LUTS and flank pain [18]. Tamsulosin is well tolerated with side effects of asthenia in 0–3% of patients (i.e., weakness) and dizziness in 1–2% of patients in a study of 0.2, 0.4, and 0.6 mg dosing, and the 0.4 mg dose was found to be most effective and comparable to placebo [19]. However, tamsulosin should be avoided in patients with cataracts who may require ophthalmologic surgery due to the risk of floppy iris syndrome, which is much higher for tamsulosin than for other alpha blockers such as alfuzosin [20]. However, fortunately tamsulosin has been found to be safe in pregnant women who have limited options for analgesia based on a limited patient study [21].

Another class of medication that has shown a benefit to patients after URS and stent placement are anticholinergics such as oxybutynin. Patients should be cautioned about the typical anticholinergic side effects seen with medications like oxybutynin that include dry mouth (most common side effect), dry eyes, and constipation [22]. Anticholinergics should be avoided in the elderly due to concern for central nervous system side effects, with one exception. Trospium displays anticholinergic properties but has the lowest penetration of the blood-brain barrier in the anticholinergic class and can therefore be tolerated by many elderly individuals [23].

Anticholinergics are also a poor option in men who have benign prostatic hyperplasia (BPH) and lower urinary tract symptoms (LUTS) with elevated post-void residual urine volumes (i.e., >150 mL) due to the theoretical potential for urinary retention. Through a similar effect as anticholinergic medication, although not an anticholinergic, belladonna and opium suppositories can also limit bladder contraction and spasms through a local narcotic mechanism. A recent randomized, double-blind placebo-controlled study demonstrated that immediate postoperative administration of a belladonna and opium suppository does improve quality of life and urinary symptoms after URS and stent placement [24]. Much investigation has also gone into the beta-3 receptor agonist mirabegron and benefits for patients with stone disease. Prior studies have confirmed the presence of β-1, β-2, and β-3 adrenergic receptors in human ureteral smooth muscle, and the same authors determined β-2 and β-3 receptor stimulation causes ureteral smooth muscle relaxation [25, 26]. Multiple prospective, randomized controlled trials (NCT02744430, NCT02095665, NCT02462837) are currently underway assessing mirabegron's effectiveness in medical expulsive therapy or in relieving stent-related symptoms. Anecdotally, we have noted success using this medication for stent discomfort. This medication has minimal side effects, but caution is advised in patients with uncontrolled hypertension as it can increase blood pressure [27].

Finally, phenazopyridine is a medication that can improve dysuria following URS and stent placement through a local anesthetic effect. The anesthetic effect of the medication has not been shown to benefit patients who are also taking antibiotics after 2 days of therapy; however, these studies focused on individuals with urinary tract infections [28]. Phenazopyridine is well-tolerated, but patients should be informed that it will cause bodily fluids (tears, saliva, urine) to turn an orange hue because it is an azo dye [28]. It is our general practice to prescribe 3 days of the medication to patients with an indwelling stent after URS.

Stent Implications on Quality of Life After URS

Ureteral stent side effects are far too common and at times debilitating for patients, impacting health-related quality of life in 80% and causing sexual dysfunction in 32% [5]. The etiology of ureteral stent pain and urinary symptoms due to stents are not fully understood. Previously, it has been shown that a high percentage of patients with standard double-J ureteral stents have vesicoureteral reflux (VUR) on voiding cystourethrogram, 63% in the filling phase and 80% in the voiding phase [29]. The VUR associated with indwelling stents most likely contributes to the pain noted with urination, especially in high-pressure voiders such as men with benign prostatic hyperplasia. Interestingly, ureteral stent diameter has been shown by Damanio et al. to not affect stent symptoms, and in another study, ureteral stent duration did not impact pain scores [30, 31]. However, the distal curl has been linked to stent morbidity in several studies. Ho et al. found that increased stent length affects the distal curl position (not proximal), and longer stents cause more frequency and urgency [32]. Multiple studies have demonstrated that if the distal curl crosses, the midline patients have worse stent-related symptoms [33]. However, is stenting necessary and can we avoid pain post URS by eliminating the ureteral stent?

Overall, there are conflicting findings in the literature on whether or not patients experience more or less pain with or without stents after URS. Multiple studies found no difference in narcotic or analgesic use between stented and non-stented in several studies [1, 34, 35]. However, one randomized controlled trial demonstrated decreased narcotic use in patients who were not stented following uncomplicated URS for distal stones [2]. The presence of LUTS post URS is more common with stents that are in place than when they are omitted [1]. Regarding flank or suprapubic pain, this was shown to be less prevalent at postoperative day 6 in patients who were stentless after URS compared to those who were stented [3]. However, it appears that omitting a stent after URS does not completely decrease morbidity, as there are possibly more hospital readmissions with stentless URS [1, 2, 34]. Schuster et al. previously reported postoperative outcomes from 322 URS procedures with a 13.3% ER visit rate [4]. Patients who returned to the ER had operative times that were 13 min longer on average, but there were no differences in stent placement compared to those who did not return to the ER.

When stents are left in place, stent material appears to have little impact on comfort. Previous studies have compared soft and firm types of stent materials and found no differences in USSQ scores at 1 and 4 weeks postoperatively [5]. Lee et al. conducted a randomized study of five different types of stents and found that Bard inlay stents had less urinary symptoms on the USSQ, but there were no differences in pain, general symptoms scores, or narcotic use [36]. Another study found that stents with a softer distal bladder coil (Polaris™) did not lead to lower pain scores [37]. A randomized multicenter trial by Krambeck et al. found no differences in unplanned physician contact, change in pain medication, or early stent removal in patients with toradol-eluting stents compared to standard double-J stents [38]. A triclosan-eluting stent was developed and shown to reduce pain and urinary symptoms with activity, but there were no differences noted when the patient was at rest [39]. In the triclosan study, a unique symptom questionnaire was employed rather than the validated USSQ, and pain medication use was not assessed. The bottom line is a home run stent has yet to be invented.

Another decision the urologist must consider following URS is not only whether to place a stent and what size/material but also whether to leave an externalized extraction string or discard the string and retrieve the stent via cystoscopy at a later date. Leaving the externalized string aids in extraction of the stent, eliminating the need for cystoscopy stent removal. However, opponents state patient discomfort and concern for stent dislodgement as reasons to remove the extraction string. A recent study by Barnes et al. found no differences in stent-related quality of life by USSQ, in number of ER visits or phone calls or in frequency of UTI between patients who had stents with strings compared to those without and required cystoscopic extraction [40]. Anecdotally it is our practice to leave the dangle extraction string for all uncomplicated URS cases to limit patient visits and inconvenience.

To date there is no clear guidance on how to avoid pain and discomfort after URS. The decision to stent or not is a fluid one made by the surgeon at the time of the procedure depending on the clinical scenario. There are numerous factors at play which may swing the pendulum toward stenting or not: ureteral lumen size, use of an access sheath, ureteral edema, ureteral injury, impacted stone, prolonged operation, solitary kidney, renal insufficiency, infection, patient preference, or prior experience. If a stent is omitted, this is no guarantee the patient will have less pain or require fewer pain medications. Furthermore, if a stent is placed, there is no ideal stent design, material, dwell time, or extraction method to limit pain.

Impact of Operative Factors on Quality of Life After URS

There are numerous operative variables which may differ from case to case and may impact the amount of pain and discomfort experienced by the patient. The end result is some patients do better after URS than others undergoing the same procedure but under a different set of conditions. To address the question of whether patients who undergo ureteral dilation have more pain, Hosking et al. performed URS without stenting in 93 patients of whom 88% had balloon dilation of the distal ureter. Patients had pain less than 1 day controlled with oral medication regardless of whether balloon dilation was utilized [41]. Other investigators have found that dilation of the distal ureter for uncomplicated treatment of a distal ureteral stone does not require routine stenting, and if stents are placed, patients have been found to have increased pain, urinary symptoms, and narcotic use [2]. It follows that patients who do not tolerate stents can safely be spared a stent when distal ureteral stones are treated with uncomplicated URS, which can lead to improved quality of life postoperatively.

Bilateral URS has been shown to be safe and effective with rates of pain, complications, and stone-free rates similar to unilateral or staged procedures [42]. One study evaluated 95 bilateral URS and followed these patients for 1 month postoperatively [43]. Complications were observed in 9.7% of patients postoperatively, only 5.3% of which experienced pain necessitating either an emergency room visit or rehospitalization. The authors' overall conclusion was that same session bilateral URS is efficacious and safe, but although most complications are minor, there may be slightly higher rates when compared to that reported for unilateral procedures. Ingimarsson et al. performed 117 same-session bilateral ureteroscopic procedures and compared the outcomes to 134 unilateral ureteroscopies [44]. Short-term complications were observed in 16.2% of patients, most commonly stent pain and discomfort in 5%. This is comparable to the unilateral group in which 6% of patients experienced stent pain and discomfort. Of the 71.8% patients that followed up at 6 weeks, there were no long-term complications. Stone-free rates with abdominal x-ray and ultrasound were 91.4% and 84.2% for patients imaged with CT scans. There was no overall difference in complication or readmission rates between the bilateral and unilateral groups. The authors concluded that bilateral ureteroscopy in a single session can be implemented as the standard of care for patients that present with bilateral stone disease.

Ureteral access sheaths are often used and are arguably safer given that there are lower intrarenal pressures for URS performed with an access sheath compared to URS performed without an access sheath [45]. Although limiting intrarenal pressure is important in all URS cases, it is most important in patients with a history of infected stones or urothelial carcinoma to avoid higher pressures which could promote pyelovenous or pyelolymphatic backflow. The ureteral access sheath also allows for repeated basket extraction of stone material to result in improved stone-free rates and improved visualization [46]. However, the use of a ureteral access sheath can result in temporary ureteral edema and in some cases ureteral perforations making the use of a ureteral stent often mandatory. A previous study demonstrated more than double the rate of emergency department visits (37% vs. 14%) when a stent was omitted after URS with an access sheath [47]. A study by Torricelli et al. reported that pre-stented patients who were left stentless after uncomplicated ureteroscopy using an access sheath had less pain than those who were stented [48]. Thus, although stent placement and its impact on postoperative recover from URS is complex, it seems that if an access sheath is used, stent placement is typically favorable unless special circumstances exist (e.g., pre-stented ureter, megaureter).

One would expect a longer operative time to potentially cause more postoperative pain. Ahn et al. reported outcomes on acute pain after URS in 143 consecutive patients from 2008 to 2010 and found that younger age, psychiatric illness, history of urinary tract infection, use of a stone basket, large stone size, and prolonged operative time were associated with more pain [49]. Factors that tend to prolong operative time, large stone size, and use of a basket were found to have an effect as expected in the study. A recent manuscript by the EDGE (Endourologic Disease Group for Excellence) Research Consortium found a significantly longer operative time when using a basketing vs. dusting technique (67.4 ± 53.3 vs. 35.9 ± 17.8 min, $p < 0.001$) [50]. However, there was no difference in postoperative complications or need for additional procedures between dusting and basketing. Also impacting operative time is stent placement which has been reported at a mean of 12 min [3]. Thus, when considering URS for larger stone burdens, the treating physician should consider longer operative times as a potential risk factor for poorly controlled postoperative pain.

Patient Factors and Rates of Emergency Room Visits, Readmissions, and Phone Calls After URS

Several baseline patient characteristics may influence recovery after URS. Patient-specific risk factors for significant pain after URS have been identified as younger age, history of psychiatric illness, and urinary tract infection [49]. A study by Penniston et al. showed that, among patients with nephrolithiasis, women have a lower healthcare-related quality of life than men after undergoing URS [51]. The authors stated in their limitations that differences in severity of stone disease between genders may have influenced their results. Also, they did point out that more women had a history of depression and musculoskeletal complaints than men in their study which likely influenced the quality of life score domains which were different between sexes (physical functioning, general health, vitality, and mental health). However, a recent publication by Ozsoy et al. demonstrated no gender differences in success or complication rates after URS [52]. As mentioned previously, ureteral access sheath use without stenting patients can result in 2.5 times the rate of ER visits compared to those with sheaths that were stented [47]. From a meta-analysis of 10 different studies with a total of 891 subjects, patients who were stented had a 4% lower rate of urologic complications, but this finding was not significant ($p = 0.175$) [53]. Morgan et al. reported that two-thirds of patients made postoperative contact with a healthcare provider after URS with 79% for medical reasons with pain as the primary complaint [54]. On multivariate analysis, only younger age and use of a larger ureteral access sheath were predictive factors of healthcare provider contact. The authors compared URS to TURBT in the same study and found that patients undergoing the URS were 2.5 times more likely to have a pain-related postoperative encounter than those who had TURBT. These results indicate that in certain groups of the population, quality of life is significantly decreased after URS, regardless of surgical factors.

Convalescence

The time needed to recover and return to work or regular activities is often a major patient determining factor when considering treatment options for symptomatic stone disease. A systematic review and meta-analysis compared URS to extracorporeal shockwave lithotripsy (ESWL) and percutaneous nephrolithotomy (PCNL). Pearle et al. looked at patients who underwent URS or ESWL for less than 10 mm lower pole stones and found that the latter had superior quality of life, shorter convalescence, and less analgesic requirement (5.6 vs. 14.7 pain pills, $p = 0.015$) [55]. For URS vs. ESWL, mean convalescence variables assessed were all lower and better for SWL: 5.3 ± 6.1 vs. 1.9 ± 1.7 days to driving, 7.9 ± 9.8 vs. 3.2 ± 3.0 days to return to nonstrenuous activity, 8.5 ± 8.3 vs. 3.3 ± 2.7 days to return to work, and 15.6 ± 11.6 vs. 8.1 ± 10.8 days until 100% recovered. A larger number of patients were willing to have a future ESWL than URS (90% vs. 63%, $p = 0.031$). Of note, 89% of the patients in the URS group were stented. Singh et al. had similar findings except satisfaction with URS was higher than ESWL with more patients willing to undergo repeat URS than ESWL (84% vs. 50%, $p = 0.002$) [56]. The preference for URS over ESWL in the Singh study may be because the URS patients had higher stone-free rates (83% vs. 49%), and the procedure was performed under epidural/spinal anesthesia with an overnight hospital stay per institutional and societal norms. Park et al. prospectively evaluated 65 patients undergoing ESWL vs. 95 undergoing URS for a single ureteral calculus ranging from 4 to 15 mm [57]. The patients who underwent URS were stented with a 6-Fr double-J stent for 2 weeks after surgery. There was no difference in patient satisfaction between the two procedures, as well as willingness to undergo the same procedure again (ESWL 64.6% vs. URS 51.6%). However, those patients treated with ESWL experienced a significantly faster return to work compared to patients treated with URS (2.48 ± 1.12 days vs. 3.02 ± 1.20 days, respectively). The authors attributed stent placement to be a main factor in prolonging convalescence in the URS cohort. Another study prospectively randomized 91 patients with large impacted proximal ureteral stones, defined as stones >1 cm in size to antegrade (44) or retrograde (47) ureteroscopic lithotripsy [58]. Stents were place in both groups for approximately 3 weeks. Retrograde ureteroscopic lithotripsy was associated with a statistically significant shorter interval to return to normal activities than PCNL antegrade URS. (2.7±0.6 days vs. 7.8±0.7). Thus, although URS seems to have a longer convalescence period than ESWL, it is significantly shorter than that experienced by those undergoing PCNL.

Sexual Function

The impact of stent placement after URS on sexual function has also been extensively studied. In one report, sexual function was decreased after URS and was not shown to improve over time after stent placement, with the authors postulating that may take more time to recover than other domains assessed by the USSQ [59]. Another study used International Index of Erectile Function-5 and Female Sexual Function Index to evaluate patients after stent placement, and both male gender and longer duration of stent dwell time were associated with lower sexual function scores on multivariable analysis [60].

Joshi et al. evaluated 85 consecutive adult patients with unilateral indwelling ureteral stents using the USSQ. Results of the USSQ revealed that at 4 weeks after stent removal, 35% of patients who were sexually active experienced pain during sex (mild pain 24%, moderate to severe pain 11%). Of the patients who reported being sexually active, 70% experienced temporary sexual dysfunction, and 14% had total sexual dysfunction. Patients' self-assessment also revealed that 18% expressed mixed feelings with overall sexual satisfaction, and 14% were completely dissatisfied with sex at the end of 4 weeks of an indwelling stent [5].

Eryildirim et al. evaluated sexual function in patients undergoing URS procedures [61]. The authors assessed 102 sexually active patients (60 male, 42 female) undergoing diagnostic and/or therapeutic URS for ureteral stone. None of these patients had stents placed after surgery. Sexual function was evaluated by using International Index of Erectile Function (IIEF) in male and Female Sexual Function Index (FSFI) forms in female cases before and at 1 month post procedure. Mean age of males was 42.07 ± 1.83, and mean age of females was 43.67±2.14. There was no statistical difference in overall sexual function in males, but when subdomains of the index were considered, men showed a statistically significant dissatisfaction with sex at 1 month post URS (IIEF-IS 9.32±0.46 vs. 6.66±051). Females showed no overall difference in sexual function, as well as no difference in the subdivisions. The authors theorized that the differences in satisfaction noted between males and females can be attributed to male lower urinary tract symptoms resulting from neuronally rich trigon mucosa irritation, anxiety, insomnia, and depression leading to sexual dysfunction.

Importance of Patient Education and Shared Decision-Making

Managing patient expectations is critical in every aspect of medicine and is particularly important for URS. Since URS is a minimally invasive procedure, there can be a patient perception that pain should be minimal to nonexistent, but in fact many patients can experience significant discomfort postoperatively and may need additional treatment. Although minimally invasive in the sense that URS is endoscopic with no incisions, it must be stressed to patients that URS can be quite painful. Taking time to educate the patient on the delicate nature of the kidney and ureter can help manage patient expectations postoperatively. The sensitive nature of the kidney and ureter is most apparent and translatable to patients from a study that found renal colic to be more painful than childbirth among women who have experienced both [62]. Stents themselves can be quite bothersome for patients, which can result in a significant number of patient encounters with the healthcare team if they are not coached and prepared on what symptoms to expect post procedure. A helpful tool available to urologists is the MUSIC (Michigan Urological Society Improvement Collaborative) stent brochure (**see** Fig. 10.2). The MUSIC brochure along with other educational tools can act as a resource to patients in the postoperative period and can be provided in the preoperative period to prepare patients.

Another factor of URS that can lead to high patient expectations is the fact that most URS is done outpatient. Patients may feel that if they can go home, then the operation must not be a big deal, and they should feel ready to return to work immediately. Some patients indeed may have such an experience, but others may require a week or so off of work as previously discussed. The bottom line is all patients are different: different anatomy, different stones, different pain thresholds, and different jobs, with different support systems. Our job as clinicians, in addition to performing their URS, is to caution them about possibilities for which they may prepare as best as possible.

It is possible and recommended to involve patients in the decision-making process for stenting. Absolute indications of course exist and include solitary kidney, transplant kidney, ureteral injury, and renal failure. Relative indications can include access sheath use, long operative time, recent urinary infection, or concern for ureteral inflammation, edema, or injury from the procedure or impaction. Some patients who fall into relative indications may be more comfortable with a slightly increased chance of readmission rate or additional procedure (stent placement) than the much

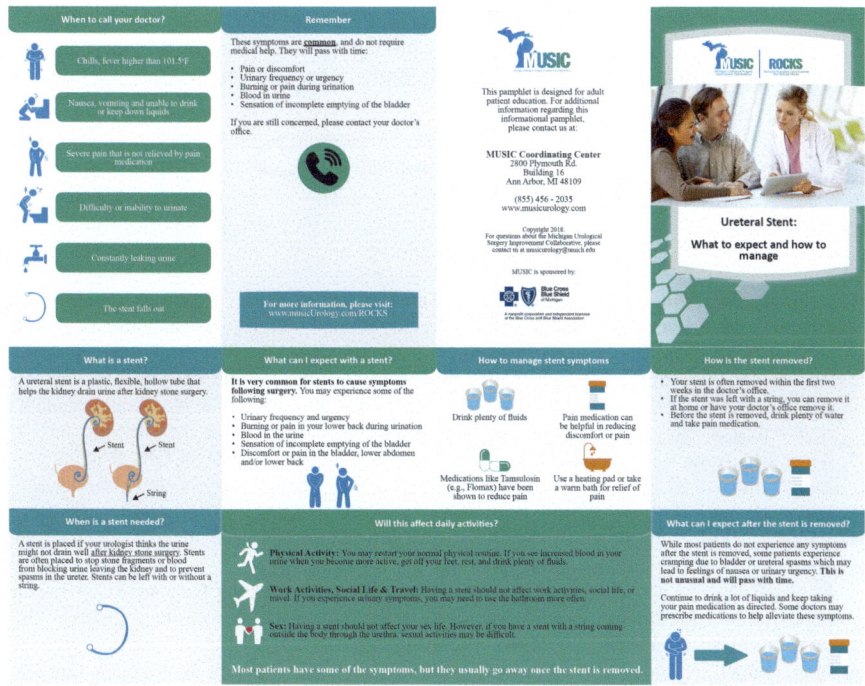

Fig. 10.2 Michigan urological society improvement collaborative. (Courtesy of Michigan Urological Surgery Improvement Collaborative (MUSIC))

higher likelihood of stent discomfort. This may depend on their own personal history as some patients tolerate stents much better than others. Another avenue for patients to participate in the decision-making process is with regard to leaving the stent completely internalized vs. attached to an externalized string. Some patients are not comfortable with the idea of having a string and are worried they may accidentally dislodge it, and these patients are better suited for an indwelling stent that can be later removed by office cystoscopy. Still, other patients have reported that office cystoscopy and stent removal were a worse experience than their initial URS, and thus these patients will be motivated to deal with an externalized string [63].

Conclusions

Quality of life after uncomplicated URS can be significantly decreased secondary to pain, decreased sexual satisfaction, and longer convalescence compared to URS. Surgeon factors such as length of surgery, use of an access sheath, stenting, and type of pain medication prescribed can greatly influence the amount of discomfort experienced by the patient post URS. Some patient factors that can lead to decreased satisfaction postoperatively include younger age and psychiatric illness. However, proper patient expectation management with appropriate education materials and utilizing shared decision-making whenever possible can help to improve overall patient satisfaction.

References

1. Denstedt JD, Wollin TA, Sofer M, Nott L, Weir M, Dah RJ. A prospective randomized controlled trial comparing nonstented versus stented ureteroscopic lithotripsy. J Urol. 2001;165(5):1419–22.
2. Borboroglu PG, Amling CL, Schenkman NS, Monga M, Ward JF, Piper NY, et al. Ureteral stenting after ureteroscopy for distal ureteral calculi: a multi-institutional prospective randomized controlled study assessing pain, outcomes and complications. J Urol. 2001;166(5):1651–7.
3. Byrne RR, Auge BK, Kourambas J, Munver R, Delvecchio F, Preminger GM. Routine ureteral stenting is not necessary after ureteroscopy and ureteropyeloscopy: a randomized trial. J Endourol. 2002;16(1):9–13.
4. Schuster TG, Hollenbeck BK, Faerber GJ, Wolf JS Jr. Complications of ureteroscopy: analysis of predictive factors. J Urol. 2001;166(2):538–40.
5. Joshi HB, Newns N, Stainthorpe A, MacDonagh RP, Keeley FX Jr, Timoney AG. Ureteral stent symptom questionnaire: development and validation of a multidimensional quality of life measure. J Urol. 2003;169(3):1060–4.
6. Penniston KL, Nakada SY. Development of an instrument to assess the health related quality of life of kidney stone formers. J Urol. 2013;189(3):921–30.
7. Penniston KL, Antonelli JA, Viprakasit DP, Averch TD, Sivalingam S, Sur RL, et al. Validation and reliability of the Wisconsin stone quality of life questionnaire. J Urol. 2017;197(5):1280–8.
8. Nelson LS, Juurlink DN, Perrone J. Addressing the opioid epidemic. JAMA. 2015;314(14):1453–4.
9. Hydrocodone/acetaminophen [Internet]. Epocrates. Available from: https://online.epocrates.com/drugs/12210/hydrocodone-acetaminophen/Monograph.
10. Pathan SA, Mitra B, Straney LD, Afzal MS, Anjum S, Shukla D, et al. Delivering safe and effective analgesia for management of renal colic in the emergency department: a double-blind, multigroup, randomised controlled trial. Lancet. 2016;387(10032):1999–2007.
11. Sobel D, Cisu T, Pham A, Stearns G, Sternberg K. PD53-07 the feasibility of discharging patients without opioids after ureteroscopy. J Urol. 2018;199(4):e1048–e9.
12. Caldwell JR. Efficacy and safety of diclofenac sodium in rheumatoid arthritis. Experience in the United States. Am J Med. 1986;80(4B):43–7.
13. Masoumi K, Forouzan A, Asgari Darian A, Feli M, Barzegari H, Khavanin A. Comparison of clinical efficacy of intravenous acetaminophen with intravenous morphine in acute renal colic: a randomized, double-blind, controlled trial. Emerg Med Int. 2014;2014:571326.
14. Sin B, Koop K, Liu M, Yeh JY, Thandi P. Intravenous acetaminophen for renal colic in the emergency department: where do we stand? Am J Ther. 2017;24(1):e12–e9.
15. Flynn K, Guidos P, Francis S, Simmering J, Polgreen P, Tracy C, et al. MP80-05 outcomes from a text messaging study performed to better predict post-ureteroscopy opioid use. J Urol. 2018;199(4):e1090–e1.
16. Raffa RB, Friderichs E, Reimann W, Shank RP, Codd EE, Vaught JL, et al. Complementary and synergistic antinociceptive interaction between the enantiomers of tramadol. J Pharmacol Exp Ther. 1993;267(1):331–40.
17. Scott LJ, Perry CM. Tramadol: a review of its use in perioperative pain. Drugs. 2000;60(1):139–76.

18. Lamb AD, Vowler SL, Johnston R, Dunn N, Wiseman OJ. Meta-analysis showing the beneficial effect of alpha-blockers on ureteric stent discomfort. BJU Int. 2011;108(11):1894–902.
19. Abrams P, Speakman M, Stott M, Arkell D, Pocock R. A dose-ranging study of the efficacy and safety of tamsulosin, the first prostate-selective alpha 1A-adrenoceptor antagonist, in patients with benign prostatic obstruction (symptomatic benign prostatic hyperplasia). Br J Urol. 1997;80(4):587–96.
20. Cheung CM, Awan MA, Sandramouli S. Prevalence and clinical findings of tamsulosin-associated intraoperative floppy-iris syndrome. J Cataract Refract Surg. 2006;32(8):1336–9.
21. Bailey G, Vaughan L, Rose C, Krambeck A. Perinatal outcomes with Tamsulosin therapy for symptomatic urolithiasis. J Urol. 2016;195(1):99–103.
22. Baigrie RJ, Kelleher JP, Fawcett DP, Pengelly AW. Oxybutynin: is it safe? Br J Urol. 1988;62(4):319–22.
23. Scheife R, Takeda M. Central nervous system safety of anticholinergic drugs for the treatment of overactive bladder in the elderly. Clin Ther. 2005;27(2):144–53.
24. Lee FC, Holt SK, Hsi RS, Haynes BM, Harper JD. Preoperative belladonna and opium suppository for ureteral stent pain: a randomized, double-blinded. Placebo-Control Stud Urol. 2017;100:27–32.
25. Park YC, Tomiyama Y, Hayakawa K, Akahane M, Ajisawa Y, Miyatake R, et al. Existence of a beta3-adrenoceptro and its functional role in the human ureter. J Urol. 2000;164(4):1364–70.
26. Matsumoto R, Otsuka A, Suzuki T, Shinbo H, Mizuno T, Kurita Y, et al. Expression and functional role of beta3 -adrenoceptors in the human ureter. Int J Urol. 2013;20(10):1007–14.
27. Nitti VW, Khullar V, van Kerrebroeck P, Herschorn S, Cambronero J, Angulo JC, et al. Mirabegron for the treatment of overactive bladder: a prespecified pooled efficacy analysis and pooled safety analysis of three randomised, double-blind, placebo-controlled, phase III studies. Int J Clin Pract. 2013;67(7):619–32.
28. Phenazopyridine hydrochloride [Internet]. Epocrates. Available from: https://online.epocrates.com/drugs/1160/Pyridium.
29. Mosli HA, Farsi HM, Al-Zimaity MF, Saleh TR, Al-Zamzami MM. Vesicoureteral reflux in patients with double pigtail stents. J Urol. 1991;146(4):966–9.
30. Damiano R, Autorino R, De Sio M, Cantiello F, Quarto G, Perdona S, et al. Does the size of ureteral stent impact urinary symptoms and quality of life? A prospective randomized study. Eur Urol. 2005;48(4):673–8.
31. Irani J, Siquier J, Pires C, Lefebvre O, Dore B, Aubert J. Symptom characteristics and the development of tolerance with time in patients with indwelling double-pigtail ureteric stents. BJU Int. 1999;84(3):276–9.
32. Ho CH, Chen SC, Chung SD, Lee YJ, Chen J, Yu HJ, et al. Determining the appropriate length of a double-pigtail ureteral stent by both stent configurations and related symptoms. J Endourol. 2008;22(7):1427–31.
33. Rane A, Saleemi A, Cahill D, Sriprasad S, Shrotri N, Tiptaft R. Have stent-related symptoms anything to do with placement technique? J Endourol. 2001;15(7):741–5.
34. Chen YT, Chen J, Wong WY, Yang SS, Hsieh CH, Wang CC. Is ureteral stenting necessary after uncomplicated ureteroscopic lithotripsy? A prospective, randomized controlled trial. J Urol. 2002;167(5):1977–80.
35. Netto NR Jr, Ikonomidis J, Zillo C. Routine ureteral stenting after ureteroscopy for ureteral lithiasis: is it really necessary? J Urol. 2001;166(4):1252–4.
36. Lee C, Kuskowski M, Premoli J, Skemp N, Monga M. Randomized evaluation of ureteral stents using validated symptom questionnaire. J Endourol. 2005;19(8):990–3.
37. Lingeman JE, Preminger GM, Goldfischer ER, Krambeck AE, Comfort ST. Assessing the impact of ureteral stent design on patient comfort. J Urol. 2009;181(6):2581–7.
38. Krambeck AE, Walsh RS, Denstedt JD, Preminger GM, Li J, Evans JC, et al. A novel drug eluting ureteral stent: a prospective, randomized, multicenter clinical trial to evaluate the safety and effectiveness of a ketorolac loaded ureteral stent. J Urol. 2010;183(3):1037–42.

39. Mendez-Probst CE, Goneau LW, MacDonald KW, Nott L, Seney S, Elwood CN, et al. The use of triclosan eluting stents effectively reduces ureteral stent symptoms: a prospective randomized trial. BJU Int. 2012;110(5):749–54.
40. Barnes KT, Bing MT, Tracy CR. Do ureteric stent extraction strings affect stent-related quality of life or complications after ureteroscopy for urolithiasis: a prospective randomised control trial. BJU Int. 2014;113(4):605–9.
41. Hosking DH, McColm SE, Smith WE. Is stenting following ureteroscopy for removal of distal ureteral calculi necessary? J Urol. 1999;161(1):48–50.
42. Mushtaque M, Gupta CL, Shah I, Khanday MA, Khanday SA. Outcome of bilateral ureteroscopic retrieval of stones in a single session. Urol Ann. 2012;4(3):158–61.
43. Watson JM, Chang C, Pattaras JG, Ogan K. Same session bilateral ureteroscopy is safe and efficacious. J Urol. 2011;185(1):170–4.
44. Ingimarsson JP, Rivera M, Knoedler JJ, Krambeck AE. Same-session bilateral ureteroscopy: safety and outcomes. Urology. 2017;108:29–33.
45. Auge BK, Pietrow PK, Lallas CD, Raj GV, Santa-Cruz RW, Preminger GM. Ureteral access sheath provides protection against elevated renal pressures during routine flexible ureteroscopic stone manipulation. J Endourol. 2004;18(1):33–6.
46. Kaplan AG, Lipkin ME, Scales CD Jr, Preminger GM. Use of ureteral access sheaths in ureteroscopy. Nat Rev Urol. 2015;13:135.
47. Rapoport D, Perks AE, Teichman JM. Ureteral access sheath use and stenting in ureteroscopy: effect on unplanned emergency room visits and cost. J Endourol. 2007;21(9):993–7.
48. Torricelli FC, De S, Hinck B, Noble M, Monga M. Flexible ureteroscopy with a ureteral access sheath: when to stent? Urology. 2014;83(2):278–81.
49. Ahn ST, Kim JH, Park JY, du Moon G, Bae JH. Acute postoperative pain after ureteroscopic removal of stone: incidence and risk factors. Korean J Urol. 2012;53(1):34–9.
50. Humphreys MR, Shah OD, Monga M, Chang YH, Krambeck AE, Sur RL, et al. Dusting versus basketing during ureteroscopy-which technique is more efficacious? A prospective multicenter trial from the EDGE research consortium. J Urol. 2018;199(5):1272–6.
51. Penniston KL, Nakada SY. Health related quality of life differs between male and female stone formers. J Urol. 2007;178(6):2435–40; discussion 40.
52. Ozsoy M, Acar O, Sarica K, Saratlija-Novakovic Z, Fajkovic H, Librenjak D, et al. Impact of gender on success and complication rates after ureteroscopy. World J Urol. 2015;33(9):1297–302.
53. Makarov DV, Trock BJ, Allaf ME, Matlaga BR. The effect of ureteral stent placement on post-ureteroscopy complications: a meta-analysis. Urology. 2008;71(5):796–800.
54. Morgan MS, Antonelli JA, Lotan Y, Shakir N, Kavoussi N, Cohen A, et al. Use of an electronic medical record to assess patient-reported morbidity following ureteroscopy. J Endourol. 2016;30(Suppl 1):S46–51.
55. Pearle MS, Lingeman JE, Leveillee R, Kuo R, Preminger GM, Nadler RB, et al. Prospective randomized trial comparing shock wave lithotripsy and ureteroscopy for lower pole caliceal calculi 1 cm or less. J Urol. 2008;179(5 Suppl):S69–73.
56. Singh BP, Prakash J, Sankhwar SN, Dhakad U, Sankhwar PL, Goel A, et al. Retrograde intrarenal surgery vs extracorporeal shock wave lithotripsy for intermediate size inferior pole calculi: a prospective assessment of objective and subjective outcomes. Urology. 2014;83(5):1016–22.
57. Park J, Shin DW, Chung JH, Lee SW. Shock wave lithotripsy versus ureteroscopy for ureteral calculi: a prospective assessment of patient-reported outcomes. World J Urol. 2013;31(6):1569–74.
58. Sun X, Xia S, Lu J, Liu H, Han B, Li W. Treatment of large impacted proximal ureteral stones: randomized comparison of percutaneous antegrade ureterolithotripsy versus retrograde ureterolithotripsy. J Endourol. 2008;22(5):913–7.
59. Giannarini G, Keeley FX Jr, Valent F, Manassero F, Mogorovich A, Autorino R, et al. Predictors of morbidity in patients with indwelling ureteric stents: results of a prospective study using the validated Ureteric Stent Symptoms Questionnaire. BJU Int. 2011;107(4):648–54.

60. Sighinolfi MC, Micali S, De Stefani S, Mofferdin A, Grande M, Giacometti M, et al. Indwelling ureteral stents and sexual health: a prospective, multivariate analysis. J Urol. 2007;178(1):229–31.
61. Eryildirim B, Tuncer M, Sahin C, Yucetas U, Sarica K. Evaluation of sexual function in patients submitted to ureteroscopic procedures. Int Braz J Urol. 2015;41(4):791–5.
62. Miah S, Gunner C, Clayton L, Venugopal S, Boucher NR, Parys B. Renal colic and childbirth pain: female experience versus male perception. J Pain Res. 2017;10:1553–4.
63. Stoller ML, Wolf JS Jr, Hofmann R, Marc B. Ureteroscopy without routine balloon dilation: an outcome assessment. J Urol. 1992;147(5):1238–42.
64. Voltaren. Epocrates. https://online.epocrates.com/drugs/1407/Voltaren-XR.
65. Ultram. Epocrates. https://online.epocrates.com/drugs/1347/Ultram.
66. Tamsulosin. Epocrates. https://online.epocrates.com/drugs/754/tamsulosin.
67. Ditropan. Epocrates. https://online.epocrates.com/drugs/652/Ditropan-XL.

Chapter 11
Postoperative Care of the Ureteroscopy Patient

Itay M. Sabler, Ioannis Katafygiotis, and Mordechai Duvdevani

Abbreviations

CT	Computer tomography
DJS	Double-J stent
MET	Medical expulsive therapy
NSAIDs	Nonsteroidal anti-inflammatory drugs
PCNL	Percutaneous nephrolithotomy
PRH	Perirenal hematoma
SFR	Stone-free rate
SWL	Shock wave lithotripsy
UC	Ureter catheter
URS	Ureteroscopy

Introduction

Ureteroscopy (URS) is the first-line therapy for ureteral and renal stones. Stone-free status may be as high as 90–100%. Stone procedures are even performed in various centers all over the world in the ambulatory setting at hospital outpatient facilities [1, 2].

In parallel to high stone-free rates and the use of miniaturized flexible instruments, the postoperative complication rates still remain a major issue. The incidence of unplanned admissions owing to post-URS complications ranges from 1.5% to 14.3% in Western countries, with the postoperative pain being the leading one [3, 4].

Important factors in postoperative care after ureterorenoscopy are also the infections and the septic complications. During endoscopic procedures, fluids infused to the collecting system elevate the intrarenal pressure. This fact in conjunction with

I. M. Sabler · I. Katafygiotis · M. Duvdevani (✉)
Department of Urology, Hadassah Hebrew University Medical Center, Jerusalem, Israel

© Springer Nature Switzerland AG 2020   141
B. F. Schwartz, J. D. Denstedt (eds.), *Ureteroscopy*,
https://doi.org/10.1007/978-3-030-26649-3_11

the treatment of infectious stones plays the key role in possible postoperative septic, life-threatening events. Careful perioperative antibiotic prophylaxis and proper upper tract drainage are mandatory and discussed in this chapter [5].

Emergencies in Immediate Postoperative Period

The advances in the equipment and the technology have allowed endourologists to perform increasingly complex procedures to treat upper urinary tract stones. Larger diameter stones are now treated with URS with acceptable complication profiles. URS is reported to have a high stone clearance, and its observed complication rate is relatively low. The recent Clinical Research of the Endourological Society (CROES) of 11,885 patients found a URS complication rate of 7.4%. The most common complications after URS were bleeding, fever, and urinary tract infections (UTIs) [6].

SIRS and Sepsis

Understanding the Risk Factors

Urosepsis is defined as sepsis caused by a urogenital tract infection. Urosepsis in adults accounts for approximately 25% of all sepsis cases. Severe sepsis/ septic shock is a critical condition, with a reported mortality rate ranging from 20% to 40%. Main risk factors are urinary obstruction, with urolithiasis being the most common cause [7]. Treatment of urosepsis has four major aspects: (1) early diagnosis, (2) early goal-oriented therapy including optimal antimicrobials with high concentrations both in the plasma and in the urinary tract, (3) identification and control of the complicating factor in the urinary tract, and (4) specific sepsis therapy. Early adequate tissue oxygenation, adequate initial antibiotic therapy, and rapid identification and control of the septic focus in the urinary tract are critical steps in the successful management of a patient with urosepsis, which includes early imaging and an optimal interdisciplinary approach encompassing emergency unit and urological and intensive care medicine specialists. An early diagnosis is crucial for survival and better clinical outcome. Emergent decompression of the collecting system is the standard of care for the initial management of urosepsis from obstructive urolithiasis or edema secondary to URS. Both retrograde ureteral stent placement and percutaneous nephrostomy (PCN) drainage were shown equally effective in alleviation of the clinical course [8]. After initiation of the proper antibiotic treatment, initial diagnosis and decision for the need of decompression of the collecting system are made. If obstruction is present, diversion is mandatory by stent or nephrostomy tube.

Various risk factors for postoperative fever, sepsis, or SIRS after URS have been identified. Without doubt, a positive preoperative urine culture and also a positive intraoperative upper collecting system urine and stone cultures consist main risk factors. Female sex, preoperative drainage, hydroureteronephrosis, large or complex stone burden, volume of irrigation fluids, increased operative time, age, and immune status have all been associated with an increased risk of postoperative infection sequela. Patients with previous urosepsis are more likely to be admitted and may need postoperative use of antibiotics compared with those undergoing elective URS [9].

Initial Management

First signs of urosepsis after endourologic procedures are tachycardia, flank pain, and fever. Later on, if unrecognized or untreated, septic shock followed by cardiovascular events may develop. NPO is advised at these steps together with anticipation of invasive procedure if initial diagnostic work-up shows signs of obstruction. A Foley urethral catheter is considered necessary to be inserted for reducing the pressure. Intravenous fluids and broad spectrum antibiotics are introduced as soon as possible. Complete laboratory tests including thorough urine and blood cultures are performed. Monitoring of vital signs and fluid balance is mandatory.

Initial Imaging

The initial imaging is by sonographic examination of the urogenital organs and can be performed in the emergency unit. As obstruction of the upper urinary tract is the predominant cause of postoperative urosepsis, sonographic examination of the kidneys for ruling out dilation of the renal pelvis is the first imaging study. Additional ultrasound of the bladder, ruling out urinary retention, is recommended in the cases without a urethral catheter. If the ultrasound investigations are inconsistent, further non-contrast CT scan is performed in order to recognize and to manage the cause of obstruction accordingly.

Upper tract drainage is indicated in cases of ongoing sepsis and radiographically proven upper urinary tract obstruction.

Perirenal Hematoma (PRH)

PRH formation is closely linked to perioperative bleeding which may be caused by a number of predisposing factors. Typically, PRH is known to occur after other stone procedures, such as PCNL or SWL, and its formation after retrograde procedure is not common. Patients under anticoagulation therapy are at increased risk. Post-URS PRH is rare, but its acute and dangerous clinical course should be recognized and managed properly to avoid long-term morbidity. Whitehurst et al. in their systematic review investigated the incidence and common predisposing factors and proposed the optimal preventative strategies and most appropriate management of PRH and its long-term sequelae. The incidence of PRH ranges between 0.15% and 8.9% worldwide [10]. The predisposing factors include a moderate to severe degree of hydronephrosis, thin renal cortex, prolonged operation, hypertension, female gender, and UTIs. Other risk factors were higher perfusion pressures, larger stone size, existing chronic kidney disease (CKD), pre- and postoperative ureteral stent usage, ureteral sheath use, and previous renal operation or SWL. Patients with PRH had a larger stone size, with a mean stone size of 1.7 cm. Conflicting are the data for body mass index (BMI) as some authors claim that low BMI is a risk factor while others described opposite findings [10].

Initial conservative PRH management is proposed as the best approach and includes blood transfusion and antibiotic therapy. Intervention is required in 50% of the patients with PRH. Other cases were managed by percutaneous drainage, emergency angiography and open surgery for clot evacuation, and even nephrectomy in unstable patients. There was also one mortality reported [10]. To summarize, controlling blood pressure, UTI prophylaxis, and treatment; maintaining a low collecting system pressure during the procedure; and reducing operative duration are the main preventive measures.

In patients with PRH formation despite these measures, conservative management may be recommended in most cases, while surgical intervention is indicated in a selected group of unstable patients [7]. Bed rest during acute period is of course mandatory in these cases.

Pain Management

Postoperative pain is one of the main complicating factors necessitating direct management even in the recovery room. The cause may be multifactorial: renal colic due to stone fragments and obstruction of the upper urinary tract (either after tubeless or uneventful URS, either stent-related flank or lower abdominal pain). Nonsteroidal anti-inflammatory drugs (NSAIDs) (including metamizoledipyrone) and paracetamol are effective in patients with acute colic and have better analgesic efficacy than opioids [11]. This is the first-line treatment for acute renal colic according to the European Urology Association guidelines. Patients receiving NSAIDs are less likely to require further analgesia for the management of the initial colic. In patients suffering from congestive heart failure, the use of diclofenac and ibuprofen may cause coronary events and increase preload [12, 13]. Additionally, another factor to count in is renal function. NSAIDs decrease renal blood flow with further increase of intrapelvic pressure. The risk increases with dose and duration of the treatment, and the lowest effective dose should be used for the shortest needed duration [14]. In summary, for patients with ureteral residual fragments that are expected to pass spontaneously and normal renal function, NSAIDs (e.g., diclofenac sodium, 100–150 mg/day, 3–10 days) may help reduce inflammation and the risk of recurrent pain [15].

The addition of spasmolytics doesn't result in better pain control and is not advised for renal colic treatment [12].

Opioids, particularly pethidine, are used widely for renal colic pain control. Their use may be associated with a high rate of nausea and vomiting compared to NSAIDs and unlikely to NSAIDs have a greater likelihood of pain recurrence and use of additional pain control medication [11].

Apart from the use of NSAIDs, corticosteroids, or opioids for immediate symptomatic control, passage of ureteral stones may be facilitated with the use of medical expulsive therapy (MET). Although the ongoing discussion MET may contribute both to spontaneous passage and the control of pain. In case of post-URS residual fragments, obstruction, and pain, painkillers may not be enough, since the goal of the treatment is to avoid second intervention if possible. Hollingsworth et al. (2016) in a recent meta-analysis concluded that medical expulsive therapy seems efficacious in reducing pain episodes of patients with ureteral stones. Interestingly, regarding stone size, no benefit of MET for smaller ureteric stones was observed. Patients with larger stones, however, had a 57% higher possibility of stone passage compared with controls. More than that, there was a 9.8% increase in the risk ratio for stone passage for every 1 mm increase in stone size [16].

Hamidi et al., in an interesting retrospective study of 397 patients who underwent unstented ureteroscopy, concluded that the administration of corticosteroids after uncomplicated unstented ureteroscopy may reduce early postoperative pain, renal colic episodes, and the need of the total analgesic consumption [17].

In summary, standardized postoperative pain control protocol should be developed in every endourologic department. If analgesia cannot be achieved by medications or there is evidence of obstruction of the upper urinary tract and/or renal function deterioration, drainage, using stenting, percutaneous nephrostomy, or stone removal with additional procedure are indicated [12].

Postoperative Upper Urinary Tract Drainage

Intraoperative upper urinary tract drainage may also affect the postoperative course. The main options of drainage are either the temporarily placed ureter catheter (UC) or a mono-J stent usually attached to the urethral catheter or a long-term-placed double-J stent (DJS). According to EAU guidelines, routine stenting is not necessary before URS. However, pre-stenting may improve the stone-free rates (SFR) and reduce intraoperative complications [18]. In general, randomized prospective trials have found that routine stenting after uncomplicated URS and complete stone removal is not necessary. A stent might also be associated with higher postoperative morbidity [19]. Stents should be inserted in patients who are at increased risk of complications: obvious intraoperative ureteral trauma, suspected residual fragments, bleeding, history of sepsis, and in all doubtful cases, to avoid stressful emergencies.

The ideal duration of postoperative stenting is not known. The majority of urologists prefer to retain the stent for 1–2 weeks after URS, while others prefer to remove the stent only after abdominal computer tomography 4–6 weeks after the procedure confirming stone-free status. The different approaches, most probably, are due to different types of stone treatment: fragmentation or dusting. "Dusters" need to ensure stone fragments expulsion before removing the stent. Ureteral stents could be the source of significant long-term postoperative morbidity, including flank or suprapubic pain and lower urinary tract symptoms, and it demands additional invasive procedure for its extraction.

The proponents of tubeless approach after uncomplicated ureterorenoscopic lithotripsy state that patients without ureteral stenting tend to have similar renal function recovery and satisfactory pain reduction with less irritative symptoms compared to those treated with an ureteral stent. They suggest that it is not necessary to place a stent routinely especially after treatment of stones smaller than 1 cm [20]. A suggestion is that a ureter catheter with a shorter indwelling time (1 day) may also be used, with similar results. Decision to place ureter catheter necessitates also the placement of a urethral catheter, which is not absolutely needed in tubeless or DJS approaches. This fact may prolong hospitalization period and cause symptoms that could be avoided, but on the other hand, the period of postoperative drainage is usually short, and lower urinary symptoms subside few days later.

The main goals of a postoperative double-J stent or UC are to avoid pain, facilitate stone fragments expulsion, and prevent infections and ureteral stricture formation [4]. The prevention of upper urinary tract obstruction secondary to intramural ureteral edema due to the intraoperative manipulations is another advantage [21]. Various studies suggested that there are significant disadvantages in the placement of stents in terms of LUTS and postoperative pain with no benefit in stone-free rates, infections rates, morbidity, and analgesia requirements. These studies conclude that there is no routine need for ureteral drainage after uncomplicated intracorporeal lithotripsy [22–24]. Decreasing instrumentation size and the stent-related symptoms in up to 50% of cases led to the conclusion that there is no need for routine upper tract drainage after uncomplicated procedures with efficient stone dusting [25]. Avoiding postoperative drainage constitutes ureterorenoscopy a viable ambulatory option, and the discharge of the patient is possible at the same day without the need for further upper urinary tract manipulation. Additionally, there is no difference in the occurrence of urinary frequency, urgency, or dysuria between the stented and tubeless groups on postoperative day one, but all these symptoms are significantly reduced in the non-stented group further on. A recent meta-analysis of 22 randomized controlled trials (RCT) by Hai Wang et al. concluded that stenting failed to improve stone-free rates and, instead, resulted in additional complications [26]. However, ureteral stents contributed in the prevention of re-hospitalization. In another study no significant differences in the visual analog scale (VAS), stricture formation, fever, or hospital stay were found between stented and non-stented groups. Stenting was independent on the stone size and location [27]. The decision for stenting and proper postoperative monitoring should be made on basis of each individual case [28]. To summarize, the advances in stent technology, with a particular focus on identifying the nature and source of stent morbidity, should eventually minimize bothersome symptoms and improve surgical care in postoperative ureterorenoscopy period.

Perioperative Antibiotic Treatment

Diagnostic and therapeutic upper urinary tract endoscopic procedures, especially stone treatment, have an increased risk of urinary tract infections and urosepsis. Risk factors are considered the trauma to the mucosa, bleeding, duration of the operation, increased intrarenal pressure, and manipulation or resection of infected material and stones. Knopf et al. described the use of antimicrobial prophylaxis by fluoroquinolone administration and showed that it significantly reduced post-procedural UTIs in healthy patients with ureteral stones and sterile preoperative urine [29]. If an infection or infectious material is suspected, culture and a full perioperative treatment course of an appropriate antimicrobial agents are recommended before the procedure.

The risk of infectious endocarditis (IE) after urologic procedures is low. Previous guidelines from the American Heart Association (AHA) had recommended routine prophylaxis, but the current recommendation is that the use of prophylactic antibiotics solely to prevent IE is not recommended. However, instrumentation in the GU tract may result in transient enterococcal bacteremia [30]. There is no data to demonstrate the link between bacteremia and IE or that administration of antimicrobial prophylaxis prevents IE. Regardless, the guidelines state that for patients with specific concomitant conditions (prosthetic cardiac valve, previous IE, congenital heart disease, cardiac transplantation) and an active infection or colonization that are planned to be submitted to GU tract manipulation, antibiotic therapy to sterilize the urine may be reasonable. In these patients amoxicillin or ampicillin is suggested as a first-line antibiotic for the management of enterococci or vancomycin in case of allergy or culture-directed agents as possible [30].

According to the guidelines, urinary tract infections should always be treated if stone removal is planned. In patients with clinically significant infection and obstruction, drainage should be performed for several days before stone removal. A urine culture should be performed before treatment [31].

For the prevention of infection following URS and percutaneous stone removal, no clear-cut evidence exists. In a review including a large number of patients submitted to PNL, it was reported that in patients with negative baseline urine culture, antibiotic prophylaxis significantly reduced the rate of postoperative fever and other complications [32].

The need for postoperative antibiotics is still a contradictory subject. There is a trend in various centers to continue prophylactic antibiotic treatment even in cases of sterile preoperative cultures. The suggested duration of such treatment may vary from 3 to 5 days postoperatively and depends on local microbiologic conditions. The commonly used antibiotics, acting effectively in urinary tract, are mostly quinolones, cephalosporins, and trimethoprim/sulfamethoxazole with or without penicillin (amoxicillin). These antibiotics have a compatible side effects profile and are potent suppressors of urinary bacteria. Despite that, a single preoperative dose should be sufficient according to current guidelines, and each endourologist may choose the appropriate antimicrobial prophylaxis strategy. Preoperative bacteriuria should be treated according to culture results and sensitivity test and should be initiated as soon as possible and continued at least 3 days after the procedure.

Postoperative sepsis must be treated aggressively, and initial work-up includes urine and blood cultures, renal function, CBC, CRP and maximal drainage of lower and upper urinary tracts, intravenous fluids, and antibiotics initiated with first sign of sepsis. Thorough cardiovascular monitoring, intravascular fluid balance, and possible ICU admission should be the next step in acute management.

Conclusions

Postoperative care of the patient submitted to a URS procedure is multifactorial. It depends on the type of instrumentation (rigid, flexible), on the size of the ureteroscope, on the type of the procedure (diagnostic, therapeutic for stone or tumor), on the anatomic location the procedure is focused (ureter or kidney), on the duration of the operation, on the use or not of upper urinary tract drainage, and finally on the occurrence of intraoperative complications. All these factors must be taken into consideration, and regardless the guidelines the postoperative follow-up of a patient submitted to a URS is individualized. Apart from the administration of antibiotics and perhaps the use of a stent, there are not specific guidelines for the postoperative care of the URS patient, and more studies are needed in order for a standardized protocol to be proposed. URS is a common but very important operation performed with delicate instruments requiring specialized endourologist maneuvers, and the postoperative care is also a crucial part of the procedure that can last till 4–6 weeks after the initial procedure where an inserted stent is planned to be removed or a second auxiliary procedure is to be performed.

References

1. Tan HJ, Strope SA, He C, Roberts WW, Faerber GJ, Wolf JS. Jr immediate unplanned hospital admission after outpatient ureteroscopy for stone disease. J Urol. 2011;185:2181–5.
2. Pearle MS, Calhoun EA, Curhan GC, Urologic diseases of America Project. Urologic diseases in America project: urolithiasis. J Urol. 2005;173:848–57.
3. Cheung MC, Lee F, Leung YL, Wong BB, Chu SM, Tam PC. Outpatient ureterscopy: predictive factors for postoperative events. Urology. 2001;58:914–8.
4. Bromwich EJ, Lockyer R, Keoghane SR. Day-case rigid and flexible ureteroscopy. Ann R Coll Surg Engl. 2007;89:526–8.

5. Lo CW, et al. Effectiveness of prophylactic antibiotics against post-ureteroscopic lithotripsy infections: systematic review and meta-analysis. Surg Infect (Larchmt). 2015;16:415–20.
6. Wagenlehner FM, Lichtenstern C, Rolfes C, et al. Diagnosis and management for urosepsis. Int J Urol. 2013;20:963–70.
7. Somani BK, Giusti G, Sun Y, et al. Complications associated with ureterorenoscopy (URS) related to the treatment of urolithiasis: the clinical research office of endourological society URS global study. World J Urol. 2017;35(4):675–81.
8. Pearle MS, Pierce HL, Miller GL, et al. Optimal method of urgent decompression of the collecting system for obstruction and infection due to ureteral calculi. J Urol. 1998;160:1260–4.
9. Ramy F, Youssef MD, Andreas Neisius MD, Zachariah G, et al. Clinical outcomes after ureteroscopic lithotripsy in patients who initially presented with urosepsis: matched pair comparison with elective ureteroscopy. J Endourol. 2014;28(12):1439–43.
10. Whitehurst LA, Somani BK. Perirenal hematoma after ureteroscopy: a systematic review. J Endourol. 2017;31(5):438–45.
11. Pathan SA, et al. Delivering safe and effective analgesia for management of renal colic in the emergency department: a double-blind, multigroup, randomised controlled trial. Lancet. 2016;387(10032):1999–2007. https://www.ncbi.nlm.nih.gov/pu
12. Türk C, Neisius A, Petrik A, Seitz C, Skolarikos A, Tepeler A, et al. EUA Nephrolithiasis guidelines 2017. Retrieved from: https://uroweb.org/guideline/2017. Nephrolithiasis guidelines/accessed 11.06.2017.
13. Krum H, et al. Blood pressure and cardiovascular outcomes in patients taking nonsteroidal nti-inflammatory drugs. Cardiovasc Ther. 2012;30(6):342–50.
14. Bhala N, et al. Vascular and upper gastrointestinal effects of non-steroidal anti-inflammatory drugs: meta-analyses of individual participant data from randomised trials. Lancet. 2013;382(9894):769–79.
15. Holdgate A, et al. Systematic review of the relative efficacy of non-steroidal anti-inflammatory drugs and opioids in the treatment of acute renal colic. BMJ. 2004;328(7453):1401.
16. Hollingsworth JM, et al. Alpha blockers for treatment of ureteric stones: systematic review and meta-analysis. BMJ. 2016;355:i6112.
17. Hamidi N, Ozturk E, Yikilmaz TN, Atmaca AF, Basar H. The effect of corticosteroid on postoperative early pain, renal colic and total analgesic consumption after uncomplicated and unstented ureteroscopy: a matched-pair analysis. World J Urol. 2018;36(6):979–84.
18. Assimos D, et al. Preoperative JJ stent placement in ureteric and renal stone treatment: results from the Clinical Research Office of Endourological Society (CROES) ureteroscopy (URS) Global Study. BJU Int. 2016;117:648.
19. Song T, et al. Meta-analysis of postoperatively stenting or not in patients underwent ureteroscopic lithotripsy. Urol Res. 2012;40(1):67–77.
20. Chen YT, Chen J, Wong WY, Yang SS, Hsieh CH, Wang CC. Is ureteral stenting necessary after uncomplicated ureteroscopic lithotripsy? A prospective, randomized controlled trial. J Urol. 2002;167(5):1977–80.
21. Gettman MT, Segura JW. Management of ureteric stones: issues and controversies. BJU Int. 2005;95:85–93.
22. Gunlusoy B, Degermenci T, Arslan M, et al. Is ureteral catheterization necessary after ureteroscopic lithotripsy for uncomplicated upper ureteral stones? J Endourol. 2008;22:1645.
23. Shen P, Li Y, Yang J, et al. The results of ureteral stenting after uretroscopic lithotripsy for ureteral calculi: a systematic review and meta-analysis. J Urol. 2011;186:1904–9.
24. Denstedt JD, Wollin TA, Sofer M, et al. A prospective randomized controlled trial comparing nonstented versus stented ureteroscopic lithotripsy. J Urol. 2001;165:1419–22.
25. Pengfei S, Yutao L, Jie Y, et al. The results of ureteral stenting after ureteroscopic lithotripsy for ureteral calculi: a systematic review and meta-analysis. J Urol. 2011;186:1904–9.
26. Knudsen BE, Beiko DT, Denstedt JD, et al. Stenting after ureteroscopy: pros and cons. Urol Clin North Am. 2004;31:173–80.

27. Wang H, Man L, Li G, et al. Meta-analysis of stenting versus non-stenting for the treatment of ureteral stones. PLoS One. 2017;12(1):e0167670.
28. Sabler IM, et al. Does retrograde treatment of upper urinary tract stones necessitate postoperative upper urinary tract drainage? Conclusions from over 500 single center consecutive cases. J Endourol. 2018;32(6):477–81.
29. Knopf HJ, Graff HJ, Schulze H. Perioperative antibiotic prophylaxis in ureteroscopic stone removal. Eur Urol. 2003;44(1):115–8.
30. Wilson W, Taubert K, Gewitz M, et al. Prevention of Infective Endocarditis: guidelines from the American Heart Association: a guideline from the American Heart Association Rheumatic Fever, Endocarditis, and Kawasaki Disease Committee, Council on Cardiovascular Disease in the Young, and the Council on Clinical Cardiology, Council on Cardiovascular Surgery and Anesthesia, and the Quality of Care and Outcomes Research Interdisciplinary Working Group. Circulation. 2007;116:1736–54.
31. Mariappan P, et al. Stone and pelvic urine culture and sensitivity are better than bladder urine as predictors of urosepsis following percutaneous nephrolithotomy: a prospective clinical study. J Urol. 2005;173:1610.
32. Gravas S, et al. Postoperative infection rates in low risk patients undergoing percutaneous nephrolithotomy with and without antibiotic prophylaxis: a matched case control study. J Urol. 2012;188:843.

Chapter 12
Complications of Ureteroscopy

Vincent De Coninck, Etienne Xavier Keller, and Olivier Traxer

Classification Systems of Complications

Complications of ureteroscopy can be classified following the modified Clavien classification system (MCCS) and the modified Satava classification system [1–3]. Standardized systems for classifying complications are necessary to compare results among different studies and to conduct meta-analyses (Tables 12.1 and 12.2).

Intraoperative Complications

Ureteral Avulsion

Ureteral avulsion is one of most devastating complications during ureteroscopy. It is relatively rare, with a reported incidence up to 0.4%. While it may be assumable that avulsion occurs more commonly in the proximal ureter due to its less well-defined muscular wall, a relationship with stone location within the ureter has not yet been found [4].

The most known mechanism of ureteral avulsion is when stones are tried to be removed with a basket with excessive force while they are too large to be passed through the ureteral lumen. To avoid this complication, stones should not be entrapped in the basket until they are reduced to small fragments. When a basket is

V. De Coninck · E. X. Keller · O. Traxer (✉)
Sorbonne Université, Service d'Urologie, AP-HP, Hôpital Tenon, Paris, France

Sorbonne Université, GRC n°20, Groupe de Recherche Clinique sur la Lithiase Urinaire, Hôpital Tenon, Paris, France
e-mail: olivier.traxer@aphp.fr

© Springer Nature Switzerland AG 2020
B. F. Schwartz, J. D. Denstedt (eds.), *Ureteroscopy*,
https://doi.org/10.1007/978-3-030-26649-3_12

Table 12.1 Clavien classification system

Grade I: any deviation from normal postoperative course without the need for pharmacologic treatment or surgical, endoscopic, or radiologic intervention. The allowed therapeutic regimens include drugs such as antiemetics, antipyretics, analgesics, diuretics, electrolytes, and physiotherapy. This grade also includes wound infections opened at the bedside

Grade II: complications requiring pharmacologic treatment with drugs other than those allowed for grade I complications. The use of blood transfusions and total parenteral nutrition is also included

Grade III: complications requiring surgical, endoscopic, or radiologic intervention

    Grade IIIa: intervention required without general anesthesia

    Grade IIIb: intervention required with general anesthesia

Grade IV: life-threatening complications, including central nervous system complications, requiring intensive care unit stay

    Grade IVa: single organ dysfunction, including requiring dialysis

    Grade IVb: multiorgan dysfunction

Grade V: death of the patient

Modified from Dindo et al. [3], with permission of Wolters Kluwer Health, Inc.

Table 12.2 Satava classification system

Grade 1 complications (incidents without consequences)
Grade 2 complications (incidents treated with endoscopic surgery)
Grade 2a complications (incidents treated intraoperatively with endoscopic surgery)
Grade 2b complications (incidents requiring endoscopic re-treatment)
Grade 3 complications (incidents requiring open or laparoscopic surgery)

Adapted from Tepeler et al. [1], with permission of Springer Nature

impacted in the ureter, one should try to release the stones by opening the basket and pushing it gently against the ureteral wall. In case of failure, a laser fiber should be advanced through the working channel to reduce the size of the stone fragments. Another option is to cut the wires of the basket or to dismantle the handle of the basket.

A less known mechanism is the two-point or "scabbard" ureteral avulsion in which the ureter is wedged in the intramural ureter. It involves a proximal and distal discontinuity of the ureter, with a resultant scabbard, as the ureter is withdrawn as a sheath on the ureteroscope [5–7]. The authors attribute this complication to the tapered design of the endoscope, in which the larger proximal shaft becomes wedged in the intramural ureter. Ureteral avulsion may also occur during removal of a locked ureteroscope. This may occur when a flexible ureteroscope is pulled through a stenotic infundibulum in maximal deflection [8, 9]. In case of locked flexible ureteroscope, one may try to manually straighten the ureteroscope by passing a coaxial dilator alongside the ureteroscope [8]. In case of failure, one may try remove the ureteroscope without damaging the urinary tract by cutting the handle of the flexible ureteroscope or by cutting the distal part through a percutaneous access. To avoid this calamitous complication, the urologist should always be aware of the position of the ureteroscope within the confines of the collecting system by using fluoroscopy.

A ureteral avulsion can be repaired immediately at the time of recognition or in a staged session after discussing the treatment options with the patient. In case of delayed repair, an appropriate urinary drainage should be guaranteed through a ureteral stent or nephrostomy tube. Definitive surgical options include several types of ureteral reimplantation depending of the level of avulsion, ileal interposition, or renal autotransplantation.

Mucosal Erosion, Submucosal Tunnel, and Ureteral Perforation

The ureteral wall is extremely vulnerable to intraoperative injury. Thomas and Traxer proposed an endoscopic classification of ureteral wall injuries after ureteral access sheath usage in 2013 (Table 12.3) (Fig. 12.1) [10]. After using a 12/14Fr ureteral access sheath, they found ureteral wall injuries in 46% of patients. Severe injury involving the smooth muscle layers was noticed in 13% of cases. The most important risk factor for severe ureteral access sheath-related ureteral injury was absence of pre-stenting before surgery, followed by male gender and increasing age. In the same year, Schoentaler et al. proposed a simple grading system for the description of ureteral lesions after ureteroscopy (Table 12.4) [11]. Urologists from different countries validated this scale with a video-based multicenter evaluation.

Mucosal ureteral erosions, false passages (or submucosal tunneling), and ureteral perforations usually occur during lithotripsy, stone extraction, ureteroscope ascending, intramural ureteral dilation, or ureteral access sheath of guidewire placement. Reported incidence of mucosal erosions and false passage after ureteroscopy is up to 10%. Perforations occur in up to 7% of ureteroscopic procedures. They may be associated with an extravasation of irrigant agent or urine,

Table 12.3 Endoscopic classification of ureteral wall injury after RIRS using ureteral access sheath [10]

Grade 0 (low) no lesion found or only mucosal petechiae
Grade 1 (low) ureteral mucosal erosion without smooth muscle injury
Grade 2 (high) ureteral wall injury, including mucosa and smooth muscle, with adventitial preservation (periureteral fat not seen)
Grade 3 (high) ureteral wall injury, including mucosa and smooth muscle, with adventitial perforation (periureteral fat seen)
Grade 4 (high) total ureteral avulsion

From Traxer and Thomas [10], with permission of Wolters Kluwer Health, Inc.

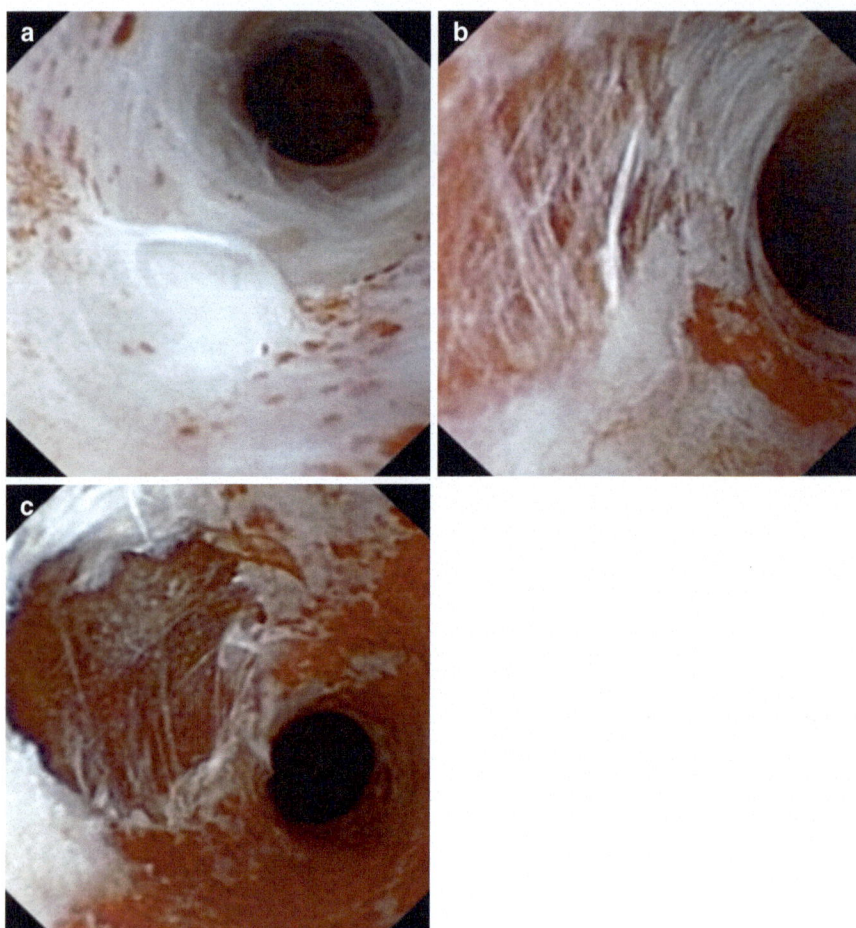

Fig. 12.1 Endoscopic views of ureteral wall injuries. (**a**) Grade 1. (**b**) Grade 2. (**c**) Grade 3. (From Traxer and Thomas [10], with permission of Wolters Kluwer Health, Inc.)

Table 12.4 Post-Ureteroscopic Lesion Scale (PULS) [11]	
	Grade 0 no lesion (uncomplicated URS)
	Grade 1 superficial mucosal lesion and/or significant mucosal edema/hematoma
	Grade 2 submucosal lesion
	Grade 3 perforation with less than 50% partial transection
	Grade 4 more than 50% partial transection
	Grade 5 complete transection
	From Schoenthaler et al. [11]. With permission of Springer Nature

Fig. 12.2 Ureteral perforation confirmed by retrograde ureterography

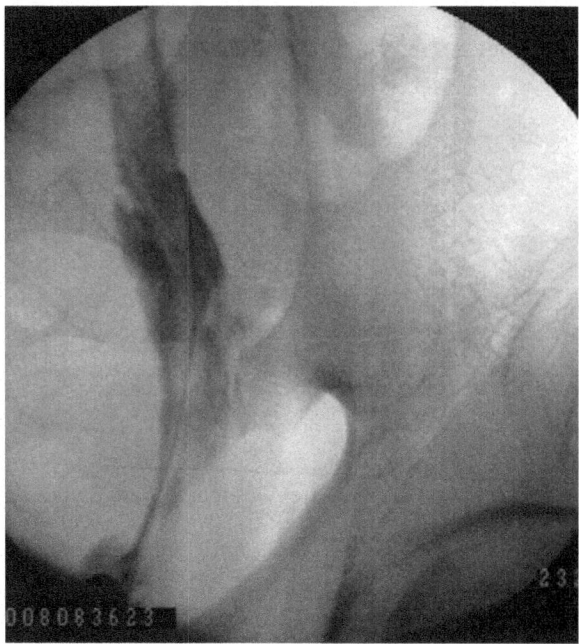

with a reported incidence of up to 4% [12–14] (Fig. 12.2). Schuster et al. reported that perforations are associated with longer operative time [15].

One may expect that false passages occur more likely at the distal ureter at the medial and posterior side due to the bulky transitional layer, thick muscular backing, and oblique insertion in the bladder. Avulsion may occur more commonly in the proximal ureter where the muscular wall is less well defined. However, this hypothesis has not yet been confirmed [4].

Mucosal ureteral erosions, false passages, and ureteral perforations may also be further complicated by submucosal or extra-ureteral stone migration. This was reported by Georgescu et al. in 0.15% of semirigid ureteroscopies for ureteral stones [16]. Ideally, every effort should be made to remove residual submucosal fragments or in order to prevent later stricture formation.

Most authors suggest continuing the intervention despite the lesions and leaving a ureteral stent afterward in a retrograde or antegrade way. In case of extensive extravasation, a conversion may be appropriate with drainage of the extravasation, ureteral stent insertion, and ureterorrhaphy [12, 16–18].

Bleeding After Endoureterotomy or Endopyelotomy

Performing an endoureterotomy or endopyelotomy is simple and effective technique in the treatment of ureteral or ureteropelvic junction stenosis. These can be performed by laser incision or using Acucise balloon. To avoid hemorrhagic complications, the site of incision should be carefully chosen to avoid crossing vessel injury (Fig. 12.3). It is of utmost importance to perform a contrast-enhanced CT before these interventions to evaluate how the ureter runs in relation to the vessels. Just before incision, air can be injected to define the anterior part of the ureter (12 o'clock), especially when using a digital ureteroscope or non-pendulum camera. Aberrant anatomical vessels or incisions performed at wrong locations may result in life-threatening hemorrhagic complications [19, 20]. Depending on the damaged vessels, treatment may consist of urgent embolization or endovascular or open repair.

Instrument Malfunction or Breakage

Reported incidence of instrument malfunction or breakage is up to 5%. The type and mechanism of breakage will determine the grade of associated complications. In most cases, problems like energy generator malfunction, dilation balloon breakage, or loss of view have a limited influence on the patient. In case of rupture of a lithotripsy probe, laser fiber, basket, forceps, or ureteroscope (Fig. 12.4), every effort should be made to remove the broken tool in the most conservative way possible (Fig. 12.5).

Bleeding

Intraoperative bleeding frequently occurs during ureteroscopy. Ureteral wall trauma is usually iatrogenic after inappropriate instrument usage. It may also occur as a consequence of forniceal rupture because of increases intrarenal pressure. Minor bleeding usually stops spontaneously after a couple of minutes of low-pressure irrigation. In case of prolonged poor vision caused by bleeding, it may be better to place a ureteral stent and postpone the intervention.

Following the MCCS, Mandal et al. considered hematuria lasting less than 6 h not as a complication. Hematuria resolving spontaneously by 48 h was considered as "transient hematuria." "Persistent hematuria" was defined as it lasted for more than 48 h and when additional medication or interventions were needed [2]. Transient hematuria and persistent hematuria are reported with an incidence up to 20% and 3%, respectively. This may result in urinary clot retention. In up to 1% of ureteroscopic cases, a blood transfusion is given [4]. Seldom, endourological of angiographic techniques are necessary to treat life-threatening bleeding [21].

To prevent mucosal tears, submucosal trauma, or more severe ureteral injuries, it is recommended to use small-size ureteroscopes and access sheaths. Instruments should always be adapted to the patient's anatomy and not the other way around. In case of ureteral narrowing, it is recommended to place a ureteral stent and postpone the intervention for at least 1 week, allowing passive ureteral dilatation [22]. Baskets

Fig. 12.3 (**a–e**) Locations of endoureterotomy. In absence of anatomical variations, a left endopyelotomy or proximal endoureterotomy is performed with a 5 o'clock incision (posterior and lateral) to avoid damage of crossing lower pole or gonadal vessels. At the level where the ureter crosses the iliac vessels, incision should be performed at 12 o'clock position. Incision of the distal left ureter is performed at 10 o'clock position (anterior and medial) to avoid the internal iliac vessels and at 12 o'clock for the intramural part. For the right ureter, incisions are performed at 7, 12, 2, and 12 o'clock, respectively

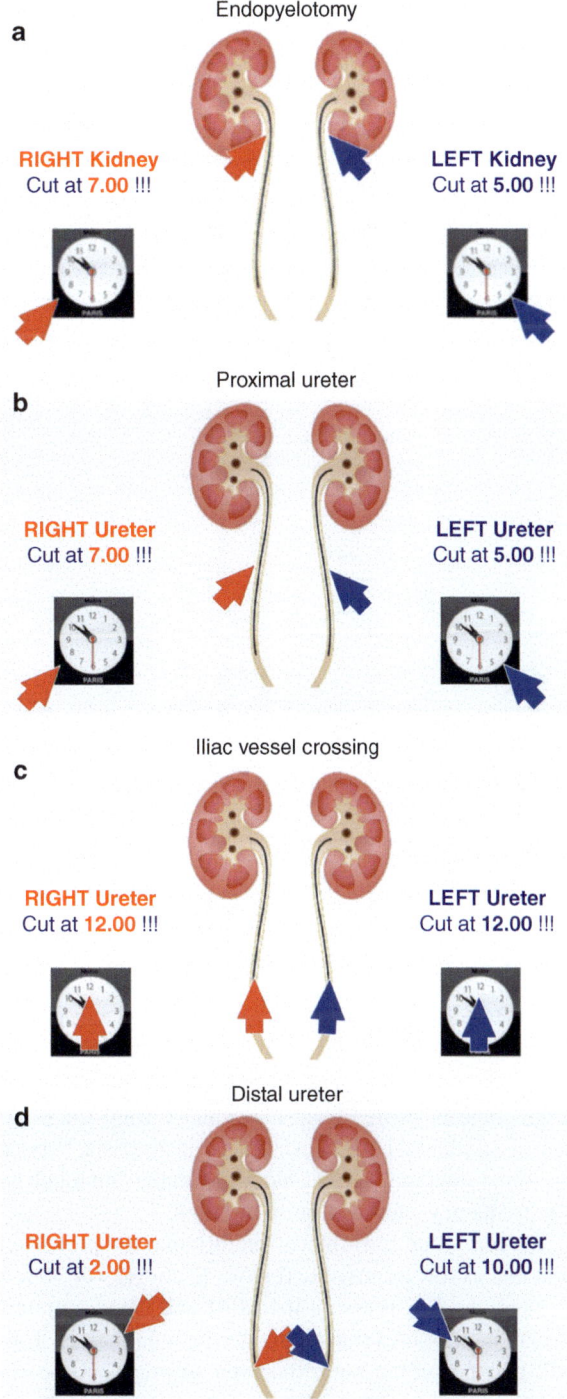

Fig. 12.3 (continued)

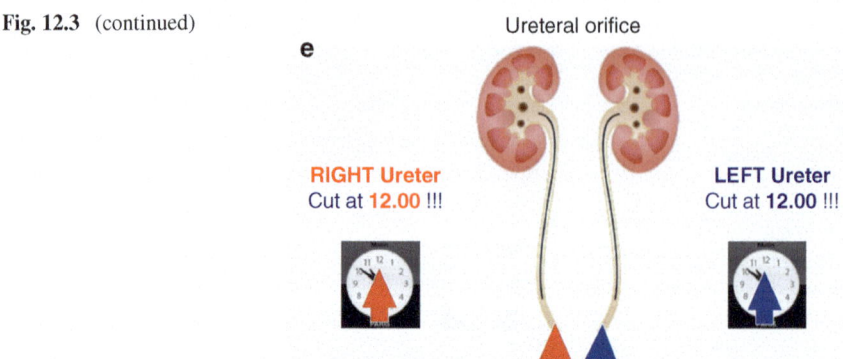

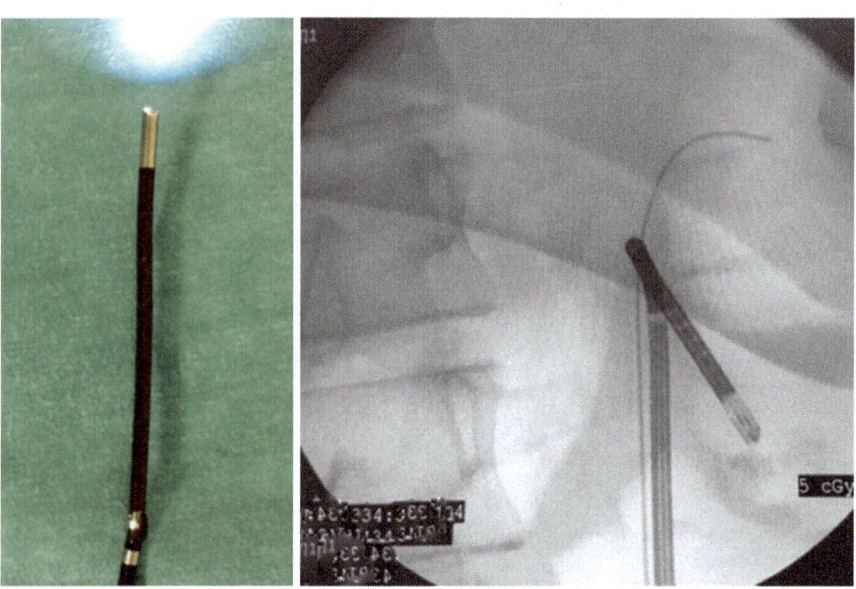

Fig. 12.4 Ureteroscope breakage while accessing difficult lower pole calyx

should be used with great care under direct vision, and ureteral stones should be fragmented or dusted from the center toward the periphery in order to reduce the risk of accidental laser activation on the mucosa. Vaporizing urothelial carcinoma of the upper tract may be less bloody with the "no touch technique" with a low energy, low frequency, and long pulse duration.

Bleeding due to forniceal rupture may be prevented by keeping the intrapelvic pressure as low as possible (below 40 cm H_2O or 30 mmHg). This may be achieved by applying low-pressure irrigation and using a ureteral access sheath that lowers irrigation pressures transmitted to the renal pelvis. The rate of decrease in pressure will depend on the outer diameter of ureteroscope and the inner diameter of the sheath [22]. Increasing irrigation pressure during bleeding may further worsen the

Fig. 12.5 Removal of
broken distal tip of laser
fiber within a basket

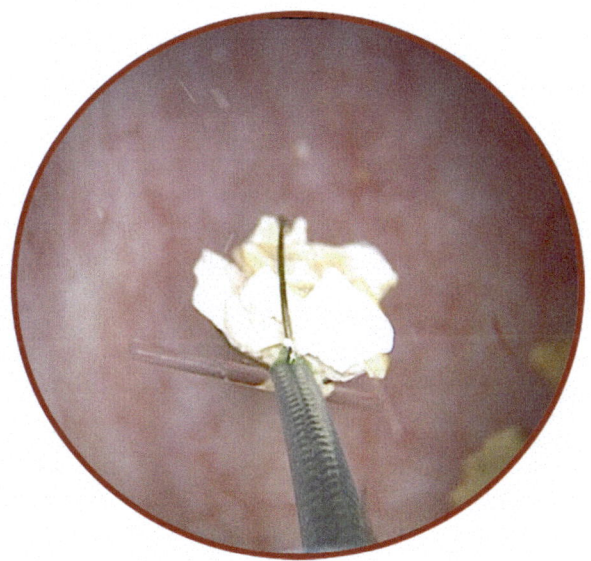

situation. As well, active aspiration should be avoided since negative intrarenal
pressure may provoke bleeding as well.

Westerman et al. studied the effect of anticoagulation and antiplatelet agents on
bleeding-related complications following ureteroscopy. They found that continuing
antiplatelet therapy in patients on chronic therapy does not increase the risk of
bleeding-related complications [23]. In contrast, continuation or bridging of
anticoagulants increases the risk of perioperative bleeding [24].

Early Postoperative Complications

Death

Even if ureteroscopy is generally considered as a safe procedure, fatal events may
occur. Most frequent reported cause of dead is urosepsis [25]. Other causes include
multiorgan failure, arrhythmia, cardiac death, and lung embolism. These complications are frequently secondary to less severe complications at first sight like infected
urolithiasis, bleeding, or perirenal hematoma [15, 21, 26]. Chang et al. reported a
gas embolism as a cause of death [27]. Possible explanatory mechanisms may be air
bubbles generated during Ho:YAG laser lithotripsy, air pushed into the upper urinary tract during repeatedly ureteroscope extraction and insertion, air bubbles during irrigation, or peripheral venous catheter-related air embolism.

Renal Pseudoaneurysm

A renal pseudoaneurysm is a serious uncommon condition that is caused by an arterial perforation that is only surrounded by connective tissue and a hematoma. This vascular lesion may become life-threatening when the arterial pressure surpasses the tamponade effect of the surrounding tissue. It has been reported after rigid and flexible ureteroscopy after endopyelotomy or lithotripsy with various energy sources techniques (laser fragmentation and electrohydraulic energy), and with or without the use of a ureteral access sheath. It may be asymptomatic or present as unexplained anemia, abdominal pain, fever, or hematuria. A renal pseudoaneurysm is diagnosed with contrast-enhanced CT or renal angiography. Treatment consists of embolization or surgery in case of treatment-refractory bleeding [28–32].

Arteriovenous Fistula

A few authors reported the initiation of intrarenal arteriovenous fistula after Ho:YAG or electrohydraulic lithotripsy. These fistulae are probably caused by damage of tissue and small interlobar arteries and veins during lithotripsy, leading to a connection between a high-pressure artery and a low-pressure vein. All cases presented with hematuria and were treated by embolization [33–35].

Urinoma, Perirenal Abscess, and Subcapsular, Perirenal, and Retroperitoneal Hematoma

Urinoma, perirenal abscess, and subcapsular, perirenal, and retroperitoneal hematoma may occur due to high intrarenal pressure during ureteroscopy and iatrogenic trauma of the pelvicalyceal system. Patients may present with lumbar pain, macroscopic hematuria, fever, septic shock, or hypovolemic shock. Diagnosis is usually made by contrast-enhanced CT or angiography (Fig. 12.6). Depending on the clinical situation, patients can be treated conservatively, with a drain, by selective embolization or by drainage with repair of the ruptured pelvicalyceal system. Seldom, patients are treated with a nephrectomy [17, 33, 36].

Urosepsis

Urosepsis occurs in up to 4% of cases following ureteroscopy. In rare cases, this complication may become fatal after ureteroscopy, especially in case of delayed initiation of supportive care, antimicrobials, and appropriate drainage or

Fig. 12.6 Contrast-
enhanced CT of
subcapsular hematoma
1 day after laser lithotripsy
of left mid-pole stone

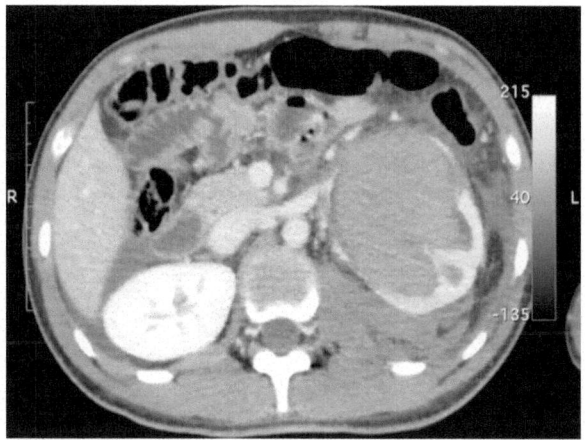

decompression of the urinary tract [33, 37]. Urosepsis after ureteroscopy mostly results from a urinary tract infection caused by *Escherichia coli*, *Proteus*, *Pseudomonas* species, *Serratia*, and group B streptococci, as well as *Candida* species [38–40]. Risk factors include immunocompromised status (e.g., post-transplantation, diabetes mellitus), elderly, anatomic abnormalities of the collecting system, recent urinary tract infection, prolonged preoperative stent dwelling time, and infectious stones [41–43].

Diagnosis relies on the recognition of symptoms associated with sepsis. Intraoperative stone culture may be more informative than preoperative urine culture [44]. Procalcitonin is a biomarker of a systemic response to infection. It accurately predicts the presence of bacteremia and bacterial load and may be a helpful biomarker to limit use of blood cultures [45]. Treatment consists of early recognition, immediate resuscitation, source control with appropriate drainage of the urinary tract, and culture-based antibiotic therapy. Preventive measures should include treating urinary tract infections prior to ureteroscopy, preoperative antibiotic prophylaxis [46–48], and sending stones for culture [44].

Ureteral Stent Migration

Ureteral stents are produced with a memory of a pigtail or double-J shape to prevent migration. Nevertheless, ureteral stent migration has a reported incidence up to 4% [49]. Migration usually occurs upward due to incorrect positioning, incorrect size selection, or ureteral peristalsis. Treatment consists of repositioning or stent removal, which may implicate another intervention when migration occurs postoperatively. Preventive measures include choosing a sufficiently long stent, placing the proximal curl in the pelvis instead of the upper calyx, and the presence of an appropriate distal curl in the bladder [50].

Preterm Labor

Urolithiasis and renal colic during pregnancy may result in obstetric complications like premature contractions and preterm labor in up to 10% of pregnant women [51]. This may result in preterm delivery [52]. A multidisciplinary approach to the pregnant patient is recommended and with both fetal monitoring and obstetrical services available.

Stone Migration and Residual Fragments

Stone migration during ureteroscopy has a reported incidence of 7%. When residual fragments are larger than 4 mm, this is associated with increased stone growth, complications, and reinterventions [53]. Stone migration may be reduced by using low-pressure irrigation, applying laser lithotripsy instead of pneumatic lithotripsy, or using anti-retropulsion devices [54–56]. Residual fragments are excluded by inspecting the whole calyceal system and the urinary tract after laser lithotripsy.

Fever and Urinary Tract Infection

Fever and urinary tract infections following ureteroscopy occur in up to 15% of cases [2]. Only in a minority cases or when not treated appropriately, they may evolve to urosepsis. Risk factors of infectious complication and fever include female gender, Crohn's and cardiovascular disease, ASA score of II or higher, preoperative bacteriuria, hydronephrosis, struvite stones, proximal ureteral stones, a high stone burden, and the placement of a urethral catheter, ureteral stent, and percutaneous nephrostomy [57, 58].

Preoperative antibiotic prophylaxis decreases the incidence of pyuria after ureteroscopy. However, it does not significantly reduce the rates of bacteriuria, postoperative urinary tract infection, and fever [58, 59]. In spite of these data, EAU and AUA guidelines recommend a single preoperative dose of antibiotics. Additional postoperative antibiotics seem not to decrease infection rates after ureteroscopic stone treatment [48].

Pain and Renal Colic

Distension of the upper urinary tract provokes pain, due to stimulation of mechanoreceptors in the ureter and kidney [60]. Pain following ureteroscopy is usually located in the flank or lower abdomen. In most cases, it can be treated conservatively with analgesics. In up to 2% following ureteroscopy, analgesic is insufficient in pain management, and ureteral stenting is required. Factors related to severe early postoperative pain after retrograde intrapelvic surgery are female gender, larger stone burden, and ureteral access sheath time [61].

Ureteral Stent Discomfort

The Clinical Research Office of the Endourological Society (CROES) reported ureteral stent discomfort in 1% of cases. This is in contrast to other reports that reported stent-related symptoms (e.g., flank pain, urgency, dysuria) in up to 88% of cases with the need of analgesics in over 70% of cases [62, 63]. These stent-related symptoms and its associated costs feed the debate about deferring routine stenting after uncomplicated ureteroscopic stone removal. Cases in which stent is probably required are larger stone size, longer operation duration, prior ipsilateral ureteroscopy, and recurrent renal colic. Use of a ureteral access sheath in itself seems not to be associated with postoperative hydronephrosis and does not require stenting at any time [36, 64].

Late Postoperative Complications

Ureteral Stricture

Ureteral strictures occur in up to 3% of patients after ureteroscopic procedures. The mechanism of stricture formation remains to be elucidated. Hypothetical mechanisms include direct mechanical trauma or perforation of the ureteral wall (e.g., guidewire, lithotripter, ureteroscope), thermal injury (e.g., laser), ischemia (e.g., impacted stone), or infection (e.g., schistosomiasis), leading to inflammatory processes in the ureteral wall [65, 66]. Kidney function deterioration, flank pain, or hydronephrosis after ureteroscopy are reminiscent of stricture formation. Treatment of the stricture may consist of dilation, incision, resection, or ureteral reimplantation [49, 67, 68]. Based on the hypothetical mechanisms of stricture formation, the incidence rate may decrease due to miniaturization of the ureteroscopic armamentarium. Impacted stones should be entirely removed in order to remove chronic inflammation leading to stricture formation.

Risk Factors for Complications Related to Ureteroscopy

Sugihara et al. reported that severe complications following ureteroscopy were associated with longer operative duration (more than 90 min), lower hospital volume (less than 15 ureteroscopic procedures per year), female gender, older age (over

80 years old), Charlson Comorbidity Index more than 1, general anesthesia, and emergent admission [69]. Other reported risk factors include impacted stones, surgeon experience, and congenital renal abnormality [36].

Conclusion

Most complications are minor and do not require intervention. Seldom, complications may be devastating. Therefore, every urologist should be aware of possible complications in order to prevent them and to manage them when encountering them.

Every patient should be screened for urinary tract infection before ureteroscopy. In case of positive urinary culture, antibiotics and appropriate drainage should be foreseen, and the intervention should be postponed.

To prevent complications, we recommend using a safely guidewire during every intervention since they do not harm and prevent worsening of certain complications. We see safety guidewires as a safety belt: it serves in a very limited number of cases, but everyone will be glad to have one in case of an accident. Once a complication happened, placing a safety guidewire may become difficult.

Force should never be used during endourological maneuvers. When a ureteroscope does not pass easily through the ureteral orifice, we recommend passive ureteral dilating by placing a ureteral stent and postponing the intervention for at least 1 week. This avoids mechanical trauma of the ureteral wall which may possibly lead to stricture formation. When ureteral narrowing persists after stenting, impacted stones or tumors should be excluded by performing a retrograde ureterography or engaging the ureter with the smallest available ureteroscope alongside a safety guidewire. As a last resort, minimal dilation up to the size of the ureteroscope can be performed.

There is sufficient evidence that a ureteral access sheath decreases intrarenal pressure and improves irrigation outflow. Data on the impact of a ureteral access sheath on complications (ureteroscope damage, postoperative pain, fever, sepsis, ureteral strictures), stone-free rates, and its cost-effectiveness are inconclusive. Therefore, inserting a UAS should not be a systematic step when performing flexible URS. The decision should be made on a patient-specific basis.

Retrieval of stone fragments with a basket should always be performed under direct ureteroscopic vision. In case of entrapment, fragments should be released from the basket or fragmented to a smaller size to prevent ureteral lesions.

The last step of ureteroscopy should include inspecting the urinary tract to exclude bleeding, mucosal wall lesions, residual or impacted stones, or ureteral narrowings. This allows to undertake preventive measures to avoid complications during the postoperative period.

Placing an indwelling stent after uncomplicated ureteroscopy is not decreasing postoperative complications. Moreover, they increase costs and hospital readmission rates and result in stent-related symptoms. Therefore, postoperative stenting should only be considered in case of increased risk of postoperative complications.

References

1. Tepeler A, Resorlu B, Sahin T, et al. Categorization of intraoperative ureteroscopy complications using modified Satava classification system. World J Urol. 2014;32:131–6.
2. Mandal S, Goel A, Singh MK, et al. Clavien classification of semirigid ureteroscopy complications: a prospective study. Urology. 2012;80:995–1001.
3. Dindo D, Demartines N, Clavien PA. Classification of surgical complications: a new proposal with evaluation in a cohort of 6336 patients and results of a survey. Ann Surg. 2004;240:205–13.
4. Perez Castro E, Osther PJ, Jinga V, et al. Differences in ureteroscopic stone treatment and outcomes for distal, mid-, proximal, or multiple ureteral locations: the Clinical Research Office of the Endourological Society ureteroscopy global study. Eur Urol. 2014;66:102–9.
5. Ordon M, Schuler TD, Honey RJ. Ureteral avulsion during contemporary ureteroscopic stone management: "the scabbard avulsion". J Endourol. 2011;25:1259–62.
6. Tanimoto R, Cleary RC, Bagley DH, Hubosky SG. Ureteral avulsion associated with ureteroscopy: insights from the MAUDE database. J Endourol. 2016;30:257–61.
7. Gaizauskas A, Markevicius M, Gaizauskas S, Zelvys A. Possible complications of ureteroscopy in modern endourological era: two-point or "scabbard" avulsion. Case Rep Urol. 2014;2014:308093.
8. Hubosky SG, Raval AJ, Bagley DH. Locked deflection during flexible ureteroscopy: incidence and elucidation of the mechanism of an underreported complication. J Endourol. 2015;29:907–12.
9. Anderson JK, Lavers A, Hulbert JC, Monga M. The fractured flexible ureteroscope with locked deflection. J Urol. 2004;171:335.
10. Traxer O, Thomas A. Prospective evaluation and classification of ureteral wall injuries resulting from insertion of a ureteral access sheath during retrograde intrarenal surgery. J Urol. 2013;189:580–4.
11. Schoenthaler M, Buchholz N, Farin E, et al. The Post-Ureteroscopic Lesion Scale (PULS): a multicenter video-based evaluation of inter-rater reliability. World J Urol. 2014;32:1033–40.
12. El-Nahas AR, El-Tabey NA, Eraky I, et al. Semirigid ureteroscopy for ureteral stones: a multivariate analysis of unfavorable results. J Urol. 2009;181:1158–62.
13. Mursi K, Elsheemy MS, Morsi HA, Ali Ghaleb AK, Abdel-Razzak OM. Semi-rigid ureteroscopy for ureteric and renal pelvic calculi: predictive factors for complications and success. Arab J Urol. 2013;11:136–41.
14. Salem HK. A prospective randomized study comparing shock wave lithotripsy and semirigid ureteroscopy for the management of proximal ureteral calculi. Urology. 2009;74:1216–21.
15. Schuster TG, Hollenbeck BK, Faerber GJ, Wolf JS Jr. Complications of ureteroscopy: analysis of predictive factors. J Urol. 2001;166:538–40.
16. Georgescu D, Multescu R, Geavlete B, Geavlete P. Intraoperative complications after 8150 semirigid ureteroscopies for ureteral lithiasis: risk analysis and management. Chirurgia (Bucur). 2014;109:369–74.
17. Geavlete P, Georgescu D, Nita G, Mirciulescu V, Cauni V. Complications of 2735 retrograde semirigid ureteroscopy procedures: a single-center experience. J Endourol. 2006;20:179–85.
18. Ibrahim AK. Reporting ureteroscopy complications using the modified clavien classification system. Urol Ann. 2015;7:53–7.
19. Kim FJ, Herrell SD, Jahoda AE, Albala DM. Complications of acucise endopyelotomy. J Endourol. 1998;12:433–6.
20. Lopes RI, Torricelli FC, Gomes CM, Carnevale F, Bruschini H, Srougi M. Endovascular repair of a nearly fatal iliac artery injury after endoureterotomy. Scand J Urol. 2013;47:437–9.
21. Somani BK, Giusti G, Sun Y, et al. Complications associated with ureterorenoscopy (URS) related to treatment of urolithiasis: the Clinical Research Office of Endourological Society URS Global study. World J Urol. 2017;35:675–81.
22. De Coninck V, Keller EX, Rodriguez-Monsalve M, Audouin M, Doizi S, Traxer O. Systematic review of ureteral access sheaths: facts and myths. BJU Int. 2018;122:959–69.

23. Westerman ME, Sharma V, Scales J, Gearman DJ, Ingimarsson JP, Krambeck AE. The effect of antiplatelet agents on bleeding-related complications after ureteroscopy. J Endourol. 2016;30:1073–8.
24. Westerman ME, Scales JA, Sharma V, Gearman DJ, Ingimarsson JP, Krambeck AE. The effect of anticoagulation on bleeding-related complications following ureteroscopy. Urology. 2017;100:45–52.
25. Cindolo L, Castellan P, Scoffone CM, et al. Mortality and flexible ureteroscopy: analysis of six cases. World J Urol. 2016;34:305–10.
26. de la Rosette J, Denstedt J, Geavlete P, et al. The clinical research office of the endourological society ureteroscopy global study: indications, complications, and outcomes in 11,885 patients. J Endourol. 2014;28:131–9.
27. Chang CP, Liou CC, Yang YL, Sun MS. Fatal gas embolism during ureteroscopic holmium: yttrium-aluminium-garnet laser lithotripsy under spinal anesthesia – a case report. Minim Invasive Ther Allied Technol. 2008;17:259–61.
28. Jubber I, Patel PR, Hori S, Al-Hayek S. Renal pseudoaneurysm: a rare and potentially fatal complication following ureteroscopy and laser fragmentation of stones. Ann R Coll Surg Engl. 2018;100:e51–2.
29. Aston W, Whiting R, Bultitude M, Challacombe B, Glass J, Dasgupta P. Pseudoaneurysm formation after flexible ureterorenoscopy and electrohydraulic lithotripsy. Int J Clin Pract. 2004;58:310–1.
30. Angelsen A, Talseth T, Mjones JG, Hedlund H. Hypertension and pseudoaneurism on the renal artery following retrograde endopyelotomy (Acucise). Scand J Urol Nephrol. 2000;34:79–80.
31. Durner L, El Howairis MEF, Buchholz N. Renal pseudoaneurysm after flexible ureterorenoscopy – an unusual complication. Urol Int. 2017;99:484–6.
32. Ngo TC, Lee JJ, Gonzalgo ML. Renal pseudoaneurysm: an overview. Nat Rev Urol. 2010;7:619–25.
33. Cindolo L, Castellan P, Primiceri G, et al. Life-threatening complications after ureteroscopy for urinary stones: survey and systematic literature review. Minerva Urol Nefrol. 2017;69:421–31.
34. Rudnick DM, Dretler SP. Intrarenal pseudoaneurysm following ureterorenoscopy and electrohydraulic lithotripsy. J Urol. 1998;159:1290–1.
35. Tiplitsky SI, Milhoua PM, Patel MB, Minsky L, Hoenig DM. Case report: intrarenal arteriovenous fistula after ureteroscopic stone extraction with holmium laser lithotripsy. J Endourol. 2007;21:530–2.
36. Bas O, Tuygun C, Dede O, et al. Factors affecting complication rates of retrograde flexible ureterorenoscopy: analysis of 1571 procedures-a single-center experience. World J Urol. 2017;35:819–26.
37. Ferrer R, Martin-Loeches I, Phillips G, et al. Empiric antibiotic treatment reduces mortality in severe sepsis and septic shock from the first hour: results from a guideline-based performance improvement program. Crit Care Med. 2014;42:1749–55.
38. Scotland KB, Lange D. Prevention and management of urosepsis triggered by ureteroscopy. Res Rep Urol. 2018;10:43–9.
39. Gautam G, Singh AK, Kumar R, Hemal AK, Kothari A. Beware! Fungal urosepsis may follow endoscopic intervention for prolonged indwelling ureteral stent. J Endourol. 2006;20:522–4.
40. Blackmur JP, Maitra NU, Marri RR, Housami F, Malki M, McIlhenny C. Analysis of factors' association with risk of postoperative urosepsis in patients undergoing ureteroscopy for treatment of stone disease. J Endourol. 2016;30:963–9.
41. Bloom J, Fox C, Fullerton S, Matthews G, Phillips J. Sepsis after elective ureteroscopy. Can J Urol. 2017;24:9017–23.
42. Nevo A, Mano R, Baniel J, Lifshitz DA. Ureteric stent dwelling time: a risk factor for post-ureteroscopy sepsis. BJU Int. 2017;120:117–22.
43. Mitsuzuka K, Nakano O, Takahashi N, Satoh M. Identification of factors associated with postoperative febrile urinary tract infection after ureteroscopy for urinary stones. Urolithiasis. 2016;44:257–62.

44. Eswara JR, Shariftabrizi A, Sacco D. Positive stone culture is associated with a higher rate of sepsis after endourological procedures. Urolithiasis. 2013;41:411–4.
45. van Nieuwkoop C, Bonten TN, van't Wout JW, et al. Procalcitonin reflects bacteremia and bacterial load in urosepsis syndrome: a prospective observational study. Crit Care. 2010;14:R206.
46. Qiao LD, Chen S, Lin YH, et al. Evaluation of perioperative prophylaxis with fosfomycin tromethamine in ureteroscopic stone removal: an investigator-driven prospective, multicenter, randomized, controlled study. Int Urol Nephrol. 2018;50:427–32.
47. Knopf HJ, Graff HJ, Schulze H. Perioperative antibiotic prophylaxis in ureteroscopic stone removal. Eur Urol. 2003;44:115–8.
48. Chew BH, Flannigan R, Kurtz M, et al. A single dose of intraoperative antibiotics is sufficient to prevent urinary tract infection during ureteroscopy. J Endourol. 2016;30:63–8.
49. Cheung MC, Lee F, Leung YL, Wong BB, Chu SM, Tam PC. Outpatient ureteroscopy: predictive factors for postoperative events. Urology. 2001;58:914–8.
50. Slaton JW, Kropp KA. Proximal ureteral stent migration: an avoidable complication? J Urol. 1996;155:58–61.
51. Zhang S, Liu G, Duo Y, Wang J, Li J, Li C. Application of ureteroscope in emergency treatment with persistent renal colic patients during pregnancy. PLoS One. 2016;11:e0146597.
52. Johnson EB, Krambeck AE, White WM, et al. Obstetric complications of ureteroscopy during pregnancy. J Urol. 2012;188:151–4.
53. Chew BH, Brotherhood HL, Sur RL, et al. Natural history, complications and re-intervention rates of asymptomatic residual stone fragments after ureteroscopy: a report from the EDGE Research Consortium. J Urol. 2016;195:982–6.
54. Maghsoudi R, Amjadi M, Norizadeh D, Hassanzadeh H. Treatment of ureteral stones: a prospective randomized controlled trial on comparison of Ho:YAG laser and pneumatic lithotripsy. Indian J Urol. 2008;24:352–4.
55. Hendlin K, Weiland D, Monga M. Impact of irrigation systems on stone migration. J Endourol. 2008;22:453–8.
56. Kroczak T, Ghiculete D, Sowerby R, et al. Dual usage of a stone basket: stone capture and retropulsion prevention. Can Urol Assoc J. 2018;12:280–3.
57. Sohn DW, Kim SW, Hong CG, Yoon BI, Ha US, Cho YH. Risk factors of infectious complication after ureteroscopic procedures of the upper urinary tract. J Infect Chemother. 2013;19:1102–8.
58. Hsieh CH, Yang SS, Lin CD, Chang SJ. Are prophylactic antibiotics necessary in patients with preoperative sterile urine undergoing ureterorenoscopic lithotripsy? BJU Int. 2014;113:275–80.
59. Martov A, Gravas S, Etemadian M, et al. Postoperative infection rates in patients with a negative baseline urine culture undergoing ureteroscopic stone removal: a matched case-control analysis on antibiotic prophylaxis from the CROES URS global study. J Endourol. 2015;29:171–80.
60. Pedersen KV, Drewes AM, Frimodt-Moller PC, Osther PJ. Visceral pain originating from the upper urinary tract. Urol Res. 2010;38:345–55.
61. Oguz U, Sahin T, Senocak C, et al. Factors associated with postoperative pain after retrograde intrarenal surgery for kidney stones. Turk J Urol. 2017;43:303–8.
62. Al-Kandari AM, Al-Shaiji TF, Shaaban H, Ibrahim HM, Elshebiny YH, Shokeir AA. Effects of proximal and distal ends of double-J ureteral stent position on postprocedural symptoms and quality of life: a randomized clinical trial. J Endourol. 2007;21:698–702.
63. Giannarini G, Keeley FX Jr, Valent F, et al. Predictors of morbidity in patients with indwelling ureteric stents: results of a prospective study using the validated Ureteric Stent Symptoms Questionnaire. BJU Int. 2011;107:648–54.
64. Barbour ML, Raman JD. Incidence and predictors for ipsilateral hydronephrosis following ureteroscopic lithotripsy. Urology. 2015;86:465–71.
65. Roberts WW, Cadeddu JA, Micali S, Kavoussi LR, Moore RG. Ureteral stricture formation after removal of impacted calculi. J Urol. 1998;159:723–6.

66. Sharfi AR, Rayis AB. The continuing challenge of bilharzial ureteric stricture. Scand J Urol Nephrol. 1989;23:123–6.
67. Elashry OM, Elgamasy AK, Sabaa MA, et al. Ureteroscopic management of lower ureteric calculi: a 15-year single-centre experience. BJU Int. 2008;102:1010–7.
68. Fuganti PE, Pires S, Branco R, Porto J. Predictive factors for intraoperative complications in semirigid ureteroscopy: analysis of 1235 ballistic ureterolithotripsies. Urology. 2008;72:770–4.
69. Sugihara T, Yasunaga H, Horiguchi H, et al. A nomogram predicting severe adverse events after ureteroscopic lithotripsy: 12 372 patients in a Japanese national series. BJU Int. 2013;111:459–66.

Chapter 13
Management of Urolithiasis in Pregnancy

Jennifer Bjazevic and John D. Denstedt

Introduction

Stone disease in pregnancy represents a challenging and complex clinical situation. A thoughtful and individualized approach to diagnosis and management is required given the unique and significant risks present to both the mother and the fetus. Collaboration with a multidisciplinary team consisting of a urologist, radiologist, obstetrician, neonatologist, and anesthesiologist is necessary in order to provide safe and optimized patient care. Multiple advances in diagnostic imaging, endourological care and equipment, fetal monitoring, and obstetrical care have led to significant improvements in patient care and outcomes. Specifically, there has been a paradigm shift for the management of acute stone disease in pregnancy over the past 20 years. Definitive surgical treatment with ureteroscopy has now become the preferred treatment option for patients who fail expectant management, whereas temporized drainage with a ureteric stent or nephrostomy tube has become a second-line option.

Epidemiology

Urolithiasis is a highly prevalent condition afflicting approximately 10% of individuals, and multiple reports suggest that the incidence of urinary stone disease has been increasing worldwide [1–5]. However, the rising incidence of nephrolithiasis appears more pronounced in women. For instance, in the United States over the past 30 years, there has been an annual increase in the rate of female stone disease by

J. Bjazevic · J. D. Denstedt (✉)
Department of Surgery, Division of Urology, Schulich School of Medicine & Dentistry,
Western University, London, ON, Canada
e-mail: John.Denstedt@sjhc.london.on.ca

© Springer Nature Switzerland AG 2020
B. F. Schwartz, J. D. Denstedt (eds.), *Ureteroscopy*,
https://doi.org/10.1007/978-3-030-26649-3_13

1.9%; along with this hospital admissions for urolithiasis in women have risen by 52% [6, 7].

The true incidence of urolithiasis in pregnancy remains unverified as rates reported in the literature vary widely from 1 out of every 200 to 3800 pregnancies, with an estimated incidence of 1:1500 (0.07%) [8, 9]. Recent reports demonstrate no change in the incidence of urolithiasis in pregnant women over the past 20 years [10]. Overall, pregnant women have the same risk of stone formation as their non-pregnant counterparts with similar age and demographic characteristics [11]. However, a recent study of the National Health and Nutrition Examination Survey (NHANES) data showed that the prevalence of stone disease among reproductive-aged women increased significantly with prior pregnancy and was correlated with the number of previous pregnancies [12]. While stone disease during pregnancy is not common, it is an important clinical situation given the potential serious risks posed to both the mother and the fetus and requires careful consideration of diagnostic and treatment strategies.

Etiology

There are significant alterations that occur to both genitourinary anatomy and physiology during pregnancy which may impact potential stone formation, such as increased urinary stasis and changes to urinary constituents. Gestational hydronephrosis is exceedingly common and is present in up to 90% of women by the third trimester [13]. Multiple factors contribute to the development of hydronephrosis in pregnancy such as hormonal alterations, elevated renal function, and most significantly extrinsic compression from the gravid uterus. Increased levels of progesterone during pregnancy cause relaxation of the smooth muscles of the urinary collecting system and decrease peristalsis, resulting in subsequent dilatation of the renal pelvises, calyces, and ureters [14]. In addition, renal function increases significantly during the first trimester with the glomerular filtration rate (GFR) rising by 40–65%. This results from the combination of an elevated cardiac output and circulating blood volume along with a decrease in systemic vascular resistance [15]. However, the most substantial factor contributing to gestational hydronephrosis is extrinsic compression of the ureter at the level of the pelvic brim by the gravid uterus [13]. For this reason, physiologic dilatation of the ureter below the pelvic brim does not occur [16]. The degree of hydronephrosis is characteristically greater on the right side secondary to dextrorotation of the uterus and shielding of the left ureter by the sigmoid colon [17].

Physiologic hydronephrosis of pregnancy can develop as early as 6 weeks of gestation and persist until 6 weeks postpartum [13]. It is typically not associated with significant obstruction and remains asymptomatic; however, in certain instances it may result in significant flank pain and even forniceal rupture [13]. Gestational hydronephrosis may increase the potential for stone formation by causing urinary stasis and increasing contact time with urinary lithogenic constituents. In addition, the resulting dilatation of the collecting system may allow for easier migration of renal stones into the ureter, providing a potential explanation for the observation that ureteric calculi are twice as common as renal calculi during pregnancy [18].

Renal physiology is also considerably altered during pregnancy, which results in important changes to the urinary milieu. As mentioned previously, GFR increases substantially during the first trimester, thereby increasing renal filtration. This results in a corresponding rise of multiple lithogenic constituents of the urine including calcium, oxalate, uric acid, and sodium [19, 20]. Placental production of 1,25-dihydroxychloecalciferol (1,25-vit D) also contributes to hypercalciuria by suppressing parathyroid hormone levels and increasing the gastrointestinal absorption and bone resorption of calcium [9, 19]. All of these actions of 1,25-vit D act to increase the filtration and decrease the resorption of calcium by the kidney, thereby causing hypercalciuria [19]. Furthermore, many pregnant women consume additional calcium supplementation based on recent evidence that it may significantly reduce the risk of preterm birth, preeclampsia, and maternal morbidity and mortality [21]. Previous investigation has demonstrated a trend toward an increased risk of stone disease with calcium supplementation during pregnancy [22]. However, additional high-quality research into the impact of calcium supplementation on the risk of stone disease during pregnancy as well as maternal and fetal outcomes is required. Currently, the risk and benefits of calcium supplementation during pregnancy must be carefully balanced and individualized, especially in women at high risk of urolithiasis.

While many alterations to renal physiology during pregnancy result in the increased potential for stone formation, these are balanced by a corresponding number of changes which act to inhibit this. For instance, the increase in GFR increases urine volume and thereby decreases the risk of stone formation [23]. The elevation in pro-lithogenic urinary factors is balanced by a similar increase in the excretion of many stone inhibitors such as citrate, magnesium, glycosaminoglycans, nephrocalcin, uromodulin, and thiosulfate, all of which act to inhibit crystal growth and aggregation [24]. Elevation in urinary citrate levels also increases the urinary pH, thereby preventing calcium oxalate and uric acid stone formation [20]. However, this alkalinization of the urine can increase the risk of calcium phosphate stone formation, and indeed studies have shown an increased incidence of calcium phosphate stones in pregnant women [25]. Many complex changes occur to renal anatomy and physiology throughout pregnancy; the net effect of these changes ultimately results in no overall difference to the risk of stone formation during pregnancy.

Clinical Presentation

The diagnosis of urinary stone disease during pregnancy can be difficult due to the high prevalence of symptoms in pregnancy that mimic acute renal colic [26]. For instance, flank and abdominal pain, nausea and vomiting, hematuria, and lower urinary tract voiding systems are all commonly reported by pregnant women. Up to

84% of women report some back and abdominal pain during pregnancy secondary to the stretching of ligaments and musculature [18]. Nausea and vomiting caused from elevated levels of progesterone are most commonly present within the first trimester but can persist for the entire pregnancy [18]. Fifty-two percent of women without urolithiasis present with microscopic or gross hematuria during their pregnancy, which can result from the rupture of small renal pyramid veins caused by renal enlargement [27]. Up to 30% of cases of urolithiasis during pregnancy will be misdiagnosed, and a high index of suspicion is required to ensure a prompt and accurate diagnosis [27].

Urinary stone disease during pregnancy most commonly occurs within the second (39%) and third (45%) trimesters [25]. Approximately 30% of patients will have a prior history of urolithiasis, and 3.7% of patients will have experienced a previous stone episode during pregnancy [25]. The most common presenting symptoms include flank or abdominal pain (85%), microscopic (95%) or gross (20%) hematuria, pyuria (42%) and worsening lower urinary tract voiding symptoms [26, 28]. Patients can also present with complications from urolithiasis including urosepsis, hypertension, preeclampsia, premature rupture of membranes, premature labor, and pregnancy loss though this occurs less frequently [29]. The published rate of complications from urinary stone disease in pregnancy varies widely from 0% to 67%. However, multiple studies have demonstrated no association between acute renal colic in pregnancy and adverse perinatal outcomes [29, 30].

Investigations

All pregnant patients presenting with symptoms suggestive of renal colic should undergo a detailed history and physical examination. Laboratory investigations should include a complete blood count (CBC), serum electrolytes, and measurement of renal function with urea and creatinine. In addition, serum uric acid and calcium levels may also be helpful as elevations in these may further predispose to the development of stone disease. It is important to also obtain a urinalysis and urine culture. Asymptomatic bacteriuria should be treated in pregnancy given the higher risk of developing pyelonephritis secondary to gestational hydronephrosis and urinary stasis [31]. If an extensive metabolic evaluation including 24-h urine studies is clinically indicated, this should be delayed until the end of pregnancy and weaning of breastfeeding as urine chemistries may be significantly altered by the hormonal changes that occur [9].

Given the unreliability of history and physical examination alone in accurately diagnosing renal colic in pregnancy, adjunctive diagnostic imaging is necessary in order to confirm the correct diagnosis. To date, multiple imaging modalities have been assessed and utilized for diagnosis of urinary stone disease in pregnancy including ultrasonography (US); X-ray of kidneys, ureters, and bladder (KUB); intravenous pyelogram (IVP); computed tomography (CT); and magnetic resonance urography (MRU). CT is the gold standard for the diagnosis of urinary stone disease

Table 13.1 Estimated fetal radiation doses and sensitivity and specificity of detecting urolithiasis of common imaging modalities [26, 42, 46]

Imaging study	Radiation dose (mGy)	Sensitivity (%)	Specificity (%)
Ultrasound	0	34–86	86
IVP (3 film)	1.7–10	87	94
X-ray KUB	1.4–4.2	44–77	80–87
CT (conventional)	8–49	>96	>98
CT (low dose)	≤7	>96	>96
MR urography	0	84	100

IVP intravenous pyelogram, *KUB* kidneys, ureters, bladder, *CT* computed tomography, *MR* magnetic resonance

in the nonpregnant population; however, this exposes the mother and developing fetus to potentially harmful ionizing radiation [32, 33]. Consequently, the need for an accurate and timely diagnosis must be carefully weighed against the potential risks of radiation exposure to the mother and fetus.

The estimated fetal doses of radiation for common imaging modalities vary from 0 mGy for US and MRU to 49 mGy for a conventional CT scan (Table 13.1) [33]. The American College of Obstetricians and Gynecologists (ACOG) recommends that radiation doses of less than 50 mGy during pregnancy are safe for the fetus and not associated with an increased risk of miscarriage or fetal anomalies [34]. While the judicious use of CT during pregnancy is likely to be safe given the small radiation dose, every effort should be made to minimize radiation exposure in this population, and modalities with no ionizing radiation should be utilized whenever possible.

For pregnant patients with potential renal colic, US is the preferred initial imaging modality for evaluation. It has many advantages including that it is inexpensive, easily obtained, has no ionizing radiation, and is safe to both the mother and the fetus. However, the sensitivity of ultrasound to accurately detect urolithiasis during pregnancy is operator dependent and highly variable ranging from 34% to 86%, with a specificity of 86% [26]. Gestational hydronephrosis can complicate the diagnosis as it can be challenging to discriminate between acute ureteric obstruction and physiologic hydronephrosis if a definitive stone is not visible (Fig. 13.1a, b) [8, 14]. Further difficulty with ultrasound can occur secondary to the patient's body habitus, position of the fetus, or specific location of the calculi within the ureter. The location of hydroureteronephrosis can help distinguish between pathologic and physiologic obstruction; for example, severe left hydronephrosis or hydroureter distal to the iliac vessels is suggestive of acute ureteric obstruction from a calculus [35].

A number of adjunct techniques have been employed in order to try and improve the accuracy of US including urinary jets, endovaginal ultrasound, and resistive indices (RI). Non-visualization of a urinary jet is suggestive of an obstructing calculus (Fig. 13.1c). However, up to 13% of pregnant patients without urolithiasis will still have absence of their urinary jet, and it is more commonly absent on the right [36]. Visualization of the urinary jet can be optimized by pre-hydrating the patient before US [37]. Asymmetry of urinary jets is noted in 65% of patients with

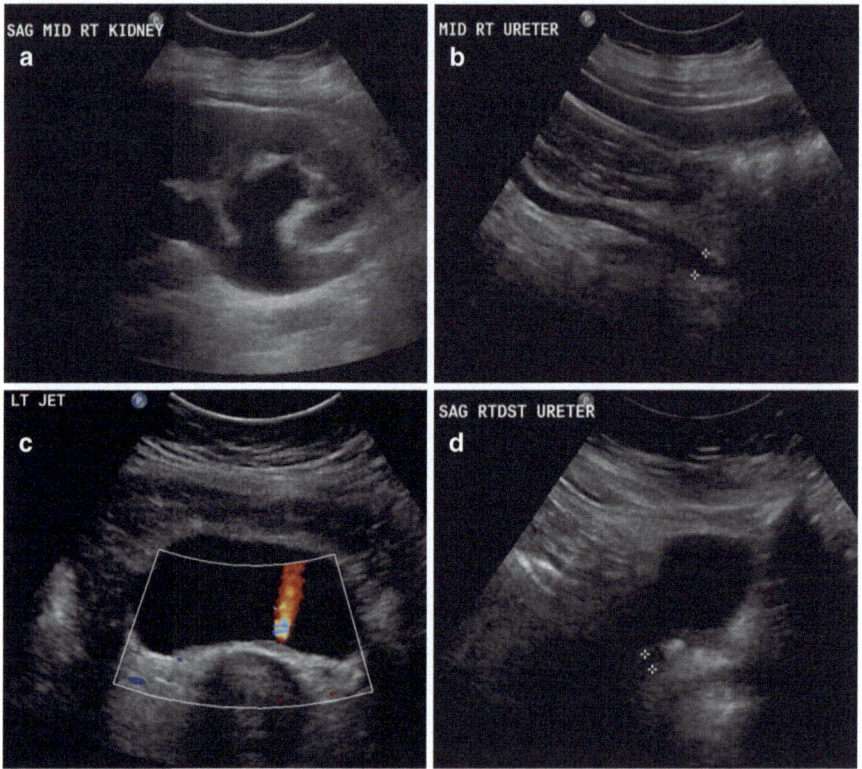

Fig. 13.1 Ultrasound images of right distal ureteric calculi in pregnancy. (**a**) Retroperitoneal ultrasound demonstrating right hydronephrosis. (**b**) Retroperitoneal ultrasound demonstrating right proximal hydroureter. (**c**) Endovaginal ultrasound demonstrating absence of right ureteral jet. (**d**) Endovaginal ultrasound demonstrating echogenic right distal ureteric calculi with ureter dilated proximal to the calculi

urolithiasis, though this can be difficult to accurately interpret [38, 39]. Endovaginal US can aid in the visualization of distal ureteric calculi and urinary jets but is contraindicated with prolapsed or ruptured membranes (Fig. 13.1d) [35].

The measurement of RI with Doppler US has been utilized to differentiate between physiologic and pathologic obstructions. RI is defined as the peak diastolic velocity subtracted from the peak systolic velocity and divided by the peak systolic velocity, with an RI of 0.70 or greater, suggestive of pathologic obstruction [40]. However, RI is a non-specific measurement, and there remains controversy regarding the absolute value to serve as a cutoff for obstruction. In addition, RI may be elevated in normal non-obstructed kidneys and can be normal during the early phase of obstruction when there is elevated renal blood flow and vascular dilatation [41]. The combination of an elevated RI and absence of a ureteric jet has been shown to increase the accuracy of US in predicting a ureteric calculus from 56.2% to 71.9% [40].

In certain cases the diagnosis of urolithiasis cannot be definitely made with history, physical examination, and US imaging alone, and consideration must be given to alternative imaging modalities. While every effort should be made to

Fig. 13.2 Low-dose CT
images of proximal right
ureteric calculi in
pregnancy. (**a**) Right
hydronephrosis. (**b**) Calculi
in proximal right ureter
with hydroureter

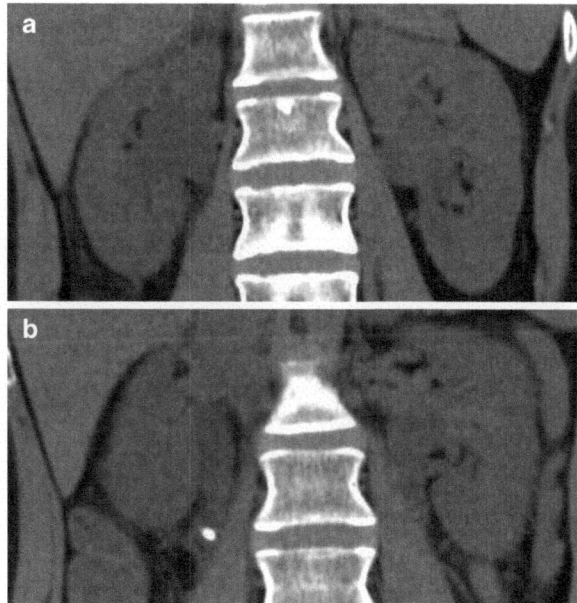

minimize ionizing radiation exposure in the pregnant population, concerns regarding radiation exposure should not prevent a medically indicated diagnostic exam from being performed. Traditionally, KUB or IVP have been second-line imaging modalities when initial evaluation with US has failed to yield a definitive diagnosis. However, with the advent of modern low-dose CT scanning techniques, KUB and IVP have fallen out of favor. Low-dose CT scans provide a highly sensitive and specific test (>96%) for the detection of urolithiasis, with levels of radiation comparable to a KUB or IVP (Fig. 13.2) [42]. In addition, low-dose CT does not require the administration of intravenous iodinated contrast which has been associated with fetal hypothyroidism [33]. The use of diagnostic CT in pregnancy is becoming increasingly more common and has increased by 25% per year from 1997 to 2006 [43].

A previous multi-institutional study comparing imaging modalities for the detection of urolithiasis in pregnancy demonstrated that low-dose CT had the highest positive predictive value (96%) [44]. In addition, a recent study examining the use of low-dose CT scans in pregnancy confirmed a very low radiation exposure of only 7.1 mGy [34]. In order to maintain the sensitivity and specificity of low-dose CT scans, above 90% patients should have a BMI of less than 30 [45]. Newer software is currently being investigated that may allow for further reductions in radiation exposure for low-dose CT scans. Currently, the American Urological Association (AUA) recommends low-dose CT scan (<5 mGy) as an appropriate second-line imaging modality for pregnant women in the second and third trimester when initial ultrasound is nondiagnostic [45]. This is based on the recommendation from ACOG that the radiation dose associated with this is well below the suggested threshold of 50 mGy and is not associated with fetal anomalies or loss [33].

Fig. 13.3 MRI image
demonstrating right
physiological
hydronephrosis of
pregnancy

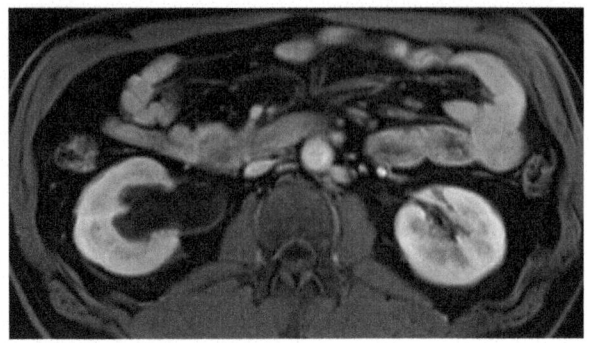

Recent evidence has demonstrated that magnetic resonance urography with a T2-weighted half-Fourier acquisition single-shot turbo-spin echo (HASTE) protocol can be utilized for the diagnosis of urinary stone disease in pregnancy (Fig. 13.3). A previous small series evaluating the use of HASTE MRU in the diagnosis of acute ureteric obstruction in pregnancy revealed a high sensitivity (84%), specificity (100%), and diagnostic accuracy (100%) [46]. MRU has multiple advantages including the avoidance of ionizing radiation, the ability to detect non-urologic causes of symptoms, a short acquisition time of approximately 15 min, and no known harmful effects to the fetus [47]. However, its use is limited by high cost, limited availability, and the contraindication of use in patients with metallic implants. Stones do not have a specific signal on MRU which makes their detection somewhat difficult. However, specific findings of ureteric obstruction include direct visualization of a stone at the point of ureteric constriction, renal stranding, perirenal extravasation, renal or ureteric edema, and the "double-kink" sign where there is ureteric constriction present both at the pelvic brim and ureterovesical junction [47]. Gadolinium contrast is not required for MRU and should be avoided in pregnancy as it crosses the placenta and has been associated with neonatal death [48].

The accurate and safe diagnosis of urinary stone disease in pregnancy remains challenging despite significant advances in diagnostic imaging. Low-dose CT has been demonstrated to have the highest positive predictive value for detecting urolithiasis during pregnancy at 96% compared with MRU and US which had positive predictive values of 80% and 77%, respectively [44]. A recent study evaluating renal colic in pregnancy demonstrated a high overall rate of negative ureteroscopy of 14% [44]. The type of preoperative imaging modality utilized significantly affected the rate of negative ureteroscopy. The rate was highest for US alone (23%), followed by US plus MRU (20%), and lowest for US plus low-dose CT (4.3%) [44].

The AUA has published recommendations for diagnostic imaging in the setting of renal colic in pregnancy. US is recommended as the first-line modality for all pregnant women suspected of renal colic given its safe, well-established use in pregnancy and wide availability [45]. If initial US is nondiagnostic, then consideration should be given to non-contrast MRU in the first trimester, or low-dose CT in the second and third trimesters, prior to proceeding with surgical intervention [45]. The clinician must carefully assess the clinical scenario and thoroughly consider potential risks and benefits of different imaging modalities prior to proceeding. Multidisciplinary collaboration between urology, obstetrics, and radiology is helpful in ensuring comprehensive care in this challenging patient population. Further advances in imaging techniques and improved diagnostic algorithms are required in order to prevent unnecessary intervention in this high-risk population.

Management

Management of urolithiasis in pregnancy is complex and challenging given the physiologic changes of pregnancy and the potential complications that can occur from both renal colic and the management of the stone. In the absence of any acute indications, expectant management is the first-line treatment for renal colic in pregnancy. Indications for acute intervention include active infection, progressive renal insufficiency, an obstructed solitary kidney, bilateral renal obstruction, intractable symptoms such as pain or emesis, or signs of imminent obstetrical complications such as preeclampsia or preterm labor. There are several options for intervention including temporizing drainage measures such as insertion of an indwelling ureteral stent or external nephrostomy tube and definitive surgical management with ureteroscopy (Fig. 13.4).

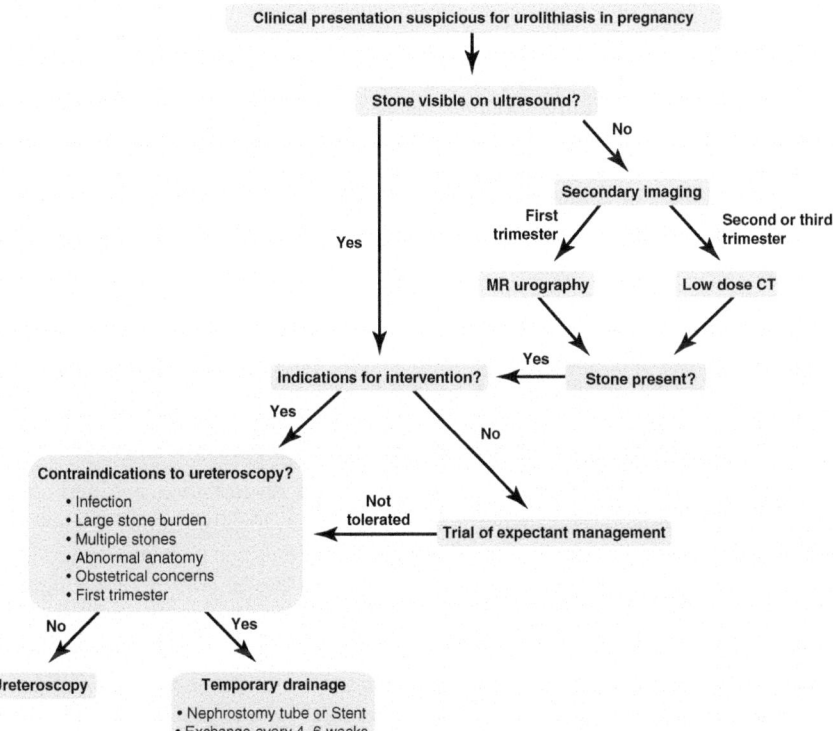

Fig. 13.4 Algorithm for the diagnosis and management of urolithiasis in pregnancy

Until the mid-2000s, temporary drainage with delay of definitive stone management until the postpartum period was the mainstay of treatment for stone disease in pregnancy. However, this is associated with many disadvantages including the requirement of multiple procedures for frequent tube changes and associated symptoms and discomfort from the drainage tube. Recent technological advances in ureteroscopy including smaller caliber ureteroscopes and the wide adoption of holmium:yttrium-aluminum-garnet (Ho:YAG) lasers have allowed ureteroscopy to become an accepted alternative for patients who fail expectant management. Surgical intervention is best performed during the second trimester of pregnancy when the risk of preterm labor and miscarriage is the lowest [49]. Other treatment modalities of urolithiasis including shockwave lithotripsy (SWL) and percutaneous nephrolithotomy (PCNL) are currently contraindicated in pregnancy. Once again, a multidisciplinary approach with the involvement of a urologist, obstetrician, radiologist, neonatologist, and potentially an anesthesiologist if surgical management is planned is highly recommended in order to optimize care for both the mother and fetus.

The first-line treatment for uncomplicated ureteric calculi in pregnancy is expectant management with a trial of spontaneous passage. It has previously been estimated that the rate of spontaneous passage for symptomatic upper tract urinary calculi in pregnancy is 70–80% [28]. In addition, a higher rate of spontaneous passage has been demonstrated in pregnant women compared to their nonpregnant counterparts (81% vs 46%) [18, 25]. This is thought to be secondary to the effects of progesterone during pregnancy which cause smooth muscle relaxation of the urinary collecting system and subsequent ureteral dilatation [28]. However, this elevated rate of spontaneous passage has recently been questioned with a more recent study demonstrating a spontaneous passage rate of only 47% [27]. This suggests that the initial high rates of spontaneous passage may have been an overestimate secondary to erroneous diagnosis and incomplete follow-up. Similar to the nonpregnant population, the rate of spontaneous passage is correlated with the location of the stone, and a previous study has demonstrated a higher spontaneous passage rate for distal ureteric calculi (44.1%) compared with proximal ureteric or ureteropelvic junction stones (27.3%) [40]. Observation with serial US examinations is recommended throughout the duration of the pregnancy while expectant management is being undertaken. If the stone fails to pass during pregnancy, approximately 50% of patients will pass their stone within the 1st month postpartum [28]. Once the patient has delivered, routine management of the stone can be undertaken if it has not already passed.

Expectant management requires aggressive fluid resuscitation and appropriate symptom management with analgesia and antiemetics. Ideally, fluid resuscitation is performed through oral supplementation; however, fluids can be administered intravenously if there is significant nausea or emesis. Careful consideration must be given to the potential adverse effects to the mother and fetus of any medications administered during pregnancy. For this reason, consultation with obstetrics and pharmacy is highly recommended. Nonsteroidal anti-inflammatory drugs (NSAIDs) are classically recommended as first-line treatment for analgesia in urolithiasis in the nonpregnant population given their effectiveness in managing renal colic and nonnarcotic quality. However, the use of NSAIDs is contraindicated in pregnancy due to the risk of premature closure of the patent ductus arteriosus during the third trimester and their association with fetal pulmonary hypertension, oligohydramnios, cardiac malformations, and miscarriage [50]. Oral agents including codeine and oxycodone have been associated with teratogenic effects in the first trimester and are not recommended for use in pregnancy [51]. For less severe pain, acetaminophen is a safe option with no known adverse effects to the mother or fetus [28]. For more severe pain, small, frequent doses of opioids such as morphine are utilized and are considered to be the mainstay of analgesia during pregnancy [51]. However, chronic use can result in intrauterine growth retardation, premature labor, and fetal narcotic addiction [27, 28].

Medical expulsive therapy (MET) utilizes α-blockers or calcium channel blockers to facilitate the spontaneous passage of ureteric calculi and is commonly employed in the nonpregnant population [52]. However, controversy exists regarding the use of MET as high-quality evidence exists both in support and opposition to its use, and there is currently no consensus. In addition, it is uncertain whether the smooth muscle relaxation provided by MET would be of benefit in pregnancy when there is already physiologic dilatation secondary to elevated progesterone levels [14]. Currently, both α-blockers and calcium channel blockers are classified as category B pregnancy medications and thought to be safe with no harmful effects having been demonstrated in humans to date [53].

A recent retrospective matched cohort study investigated the safety and efficacy of MET in pregnancy and found no association with adverse maternal or fetal outcomes. There was a nonstatistical increase in the rate of sudden infant death syndrome (SIDS) in the tamsulosin-treated group which was felt to be spurious; however, further investigation is required [54]. This study also demonstrated a 24% increase in the rate of spontaneous passage with MET; however, the time to spontaneous passage was longer in the MET treatment group [54]. While this recent study is promising that the use of MET in pregnancy is both safe and efficacious, more rigorous evidence is required before the use of MET in pregnancy can be widely adopted. Despite the limited and conflicting evidence available on the use of MET, a recent worldwide survey found that 97.6% of urologists utilize MET in stone disease and 44.3% specifically utilize it in the setting of pregnancy [55]. Currently the AUA and Endourological Society recommend that if the use of MET is being considered in a pregnant patient, careful patient counselling should be undertaken, and the patient should be informed that these medications have not been well studied for use in pregnancy and are being utilized for an "off-label" purpose [52].

When acute indications for stone treatment are present, temporizing drainage with either an indwelling ureteral stent or an external nephrostomy tube may be utilized. There are distinct advantages and disadvantages to each method of urinary drainage; and the selection of drainage method ultimately depends on the specific clinical scenario, availability of resources, and surgeon and patient preference. Both drainage devices carry a risk of infection, dislodgement, blockage, or encrustation [56]. Indwelling ureteric stents can cause lower urinary tract voiding symptoms as well as suprapubic and flank discomfort. Lower urinary tract symptoms caused by ureteric stents can be difficult to manage in pregnancy given that anticholinergics are contraindicated. In comparison, external nephrostomy tubes can also be associated with flank discomfort and require additional care as there is an external component to the tube. Nephrostomy tube insertion has a high success rate, results in rapid decompression of the collecting system, and avoids ureteric manipulation. For these reasons nephrostomy tube insertion may be preferred in the setting of sepsis [57]. However, the insertion of a nephrostomy tube is contraindicated in the setting of anticoagulation given the risk of renal hemorrhage.

Both nephrostomy tubes and ureteric stents can be inserted with minimal anesthesia. Insertion of a ureteric stent is typically performed under limited fluoroscopic guidance and for this reason may not be the ideal choice of drainage method during the first trimester [56]. Although insertion of ureteric stents under ultrasound guidance has been described, expertise in this technique is limited [56]. In contrast, nephrostomy tubes are typically inserted under ultrasound guidance and may be preferred during the first trimester. Evidence has demonstrated that either drainage modality has equivalent patient outcomes [57]. Due to the metabolic changes that occur during pregnancy, foreign bodies in the urinary tract are prone to accelerated encrustation. This necessitates the frequent exchange of either ureteric stents or nephrostomy tubes every 4–6 weeks during pregnancy [17].

Percutaneous nephrolithotomy is contraindicated during pregnancy due to the need for prolonged anesthetic and fluoroscopy times as well as prone positioning. Successful PCNL during pregnancy has been described utilizing a supine position and ultrasound-guided access, with no complications being reported for these cases [58, 59]. However, if PCNL is required due to a large or complex stone burden, this is best performed in the postpartum period and managed during pregnancy with temporizing drainage with either a nephrostomy tube or stent.

Shockwave lithotripsy is also contraindicated during pregnancy due to potential risks posed to the fetus including miscarriage, congenital malformations, intrauterine growth retardation, and placental displacement [60]. Case reports exist of inadvertent SWL being performed during pregnancy that have resulted in no complications. However, presently there is insufficient evidence to support the safe use of SWL during pregnancy [61].

Ureteroscopy

Definitive stone management with ureteroscopy is a safe and effective treatment option for urolithiasis in pregnancy for patients who fail expectant management. This has been made possible by recent advances in surgical technology including smaller diameter ureteroscopes, the widespread use of intracorporeal lithotripters, and improvements in flexible grasping devices, all of which allow for safe and efficient treatment of stones in all locations. Ureteroscopy in this setting is associated with high stone-free rates and low complication rates for both the mother and fetus. Contraindications include active infection, large stone burden, multiple or bilateral calculi, abnormal anatomy, obstetrical complications, inadequate obstetric, urological or anesthetic resources, or very early or late presentations [62]. In these instances, temporizing drainage with a stent or nephrostomy tube should be utilized, and definitive surgical management of the stone should be delayed. The teratogenic risks of anesthetic agents are significantly higher in the first trimester, and as such ureteroscopy is reserved for the second and third trimesters of pregnancy [50].

Ureteroscopy has been well established to be both safe and effective in pregnancy with stone-free rates comparable to ureteroscopy in nonpregnant patients. A number of case series have demonstrated that ureteroscopy has acceptable stone-free rates of 63–100%, comparable to results in the nonpregnant population (Table 13.2) [18, 63–90]. The safety of ureteroscopy has also been well documented with multiple studies showing a low rate of preterm labor of 0–1% (Table 13.2) [18, 63–90]. In addition, a recent meta-analysis revealed no difference in the incidence of complications such as ureteric injury or urinary tract infection in pregnant patients compared with nonpregnant patients undergoing ureteroscopy [62]. Furthermore, recent evidence has emerged that ureteroscopy may be the safest option for the treatment of uncomplicated ureteric calculi in pregnancy and was associated with the fewest number of complications compared with ureteric stent or nephrostomy tube drainage [91]. A recent study has also demonstrated that ureteroscopy resulted in fewer additional interventions and significantly decreased pain and urinary tract symptoms [92]. In addition, definitive management with ureteroscopy has been shown to be more cost-effective than temporizing drainage with a stent or nephrostomy tube [93].

Ureteroscopy is ideally performed during the second trimester when the risk of miscarriage or premature labor is the lowest and can be safely performed under general, spinal, or local anesthetic [49]. According to the ACOG, no teratogenic effects have been shown in humans from the use of modern anesthetic agents at standard concentrations [94]. A recent study demonstrated that total anesthetic time for patients undergoing ureteroscopy compared with stent insertion was no different, and there was no difference in the number of adverse anesthetic events [95]. Ureteroscopy should be performed by a skilled endourologist, at a center with available neonatal services, and an obstetrician with the capabilities to perform cesarean delivery [94]. Appropriate antibiotic prophylaxis should be administered preoperatively; and either a penicillin or cephalosporin is considered safe for use in pregnancy. It should be noted that aminoglycosides, fluoroquinolones, and sulfa drugs are contraindicated for use in pregnancy secondary to adverse fetal effects.

There are some important alterations to the surgical principles of ureteroscopy in pregnancy. The patient should be positioned in the lithotomy position with the right side of the abdomen elevated with a wedge in order to avoid uterine compression of the vena cava. It is important to monitor the fetus both during and after the procedure to identify any signs of fetal distress [94]. Radiation exposure to both the mother and fetus should be limited as much as possible. This can be accomplished by positioning the c-arm image source underneath the patient, using low-dose pulse imaging, and coning the imaging to include only the kidney [95]. In addition, lead shielding should be placed underneath the contralateral side of the abdomen, and only necessary images of the wire in the kidney and final stent curl should be taken [95].

Table 13.2 Compilation of series examining outcomes of ureteroscopy for the treatment of ureteral stones in pregnancy [18, 63–90]

Author	No. pts	Mean stone size (mm)	Stone treatment	Stone free (%)	Complications (no. of pts)
Denstedt et al. [63]	3	N/A	Basket	100	None
Ulvik et al. [64]	13	N/A	Basket	100	UTI (3), ureteric injury (1), premature contractions (1)
Carringer et al. [65]	4	9	Pulse dye laser	100	None
Scarpa et al. [66]	13	N/A	Ho:YAG, basket, pneumatic	76.9	None
Parulkar et al. [18]	4	N/A	Basket	100	None
Lemos et al. [67]	13	6	Basket, USL	100	None
Lifshitz et al. [68]	4	4	Basket	100	None
Shokeir et al. [69]	8	N/A	Basket, USL	62.5	UTI (1)
Watterson et al. [70]	8	N/A	Ho:YAG	77.7	None
Akpinar et al. [71]	6	8	Ho:YAG	85.7	Pain (1)
Juan et al. [72]	3	N/A	Basket, USL	100	None
Yang et al. [73]	3	N/A	EHL	100	None
Rana et al. [74]	19	11	Lithoclast	79	None
Travassos et al. [75]	9	8	Basket	100	None
Cocuzza et al. [76]	7	8	Ho:YAG, basket	N/A	None
Elgamasy et al. [77]	15	NA	Pneumatic	N/A	Premature labor (1), stent migration (1)
Polat et al. [78]	16	N/A	Pneumatic	72.7	None
Atar et al. [79]	19	8	Ho:YAG, basket	88.2	UTI (1), pain (4)
Hoscan et al. [80]	34	7	Pneumatic	85.3	UTI (3), premature contractions (1)
Isen et al. [81]	12	9	Pneumatic	N/A	None
Johnson et al. [82]	46	7.8	Ho:YAG, basket	88	Preterm labor (2)
Bozkurt et al. [83]	41	9	Pneumatic, Ho:YAG, basket	87.8	Ureteric injury (4), UTI (4), pain (6), sepsis (1)
Abdel-Kader et al. [84]	17	N/A	Pneumatic	100	None
Keshvari et al. [85]	44	N/A	Pneumatic	100	None
Wang et al. [86]	64	8	Ho:YAG	81.2	Premature contractions (1)
Adanur et al. [87]	19	9	Ho:YAG	N/A	Premature contractions (1), UTI (1), migrated stent (1)
Teleb et al. [88]	21	N/A	Pneumatic	N/A	UTI (2)
Zhang et al. [89]	117	N/A	Ho:YAG	87.5	Premature contractions (12), sepsis (1)
Tan et al. [90]	23	N/A	Ho:YAG	87	UTI (1)

N/A not available, *UTI* urinary tract infection, *Ho:YAG* holmium:yttrium-aluminum-garnet laser

Radiation exposure to the fetus carries a risk of teratogenesis, miscarriage, and carcinogenesis. The risk of teratogenicity and miscarriage depends on the gestational age at the time of exposure and is estimated to be 20 mGy in the first trimester and 50 mGy in the second and third trimesters [32]. In contrast, radiation has a stochastic effect on carcinogenesis where there is no absolute "safe threshold" of exposure. There is an estimated risk of 1 in 10,000 for the development of childhood malignancy secondary to the exposure of 10 mGy of in utero radiation [32]. It is currently recommended by the ACOG that radiation doses of less than 50 mGy during pregnancy are safe for the mother and the fetus and have not been associated with an increased risk of miscarriage or fetal anomalies [34]. Alternatively, ultrasound-guided ureteroscopy has been described where ultrasound is utilized to confirm wire and stent location within the kidney; however, expertise in this technique is limited [96].

Ureteric dilatation is generally unnecessary given the dilatation of ureters that occurs during pregnancy, and the gravid uterus does not generally impede the passage of the ureteroscope. There is limited evidence regarding the optimal method of intracorporeal lithotripsy to utilize during pregnancy. Theoretical concerns exist for the use of electrohydraulic lithotripsy stimulating uterine contractions and adverse effects of ultrasonic lithotripsy on fetal ear development [62]. Both Ho:YAG laser and pneumatic lithotripters are currently recommended and felt to be safe during pregnancy [62]. A ureteric stent is typically placed postoperatively for a short period of time in order to minimize the risk of complications. Some patients have experienced recurrent renal colic and premature uterine contractions when a postoperative ureteric stent was not inserted [97].

Conclusion

Over the past several decades, the female incidence of stone disease has risen quite dramatically, and as such the incidence of urolithiasis in pregnancy may also rise. Acute urinary stone disease in pregnancy represents a challenging clinical situation with potential serious complications to both the mother and the fetus. A comprehensive multidisciplinary approach is instrumental to providing appropriate patient care. While significant advancements have been made in the diagnosis and treatment of stone disease in pregnancy over the past several decades, further research is required in order optimize care in this vulnerable population.

References

1. Ramello A, Vitale C, Marangella M. Epidemiology of nephrolithiasis. J Nephrol. 2000; 13(Suppl 3):S45–50.
2. Scales CD, Smith AC, Hanley JM, Saigal CS. Prevalence of kidney stones in the United States. Eur Urol. 2012;62:160–5.

3. Stamatelou KK, Francis ME, Jones CA, Nyberg LM, Curhan GC. Time trends in reported prevalence of kidney stones in the United States: 1976–1994. Kidney Int. 2003;63:1817–23.
4. Yasui T, Iguchi M, Suzuki S, Kohri K. Prevalence and epidemiological characteristics of urolithiasis in Japan: national trends between 1965 and 2005. Urology. 2008;7:209–13.
5. Indridason OS, Birgisson S, Edvardsson VO, Sigvaldason H, Sigfusson N, Palsson R. Epidemiology of kidney stones in Iceland: a population-based study. Scand J Urol Nephrol. 2006;40:215–20.
6. Lieske JC, Pena de la Vega LS, Slezak JM, Bergstralh EJ, Leibson CL, Ho KL, et al. Renal stone epidemiology in Rochester, Minnesota: an update. Kidney Int. 2006;69:760–4.
7. Strope SA, Wolf JS, Hollenbeck BK. Changes in gender distribution of urinary stone disease. Urology. 2010;75:543–6.
8. Gorton E, Whiteld HN. Renal calculi in pregnancy. Br J Urol. 2007;80:4–9.
9. Srirangam SJ, Hickerton B, Van Cleyenbreugel B. Management of urinary calculi in pregnancy: a review. J Endourol. 2008;22:867–75.
10. Riley JM, Dudley AG, Semins MJ. Nephrolithiasis and pregnancy: has the incidence been rising? J Endourol. 2014;28:383–6.
11. Ross AE, Handa S, Lingeman JE, Matlaga BR. Kidney stones during pregnancy: an investigation into stone composition. Urol Res. 2008;36:99–102.
12. Reinstatler L, Khaleel S, Pais VM. Association of pregnancy with stone formation among women in the United States: a NHANES Analysis 2007 to 2012. J Urol. 2017;198:389–93.
13. Grenier N, Pariente JL, Trillaud H, Soussotte C, Douws C. Dilatation of the collecting system during pregnancy: physiologic vs obstructive dilatation. Eur Radiol. 2000;10:271–9.
14. Marchant DJ. Effects of pregnancy and progestational agents on the urinary tract. Am J Obstet Gynecol. 1972;112:487–501.
15. Dunlop W. Serial changes in renal hemodynamics during normal human pregnancy. Br J Obstet Gynaecol. 1981;88:1–9.
16. Charalambous S, Fotas A, Rizk DE. Urolithiasis in pregnancy. Int Urogynecol J. 2009;20:1133–6.
17. Loughlin KR. Management of urologic problems during pregnancy. Urology. 1994;44:159–69.
18. Parulkar BG, Hopkins TB, Wollin MR, Howard PJ, Lal A. Renal colic during pregnancy: a case for conservative treatment. J Urol. 1998;159:365–8.
19. Smith C, Kristensen C, Davis M, Abraham PA. An evaluation of the physicochemical risk for renal stone disease during pregnancy. Clin Nephrol. 2001;55:205–11.
20. Resim S, Ekerbicer HC, Kiran G, Kilinc M. Are changes in urinary parameters during pregnancy clinically significant? Urol Res. 2006;34:244–8.
21. Buppasiri P, Lumbiganon P, Thinkhamrop J, Ngamjarus C, Laopaiboon M, Medley N. Calcium supplementation (other than for preventing or treating hypertension) for improving pregnancy and infant outcomes. Cochrane Database Syst Rev. 2015; https://doi.org/10.1002/14651858.CD007079.pub3.
22. Imdad A, Bhutta ZA. Effect of calcium supplementation during pregnancy on maternal, fetal and birth outcomes. Paediatr Perinat Epidemiol. 2012;1:138–52.
23. Loughlin KR, Bailey RB. Internal ureteral stents for conservative management of ureteral calculi during pregnancy. N Engl J Med. 1986;315:1647–9.
24. Maikranz P, Lindheimer M, Coe F. Nephrolithiasis in pregnancy. Baillie Res Clin Obstet Gynaecol. 1994;8:375–86.
25. Meria P, Hadjadj H, Jungers P, Daudon M, Members of the French Urological Association Urolithiasis Committee. Stone formation and pregnancy: pathophysiological insights gained from morphoconstitutional stone analysis. J Urol. 2010;183:1412–6.
26. Stothers L, Lee LM. Renal colic in pregnancy. J Urol. 1992;148:1383–7.
27. Burgess KL, Gettman MT, Rangel LJ, Krambeck AE. Diagnosis of urolithiasis and rate of spontaneous passage during pregnancy. J Urol. 2011;186:2280–4.
28. Biyani CS, Joyce AD. Urolithiasis in pregnancy. I: pathophysiology, fetal considerations and diagnosis. BJU Int. 2002;89:811–8.

29. Lewis DF, Robichaux AG, Jaekle RK, Marcum NG, Stedman CM. Urolithiasis in pregnancy. Diagnosis, management and pregnancy outcome. J Reprod Med. 2003;48:28–32.
30. Banhidy F, Acs N, Puho EH, Czeizel AE. Maternal kidney stones during pregnancy and adverse birth outcomes, particularly congenital abnormalities in the offspring. Arch Gynecol Obstet. 2007;275:481–7.
31. Wright A, Walker R, Barrett D. The fluoroquinolones and their appropriate use in treatment of genitourinary tract infections. In: Ball T, Novicki D, editors. AUA update series. Houston: American Urologic Association; 1993.
32. Brent RL, Mettler FA. Pregnancy policy. Am J Roentgenol. 2004;182:819–22.
33. White WM, Zite NB, Gash J, Waters WB, Thompson W, Klain FA. Low-dose computed tomography for the evaluation of flank pain in the pregnant population. J Endourol. 2007;21:1255–60.
34. American College of Obstetricians and Gynecologists. Guidelines for diagnostic imaging during pregnancy and lactation. Committee Opinion No. 723. Obstet Gynecol. 2017;130:e210–6.
35. Kalyani V, Krambeck AE, Atwell T. Pearls and pitfalls in sonographic imaging of urolithiasis in pregnancy. Ultrasound Q. 2013;29:51–9.
36. Wachsberg RH. Unilateral absence of ureteral jets in the third trimester of pregnancy: pitfall in color Doppler US diagnosis of urinary obstruction. Radiology. 1998;209:279281.
37. Vallurupalli K, Atwell TD, Krambeck AE, Traynor KD, Broun D, Leroy AJ. Pearls and pitfalls in sonographic imaging of symptomatic urolithiasis in pregnancy. Ultrasound Q. 2013;29:51–9.
38. Sheafor DH, Hertzberg BS, Freed KS, Carroll BA, Keogan MT, Paulson EK, et al. Nonenhanced helical CT and US in the emergency evaluation of patients with renal colic: prospective comparison. Radiology. 2000;217:792–7.
39. Burge HJ, Middleton WD, McClennan BL, Hildebolt CF. Ureteral jets in healthy subjects and in patients with unilateral ureteral calculi: comparison with color doppler US. Radiology. 1991;180;437–42.
40. Andreoiu M, MacMahon R. Renal colic in pregnancy: lithiasis or physiological hydronephrosis? Urology. 2009;74:757–61.
41. Keogan MT, Kliewer MA, Hertzberg BS, DeLong DM, Tupler RH, Carroll BA. Renal resistive indexes: variability in Doppler US measurement in a healthy population. Radiology. 1996;199:165–9.
42. Hamm M, Knopfle E, Wartenberg S, Wawroschek F, Weckermann D, Harzmann R. Low dose unenhanced helical computerized tomography for the evaluation of acute flank pain. J Urol. 2002;167:1687–91.
43. Lazarus E, Debenedectis C, North D, Spencer PK, Mayo-Smith WW. Utilization of imaging in pregnant patients: 10-year review of 5270 examinations in 3285 patients – 1997–2006. Radiology. 2009;251:517–24.
44. White WM, Johnson EB, Zite NB, Beddies J, Krambeck AE, Hyams E, et al. Predictive value of current imaging modalities for the detection of urolithiasis during pregnancy: a multi-center, longitudinal study. J Urol. 2013;189:931–4.
45. Fulgham PF, Assimos DG, Pearle MS, Preminger GM. Clinical effectiveness protocols for imaging in the management of ureteral calculous disease: AUA technology assessment. J Urol. 2013;189:1203–13.
46. Semins MJ, Matlaga BR. Management of urolithiasis in pregnancy. Int J Women's Health. 2013;5:599–604.
47. Spencer JA, Chahal R, Kelly A, Taylor K, Eardley I, Lloyd SN. Evaluation of painful hydronephrosis in pregnancy: magnetic resonance urographic patterns in physiological dilatation versus calculous obstruction. J Urol. 2004;171:256–60.
48. Ray JG, Vermeulen MJ, Bharatha A, Montanera WJ, Park AL. Association between MRI exposure during pregnancy and fetal and childhood outcomes. JAMA. 2016;316:952–61.
49. Cheek TG, Baird E. Anesthesia for nonobstetric surgery: maternal and fetal considerations. Clin Obstet Gynecol. 2009;99:535–45.
50. Burdan F, Starosławska E, Szumiło J. Prenatal tolerability of acetaminophen and other over-the-counter non-selective 93 cyclooxygenase inhibitors. Pharmacol Rep. 2012;64:521–7.

51. Broussard CS, Rasmussen SA, Reefhuis J, Friedman JM, Jann MW, Riehle-Colarusso T, et al. Maternal treatment with opioid analgesics and risk for birth defects. Am J Obstet. 2011;204:e1–11.
52. Assimos D, Krambeck A, Miller NL, Monga M, Murad MH, Nelson CP, et al. Surgical management of stones: American Urological Association/Endourological Society Guideline, part II. J Urol. 2016;196:1161–9.
53. Weber-Schoendorfer C, Hannemann D, Meister R, Elefant E, Cuppers-Maarschalkerweerd B, Arnon J, et al. The safety of calcium channel blockers during pregnancy: a prospective, multicenter, observational study. Reprod Toxicol. 2008;26:24–30.
54. Bailey G, Vaughan L, Rose C, Krambeck A. Perinatal out- comes with tamsulosin therapy for symptomatic urolithiasis. J Urol. 2016;195:99.
55. Lloyd GL, Lim A, Hamoui N, Nakada SY, Kielb SJ. The use of medical expulsive therapy during pregnancy: a worldwide perspective among experts. J Endourol. 2016;30:354–8.
56. Jarrard DJ, Gerber GS, Lyon ES. Management of acute ureteral obstruction in pregnancy utilizing ultrasound- guided placement of ureteral stents. Urology. 1993;42:263–8.
57. Pearle MS, Pierce HL, Miller GL, Summa JA, Mutz JM, Petty BA, et al. Optimal method of urgent decompression of the collecting system for obstruction and infection due to ureteral calculi. J Urol. 1998;160:1260–4.
58. Fregonesi A, Dias FGF, Saade RD, Dechaalani V, Reis LO. Challenges on percutaneous nephrolithotomy in pregnancy: supine position approach through ultrasound guidance. Urol Ann. 2013;5:107–9.
59. Toth C, Toth G, Varga A, Flasko T, Salah MA. Percutaneous nephrolithotomy in early pregnancy. Int Urol Nephrol. 2005;37:1–3.
60. Chaussy CG, Fuchs GJ. Current state and future developments of noninvasive treatment of human urinary stones with extracorporeal shock wave lithotripsy. J Urol. 1989;141:782–9.
61. Asgari MA, Safarinejad MR, Hosseini SY, Dadkhah F. Extracorporeal shock wave lithotripsy of renal calculi during early pregnancy. BJU Int. 1999;84:615–7.
62. Semins MJ, Trock BJ, Matlaga BR. The safety of ureteroscopy during pregnancy: a systematic review and meta-analysis. J Urol. 2009;181:139–43.
63. Denstedt JD, Razvi H. Management of urinary calculi during pregnancy. J Urol. 1992;148(3 Pt 2):1072–4.
64. Ulvik NM, Bakke A, Høisaeter PA. Ureteroscopy in pregnancy. J Urol. 1995;154:1660–3.
65. Carringer M, Swartz R, Johansson JE. Management of ureteric calculi during pregnancy by ureteroscopy and laser lithotripsy. BJU. 1996;77:17–20.
66. Scarpa RM, De Lisa A, Usai E. Diagnosis and treatment of ureteral calculi during pregnancy with rigid ureteroscopes. J Urol. 1996;155:875–7.
67. Lemos GC, El Hayek OR, Apezzato M. Rigid ureteroscopy for diagnosis and treatment of ureteral calculi during pregnancy. Int Braz J Urol. 2002;28:311–5.
68. Lifshitz DA, Lingeman JE. Ureteroscopy as a first-line intervention for ureteral calculi in pregnancy. J Endourol. 2002;16:19–22.
69. Shokeir AA, Mutabani H. Rigid ureteroscopy in pregnant women. BJU. 1998;81:678–81; Lemos GC, El Hayek OR, Apezzato M. Rigid ureteroscopy for diagnosis and treatment of ureteral calculi during pregnancy. Int Braz J Urol. 2002;28:311–5.
70. Watterson JD, Girvan AR, Beiko DT. Ureteroscopy and holmium:YAG laser lithotripsy: an emerging definitive management strategy for symptomatic ureteral calculi in pregnancy. Urology. 2002;60:383–7.
71. Akpinar H, Tufek I, Alici B. Ureteroscopy and holmium laser lithotripsy in pregnancy: stents must be used post- operatively. J Endourol. 2006;20:107–10.
72. Juan YS, Wu WJ, Chuang SM, et al. Management of symptomatic urolithiasis during pregnancy. Kaohsiung J Med Sci. 2007;23:241–6.
73. Yang CH, Chan PH, La SK, et al. Urolithiasis in pregnancy. J Chin Med Assoc. 2007;67:625–8.
74. Rana AM, Aquil S, Khawaja AM. Semirigid ureteroscopy and pneumatic lithotripsy as definitive management of obstructive ureteral calculi during pregnancy. Urology. 2009;73:964–7.
75. Travassos M, Amselem I, Filho NS. Ureteroscopy in pregnant women for ureteral stone. J Endourol. 2009;23:405–7.

76. Cocuzza M, Colombo JJr JR, Lopes RI, et al. Use of inverted fluoroscope's C-arm during endoscopic treatment of urinary tract obstruction in pregnancy: a practicable solution to cut radiation. Urology. 2010;75:1505–8.
77. Elgamasy A, Elsherif A. Use of Doppler ultrasonography and rigid ureteroscopy for managing symptomatic ureteric stones during pregnancy. BJU Int. 2010;106:262–6.
78. Polat F, Yesil S, Kirac M, et al. Treatment outcomes of semirigid ureterorenoscopy and intracorporeal lithotripsy in pregnant women with obstructive ureteral calculi. Urol Res. 2011;39:487–90.
79. Atar M, Bozkurt Y, Soylemez H. Use of renal resistive index and semi-rigid ureteroscopy for managing symptomatic persistent hydronephrosis during pregnancy. Int J Surg. 2012;10:629–33.
80. Hoscan MB, Ekinci M, Tunckiran A, et al. Management of symptomatic ureteral calculi complicating pregnancy. Urology. 2012;80:1011–4.
81. Isen K, Hatipoglu NK, Dedeoglu S, et al. Experience with the diagnosis and management of symptomatic ureteric stones during pregnancy. Urology. 2012;79:508–12.
82. Johnson EB, Krambeck AE, White WM. Obstetric complications of ureteroscopy during pregnancy. J Urol. 2012;188:151–4.
83. Bozkurt Y, Soylemez H, Atar M. Effectiveness and safety of ureteroscopy in pregnant women: a comparative study. Urolithiasis. 2013;41:37–42.
84. Abdel-Kader MS, Tamam AA, Elderwy AA, et al. Management of symptomatic ureteral calculi during pregnancy: experience of 23 cases. Urol Ann. 2013;5:241–4.
85. Keshvari Shirvan M, Darabi Mahboub MR, Rahimi HR, et al. The evaluation of ureteroscopy and pneumatic lithotripsy results in pregnant women with ureteral calculi. Nephrourol Mon. 2013;5:874–8.
86. Wang Z, Xu L, Su Z, Yao C, et al. Invasive management of proximal ureteral calculi during pregnancy. Urology. 2014;83:745–9.
87. Adanur S, Ziypak T, Bedir F, Yapanoglu T, et al. Ureteroscopy and holmium laser lithotripsy: is this procedure safe in pregnant women with ureteral stones at different locations? Arch Ital Urol Androl. 2014;30:86–9.
88. Teleb M, Ragab A, Dawod T, Elgalay H. Definitive ureteroscopy and intracorporeal lithotripsy in treatment of ureteral calculi during pregnancy. Arab J Urol. 2014;12:299–303.
89. Shang S, Liu G, Duo Y, Wang J, et al. Application of ureteroscope in emergency treatment with persistent renal colic patients during pregnancy. PLoS One. 2016;11:e0146597.
90. Tan S, Chen X, Sun M, Wu B. The comparation of effects and security of double-J stent retention and ureteroscopy lithotripsy in the treatment of symptomatic ureteral calculi during pregnancy. Eur J Obstet Gynecol Reprodu Biol. 2018;227:32–4.
91. Song Y, Fei X, Song Y. Diagnosis and operative intervention for problematic ureteral calculi during pregnancy. Int J Gynaecol Obstet. 2013;12:115–8.
92. Bayar G, Bozkurt Y, Acinikli H, Dagguli M. Which treatment method should be used in pregnant patients with ureteral calculi? Two center comparative study. Arch Esp Urol. 2015;68:435–40.
93. Wymer K, Plunkett BA, Park S. Urolithiasis in pregnancy: a cost-effectiveness analysis of ureteroscopic management vs ureteral stenting. Am J Obstet Gynecol. 2015;213:691e1–8.
94. Practice ACoO. ACOG Committee Opinion No. 464: nonobstetric surgery during pregnancy. Obstet Gynecol. 2011;117:420–1.
95. Rivera ME, McAlvany KL, Brinton TS, Gettman MT. Anesthetic exposure in the treatment of symptomatic urinary calculi in pregnant women. Urology. 2014;84:1275–8.
96. Razvi H, Bensalah K, Peyronnet B, Gross A, Krambeck A, Smith A, et al. Stones in special situations. In: Denstedt J, Rosette J, editors. Stone disease. Montreal: Societe Internationale d'Urologie (SIU); 2014. p. 409–501.
97. Deters LA, Dagrosa LM, Herrick BW, Silas A, Pais VM. Ultrasound guided ureteroscopy for definitive management of ureteral stones: a randomized, controlled trial. J Urol. 2014;192:1710–3.

Chapter 14
Pediatric Ureteroscopy

John Barnard, Chad Crigger, Ali Hajiran, Osama Al-Omar, and Michael Ost

Introduction

Up to 20–25% of children presenting with an acute episode of flank pain from an upper urinary tract calculus will require surgical intervention [1–4]. Over the past 20 years, ureteroscopy (URS) has been increasingly utilized as first-line therapy in the pediatric population in children who are unlikely to pass a ureteral stone spontaneously or have failed a trial of medical or observational therapy. Current literature shows that URS is now being used more commonly than extracorporeal shock wave lithotripsy (ESWL) for the initial treatment of pediatric upper tract calculi [2]. The goals of pediatric URS are to achieve a high stone-free rate in a single operation, preserve renal function, and minimize complications. Newer generations of urologists have become increasingly comfortable and skilled at performing endoscopic procedures. With the development of improved optics, smaller caliber, flexible and semirigid endoscopes with accessory wires, ureteral access sheaths, and baskets, providers are now able to safely and effectively endoscopically manage upper tract calculi in patients younger than 6 months up to 17 years of age [5].

Indications

According to the most recent American Urologic Association/Endourology Society Guidelines regarding the surgical management of stones, clinicians should offer URS or ESWL to pediatric patients who are unlikely to pass the stones or failed observation and/or medical expulsive therapy (Evidence Level Grade B, Strong Recommendation) [6]. The guideline panel performed a meta-analysis that showed

J. Barnard · C. Crigger · A. Hajiran · O. Al-Omar · M. Ost (✉)
Department of Urology, West Virginia University Medicine, Morgantown, WV, USA
e-mail: Michael.ost@hsc.wvu.edu

© Springer Nature Switzerland AG 2020   189
B. F. Schwartz, J. D. Denstedt (eds.), *Ureteroscopy*,
https://doi.org/10.1007/978-3-030-26649-3_14

stone-free rates in pediatric patients with ureteral stones <10 mm are high for both ESWL (87%) and URS (95%).

Since the first report of successful ESWL in children was published in 1986, several studies have demonstrated its safety and effectiveness at treating upper tract calculi less than 2 cm [6–9]. However, ESWL has several limitations. The stone-free rate of a single ESWL procedure can be low due to incomplete fragmentation, residual stone fragments, unfavorable anatomy, stone composition (i.e., calcium oxalate monohydrate or cysteine), or inappropriate use of this treatment modality for larger stones [2, 10–13]. There are also concerns that the serial ESWL treatments that are often required to treat a urinary calculus expose pediatric patients to multiple anesthetics, pose a financial burden, and could possibly cause permanent damage to developing kidneys [14]. Alternatively, flexible URS with Holmium:YAG laser provides the advantages of treating any stone type at any level in the urinary tract without traumatizing the renal parenchyma [15, 16].

In a prospective, randomized trial comparing ESWL to URS, URS was associated with a higher stone-free rate after the first session (81.4% vs 53.3%) with no significant difference in the complication rate between the two groups (URS 29.6% and ESWL 33.3%) [16]. Mokhless et al. performed another prospective randomized trial in preschool children treated with URS monotherapy vs ESWL for stones 10–20 mm in size and found that URS has a higher stone-free rate (86.6% vs 70%) [17]. Tejwani et al. reviewed 2281 admissions for ESWL and URS and found that patients undergoing URS demonstrated a lower rate of additional stone-related procedures within 12 months (13.6% vs 18.8%, $p < 0.0007$) [2].

In the past, obtaining ureteral access with an endoscope was a major barrier to performing URS in children due to the anatomically smaller ureteral orifices and distal ureteral caliber. Many providers preferred to place ureteral stents for 7–14 days prior to performing ureteroscopy for passive ureteral dilation. However, this practice necessitates multiple surgical procedures with multiple exposures to general anesthetics. With the development of 4.5 French ureteroscopes with 9.5 French ureteral access sheaths and coaxial ureteral dilators, providers can gain access to the ureter and treat upper tract calculi in a single attempt. Both the American Urologic Association/Endourology Society and the European Association of Urology Guidelines state that routine stenting is not necessary before URS [6, 18]. Gocke et al. analyzed data of 251 pediatric URS cases and compared the success rates and complications between pre-stented and nonpre-stented patients. A slightly higher success rate (84.6% vs 74.1%, $p = 0.72$) and lower complication rate (8.5% vs 14.7%, $p = 0.347$) were associated with the pre-stented patients; however, the differences between the two groups were not found to be statistically significant [19]. The authors noted significant disadvantages of routine pre-stenting and concluded that surgeons should attempt to treat the stone in the first session and place a stent only in the case of a failed procedure [19].

Sequential coaxial dilation and ureteral access sheath placement have been shown to be useful in accessing the entire pediatric urinary tract [20]. Singh et al. showed that ureteral access sheaths facilitate improved stone-free rates in a single procedure repetitive upper tract access, decreased operative time reduced intrarenal pressures, and are associated with minimal morbidity in pediatric patients [20, 21]. However, the use of balloon dilation to gain access of the ureter during routine pediatric ureteroscopy remains controversial as it has been suggested to predispose children to perforation, strictures, or vesicoureteral reflux [3, 22, 23].

Equipment

As previously mentioned, the unique anatomic considerations in children require instruments that are appropriately tailored to them. Surgical therapy for pediatric stone disease has experienced a significant evolution with a miniaturization of equipment commonly used in adult stone cases and improved optics that now allow safe navigation of all portions of the pediatric collecting system. Performing ureteroscopy successfully in the pediatric patient requires a variety of specialized equipment depending on the location of the stone in question. For proximal and mid-ureteral stones, ureteroscopy using either rigid or flexible instruments is first-line treatment at centers experienced in pediatric ureteroscopy.

While pediatric cystoscopy is beyond the scope of this section, gaining urethral access in the pediatric patient requires great attention and care, particularly in boys, as the pediatric urethra can be easily injured. Several instruments are available to accommodate the various sizes that may be encountered, ranging from 4.5 to 12 Fr [24].

Much like the smaller and more delicate anatomy encountered in pediatric patients, it should be emphasized to all members of the surgical and perioperative team that the equipment is equally delicate. This requires deliberate and careful handling of instruments used in pediatric ureteroscopy.

Traditionally, semirigid ureteroscopes have relied on working channels ranging from 2.4 to 3.5 Fr; however modernized pediatric scopes now provide larger working channels. Standardly used semirigid ureteroscopes come in 6/7.5 Fr and are self-dilating with a 4.8 Fr working channel (Fig. 14.1). The smallest semirigid

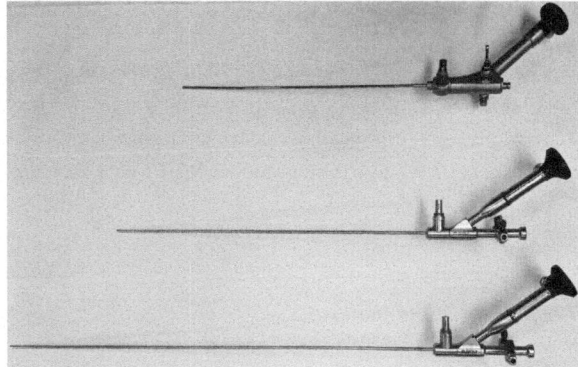

Fig. 14.1 Semirigid pediatric ureteroscopes in various sizes from 4.5/6.5 Fr and varying lengths (Karl Storz, top) and Wolf (Middle and Bottom) with offset eyepieces

ureteroscope utilizes a 4.5/6.5 Fr outer tip and 3 Fr working channel (Ultra-Thin Uretero-Renoscope 4.5/6.5 Fr; Richard Wolf GmBH, Knittlingen, Germany).

Eyepieces may either be "in-line" with the ureteroscope or offset. Eyepieces that are "in-line" are more ergonomic and typically allow easy introduction of the scope with greater control. Offset eyepieces require more attention to hand placement but allow for the passage of instruments directly in-line with the scope.

Much like their adult counterparts, pediatric flexible ureteroscopes all share similar features, including an optical housing unit, flexible deflection, and a working channel. Current models of flexible ureteroscopes allow deflection up to 270°, a feature that is particularly useful when approaching lower pole calculi (Fig. 14.2). Flexible ureteroscopes with an outer diameter of 7.5 Fr and inner 3.6 Fr working channels are the most commonly utilized configuration, though 7 Fr flexible ureteroscopes are available.

The use of guidewires is critical to any endourologic procedure, adult or pediatric. They are used for gaining access, in dilation procedures, for straightening the ureter, stent placement, and to maintain access via the safety wire. The standard Sensor guidewire measuring 0.035 in. × 150 cm utilized in adults is often used in pediatric cases. Other options include 0.018–0.025 in. × 150 cm glidewire versions when smaller wires are needed. When placing a second wire, dual-lumen ureteral access catheters, typically 10 Fr × 50 cm, can allow rapid and safe deployment of a second wire. After gaining access, ureteral access sheaths placed to protect the ureter from repeated trauma come in 9.5/11 Fr.

Whether performing retrograde ureteropyelography or being used for access, ureteral catheters are requisites in ureteroscopy. Similar to the larger 5 Fr × 70 cm catheters used in adult patients and larger adolescent pediatric patients, pediatric urology benefits from a tailored range of ureteral stents as small as 3–4 Fr × 70 cm.

Despite miniaturization, gaining safe access for primary ureteroscopy is not always easily accomplished even while using pediatric instruments. In such cases the ureter may be dilated to allow safe navigation. Pediatric dilation is most commonly performed using 8/10 Fr coaxial dilators.

Once successfully fragmented, stones are removed with a variety of baskets with numerous configurations. Common baskets include the Zero-tip™ and Ngage® baskets ranging from 1.7–3.0 Fr (Zero-tip™ Nitinol Stone Retrieval Basket, Boston Scientific, Boston, MA, USA; Ngage® Nitinol Stone Extractor, Cook Medical, Bloomington, IN, USA) (Fig. 14.3).

Prior to concluding the case, double-J ureteral stents are often deployed to facilitate continued drainage, decompression, and reduce ureteral stricture formation. An array of double-J ureteral stents are available, ranging from 3 to 6 Fr.

Contents of a basic ureteroscopic kit should include:

- Ureteroscopes:
  - 6/7.5 Fr semirigid ureteroscope
  - 5/6.5 Fr semirigid ureteroscopes
  - 7 Fr flexible ureteroscope
- Endourologic working equipment:

Fig. 14.2 Flexible
pediatric ureteroscope
showing maximal
deflection which can reach
270° allowing access to
difficult lower pole calyces

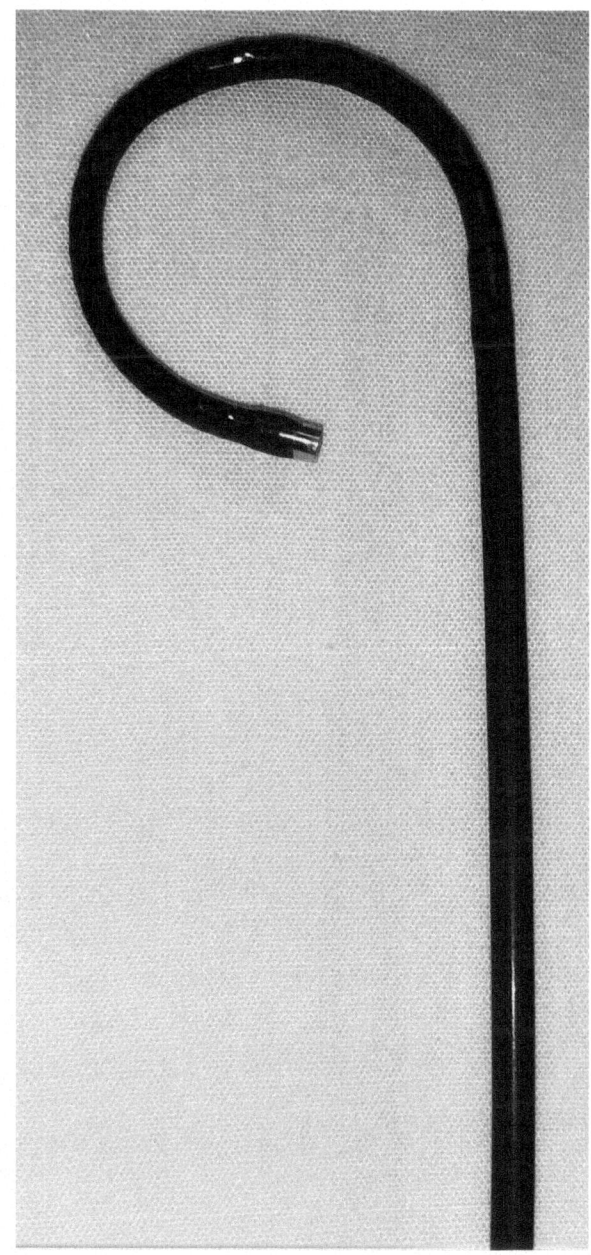

- Wires: 0.035 in Sensor™ wire, 0.018–0.025 in ZIPwire™
- Ureteral dilators: 8/10 Fr coaxial dilator
- Ureteral catheters in various sizes
- Dual-lumen ureteral access catheter: 10 Fr

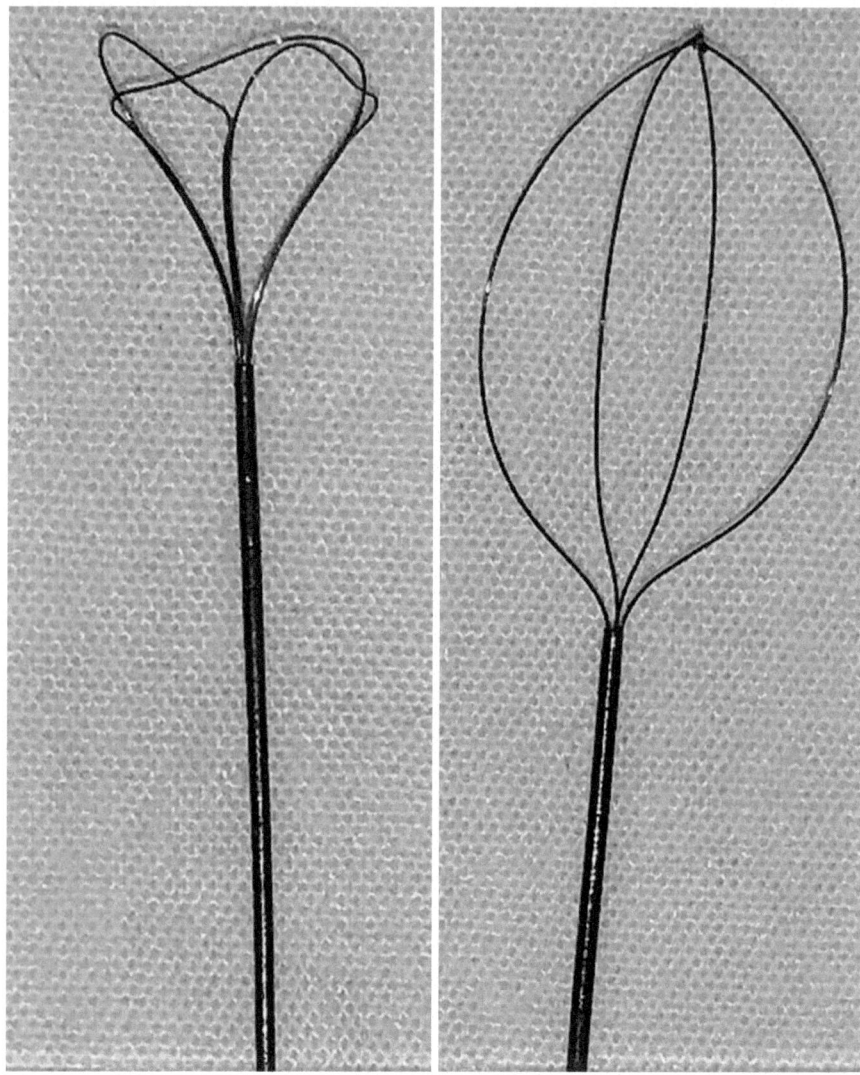

Fig. 14.3 Two common baskets include the Cook Ngage® Nitinol Stone Extractor (Left) and Boston Scientific Zero-Tip™ Nitinol Stone Retrieval Basket. The Ngage® allows for excellent control for basketing within the kidney while the Zero-Tip™ is favored for ureteral basketing by the authors

- Ureteral access sheath: 9.5/11 Fr
- Retrieval Devices: Zero-tip™ or Ngage® baskets as well as others
- Double-J Ureteral stents: including 3–6 Fr
- Irrigation device: single action pump, pressure bag, or mechanical

Technique for Lower Ureteral Calculi

Management of distal ureteral stones, defined as those located distal to the iliac vessels, is best performed via semirigid ureteroscopy due to advantages in irrigation, visualization, instrument control, and working channel diameter. To begin the procedure, a scout film should be obtained and saved prior to insertion of any instrumentation. Distal ureteral stones are difficult to visualize on fluoroscopy; however this provides documentation of any visible stone burden on plain film prior to removal.

An age-appropriate pediatric rigid cystoscope (7–12 Fr) should be inserted into the urethra and advanced into the bladder under direct vision. Panendoscopic views should be obtained to rule out an incidental bladder mass or other pathology. Both ureteral orifices should be visualized, and a safety wire (Sensor™ 0.035 in. × 150 cm PTFE/Nitinol wire with hydrophilic tip) should be inserted into the UO ipsilateral to the stone. Often, very distal stones and those right at the UVJ can make insertion of the safety wire difficult. A 5 Fr ureteral catheter can be inserted over the wire to provide stability and aid in cannulation. Alternatively, hydrophilic guidewires (ZIPwire™ 0.025–0.035 in. × 150 cm hydrophilic-coated nitinol wire) and angled tip wires can be attempted for stones which are severely impacted. After insertion of the safety wire, a 5 Fr ureteral catheter is inserted, and the wire removed so that a retrograde pyelogram can be performed (Fig. 14.4). This verifies the upper tract anatomy as well as any potential pitfalls during the case, such as submucosal passage of a wire, J-hooking of the ureter, or any other variations in anatomy. The safety wire should be reinserted and confirmed to be in the renal pelvis where it will

Fig. 14.4 Retrograde pyelogram is performed at the beginning of each case showing complete opacification of the left upper tract to delineate anatomy and provide confirmation of placement of working and safety wires

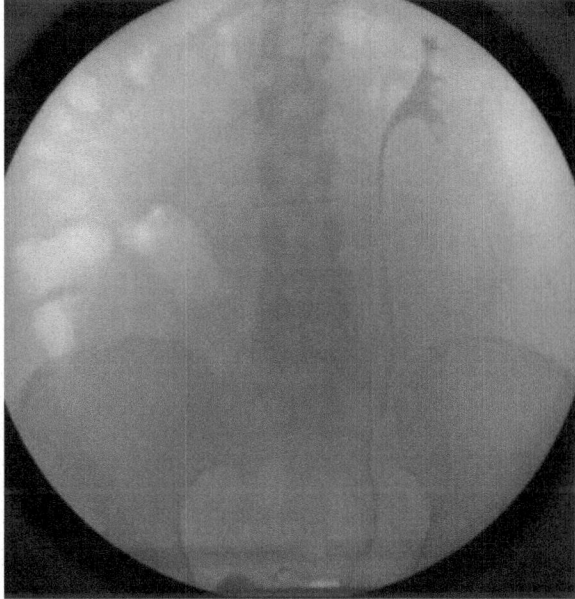

remain until the end of the case. If a hydrophilic wire was required to pass the stone, this should be replaced with a stiffer wire prior to beginning ureteroscopy. If purulent urine returns, a ureteral stent should be placed, and the patient should return after culture-directed treatment for UTI. In the event that a ureter cannot be cannulated due to severe stone impaction, a nephroureteral stent (6–8 Fr) may be required for ureteral access.

The bladder should be drained prior to initiating ureteroscopy. An age-appropriate pediatric semirigid ureteroscope (4.5–7.3 Fr) is then assembled and advanced alongside the safety wire to the level of the stone. Irrigation can be performed using a pressure bag or mechanical system for continuous flow or manually by an assistant using a hand pump. In some instances the ureter is too narrow to accommodate the ureteroscope requiring ureteral dilation. Practices vary by physician regarding the thresholds for ureteral dilation vs ureteral stent placement and aborting the procedure to return in 7–14 days after a period of passive ureteral dilation. If ureteral dilation is attempted, this can be accomplished using balloon dilating devices (which is controversial), ureteral dilating sheaths, and/or serial ureteral dilators. Dilation should be performed with care as the risk of ureteral perforation is increased, and dilation over the stone can cause extrusion making extraction difficult and increasing the chances of perforation, stone granuloma formation, and eventual development of ureteral stricture. The authors' preference is to attempt dilation with an 8/10 Fr coaxial dilator if the semirigid ureteroscope does not initially pass through the UO; however, placement of a stent is favored over balloon dilation due to less tactile feedback and increased risk of stricture formation due to ureteral injury/ischemia.

For small stones, basket retrieval can be performed; however, blind basketing and applying pressure due to tight passage through the ureter should not be attempted due to the risk of ureteral perforation and/or avulsion. Larger stones will require lithotripsy which can be accomplished by a number of devices; however, Holmium:YAG laser has emerged as the standard of care for stone fragmentation. Typically, laser lithotripsy is undertaken with a 200-μ laser fiber. Multiple techniques have been described for stone fragmentation including "dusting" or "painting" of the stone, in which it is fragmented into inconsequentially small particles which then easily pass through the urine, and "cracking" the stone into several smaller pieces which are still large enough to remove with a basketing device. For dusting, low-power and high-frequency settings (0.2 J and 30–80 Hz) are preferred, and the leading edge of the stone is contacted and "painted" continuously with the laser fiber such that it disintegrates. Irrigation washes the resulting stone powder out of the field of view. The laser fiber tip should always be in vision to prevent iatrogenic ureteral trauma. Eventually with the dusting technique, the stone will become small enough that the remaining significant stone burden can be removed with a basket device which is preferred due to the ability to send the stone for analysis. For cracking of the stone, which is preferred by the authors for distal stones due to less laser time (and less chance of iatrogenic ureteral injury) and increase in the chances of achieving stone-free status, higher-power and lower-frequency settings are used. For the authors, 0.6 J and 6 Hz is a common starting setting. The power is increased to effect by a factor of 0.2–0.4 J for harder stones with minimal changes in the frequency. The center of the stone is targeted, and the stone is lasered until it cracks into several pieces.

Basket retrieval of stone fragments can be accomplished by several devices. For distal ureteral stones, the authors prefer a 0.019 in. Zero-Tip™ basket. Stone fragments are gently grasped beginning with the most distal stones (those most proximal to the scope) and are removed extracorporeally. If a stone fragment proves too large for easy extraction, it should be dropped in the ureter and fragmented further to prevent the chances of ureteral injury or avulsion. In some instances, the basket may become entrapped around the stone, and the laser fiber must be advanced through the working channel so that the stone is fragmented while still contained within the open basket. For larger children the stone fragments can be dropped into the bladder to decrease operating time; however, at least one fragment should be sent for analysis (Fig. 14.5). All stone fragments are removed and the semirigid scope is advanced up the ureter as far as can be safely achieved to assess for retropulsion of stone fragments. Some providers prefer to deploy stone-trapping devices prior to fragmentation to prevent retropulsion (Stone Cone™, NTrap®, Leslie Parachute™, Lithocatch™, Escape™, Backstop™ gel, etc.); however, with proper lasering, basketing, and irrigation techniques, this is unnecessary and often increases operating time. If there is concern that clinically significant fragments have moved to the proximal ureter or kidney, a flexible ureteroscope can be assembled for complete ureterorenoscopy.

Following complete extraction of the stone and verifying that no clinically significant residual stone remains, the decision to leave a ureteral stent is provider specific and based on several factors. The degree of stone impaction, presence of contralateral kidney, number of passes up and down the ureter, amount of visible

Fig. 14.5 Intraoperative photo of a 4–5 mm distal ureteral stone which was extracted en bloc using a semirigid ureteroscope

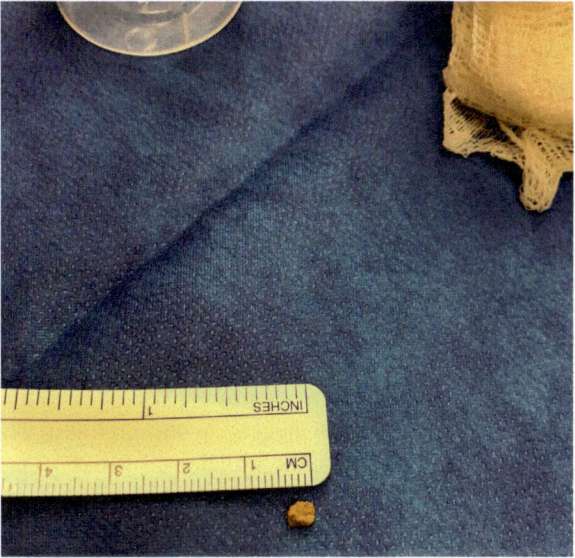

Fig. 14.6 Intraoperative fluoroscopic image confirming proper placement of right ureteral stent, with >180-degree coils noted in the renal pelvis and bladder. The distal coil is also confirmed using direct vision

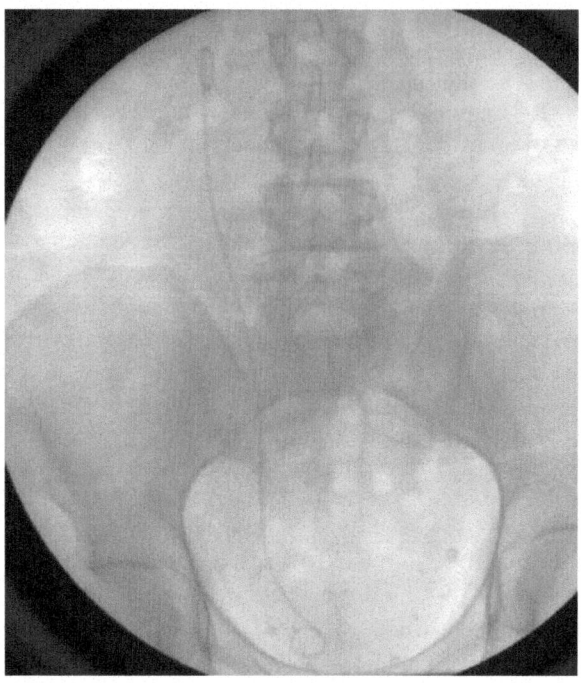

ureteral trauma, and presence of contrast extravasation on post-extraction retrograde pyelogram all contribute to the decision to leave a stent. Stentless ureteroscopy is an option in uncomplicated, low-risk patients with a healthy contralateral kidney. A double pigtail ureteral stent (4.6–6 Fr) is often left for a period of 3–7 days and can have an extracorporeal tether or be removed under sedation at follow-up procedure. Stent placement can be performed either under fluoroscopic guidance or direct vision. Care must be taken to ensure and document proper stent positioning with a spot film at the end of the case (Fig. 14.6). The distal coil should be confirmed to be within the bladder with direct visualization of at least a 180-degree coil outside the UO via the rigid cystoscope. The bladder should be drained, and the procedure terminated. Antibiotic therapy should be <24 h. The patient should be provided a limited pain control regimen, and daily Flomax can be considered for stent discomfort.

Technique for Upper Ureteral and Renal Stones

The ureteroscopic management of upper ureteral and small renal stones (<1.5 cm) introduces additional challenges to the urologist which require adjustments to surgical technique. Anatomic variations, J-hooking ureters, ureteral narrowing, and minimizing ureteral trauma must be taken into consideration. A scout film should be obtained as with lower ureteral stones to document the stone burden at the beginning of the case. Rigid cystoscopy is performed as well as retrograde pyelography to verify anatomy and placement of a safety wire. Utilizing either a dual-lumen catheter or 8/10 Fr coaxial dilator, a second wire should be placed as a working wire.

A ureteral access sheath (9.5/11 Fr is common) of age-appropriate length is advanced over the working wire and should come to rest just distal to ureteral stones and at the UPJ for renal stones. If the UO or distal ureter is stenotic, ureteral dilation can be attempted as described previously. The authors do not advise balloon dilation of the proximal or mid ureter on primary ureteroscopy due to increased risk of ureteral injury. If the access sheath will not advance beyond the mid or proximal ureter, the inner cannula should be removed and a pediatric flexible ureteroscope should be advanced through the sheath. If the ureter is stenotic, then a double pigtail stent should be placed for passive ureteral dilation, and the patient should return to care in 7–14 days for repeat ureteroscopy. Placement of the ureteral access sheath is the critical part of the case as it protects the ureter from multiple passes by the ureteroscope, straightens out J-hooking and anatomic variations, and overcomes areas of ureteral narrowing that may prohibit removal of stone fragments. Irrigation of small stone fragments, debris, and clot is also facilitated by the ureteral access sheath. Some providers will attempt to pass the ureteroscope up the working wire if the access sheath cannot be placed as a last effort to perform primary ureterosocpy. In this instance, if the proximal ureteral or renal stone is reached, the stone is typically "dusted" as previously described to minimize ureteral trauma associated with multiple passes of the ureteroscope through an unprotected ureter.

Once the ureteral access sheath is positioned, the age-appropriate pediatric flexible ureteroscope is assembled (7.0–8.5 Fr) and advanced through the sheath and into the ureter to the level of the stone. Basket retrieval and laser lithotripsy are performed as previously described. Cracking of the stone and basket retrieval of the fragmented stone burden is preferred over dusting in most cases for upper ureteral and renal stones due to the greater likelihood of achieving stone-free status. Within the ureter, 0.6 J and 6 Hz with a 200-micron fiber are the preferred starting settings, and a Zero Tip™ basket is used to retrieve the fragments. For renal stones, an N-gage® or Dakota™ basket is preferred because they allow for greater control when reaching anteriorly and precisely grasping individual fragments within the calyceal system. The stones are removed individually through the access sheath and collected to be sent for analysis. In some instances, stones will be easily manipulated within the kidney but become lodged within the narrow lumen of the ureter. As with distal stones, the basket should be removed if possible and the stone fragmented further to allow for tension free passage through the ureter. A unique issue with proximal and renal stones is the inability to pass the stone into the end of the sheath. Should this occur the stone should be fragmented at the end of the sheath to allow the basket to be removed. The sheath can then be pulled back slightly so that the fragments are in view and easily removed. Additionally, stones can become lodged within the sheath necessitating laser lithotripsy within the sheath itself. All laser firing and stone removal should be performed under direct vision at all times to minimize ureteral trauma.

At the completion of stone removal, the kidney should be completely surveyed and the ureteroscope slowly withdrawn to the level of the sheath. The sheath and scope are then withdrawn in tandem to visualize the ureter in its entirety. Care should be taken to ensure no stone fragments were trapped alongside the sheath and to rule out visible ureteral injury. One optional step when addressing a renal stone burden is to perform complete kidney mapping if a stone cannot be located, or at the end of a case to confirm no residual stone burden (Fig. 14.7). The scope should be withdrawn to the level of the UPJ, and approximately 3–5 cc of contrast medium

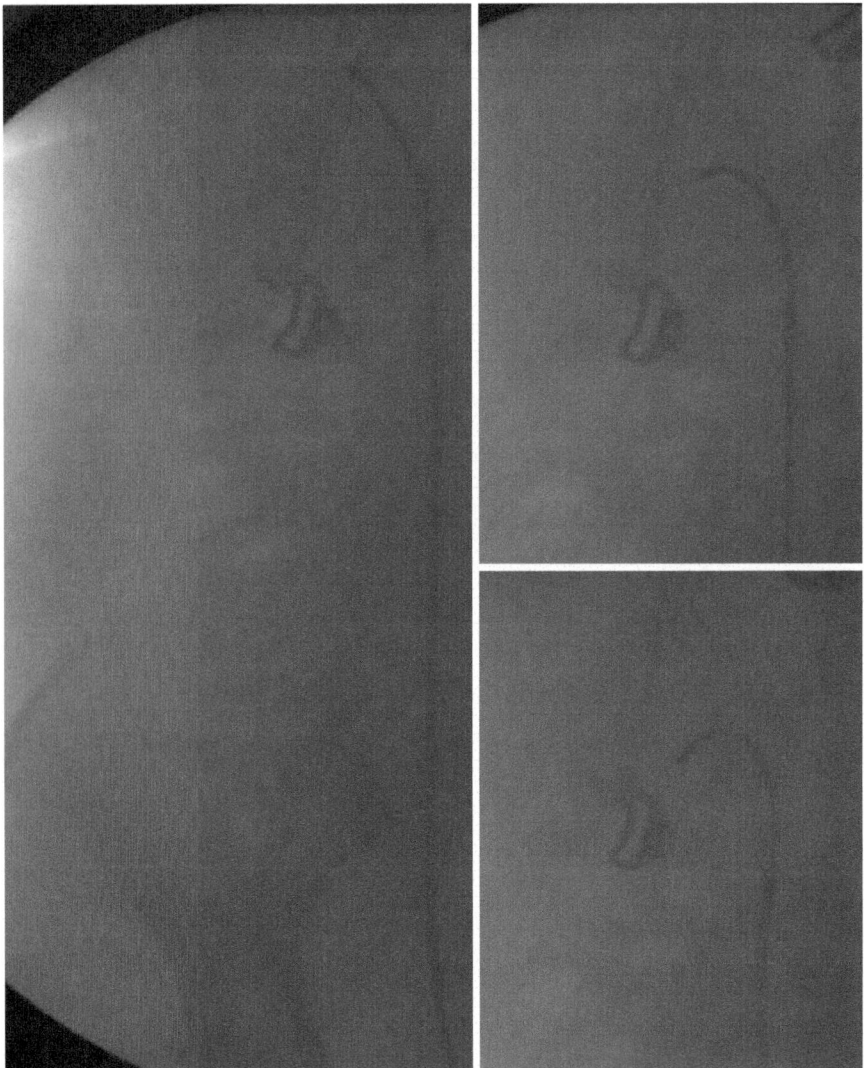

Fig. 14.7 Sequential images showing complete kidney mapping with representative images of the flexible ureteroscope surveying the upper (left), mid (top right), and lower (lower right) pole calyces. A retrograde pyelogram (not shown) can be performed prior to kidney mapping to ensure that all calyces are inspected

should be injected through the scope. Irrigation should be performed in each of the calyces to washout the contrast with a spot film taken to document complete renoscopy. The ureteroscope is then removed. Stent placement is again determined by the degree of ureteral irritation, stone manipulation, presence of a contralateral kidney, degree of stone impaction, and use of a ureteral access sheath. If a ureteral access sheath is placed to overcome ureteral narrowing, the authors prefer to leave a double pigtail stent in place for 3–7 days with or without an extracorporeal tether as previously described. Patients should then be discharged with appropriate pain control, <24 h of antibiotics, and Flomax.

Follow-up for uncomplicated ureteroscopy should include a renal ultrasound in several weeks to rule out silent obstruction from residual stone fragments or development of ureteral stricture. Additionally, all pediatric patients should be offered metabolic workup to decrease the risk of future stone formation. The authors prefer to see the patients in 6 weeks to 3 months after surgery with a Renal US and referral to pediatric nephrology for metabolic workup.

Complications

The most common complications that occur during pediatric ureteroscopy involve ureteral injuries of varying degrees of severity, from small submucosal tunnels and flaps to partial and complete ureteral avulsions (Fig. 14.8). Injuries can occur during retrograde advancement of guidewires, lasers, baskets, endoscopes, or ureteral

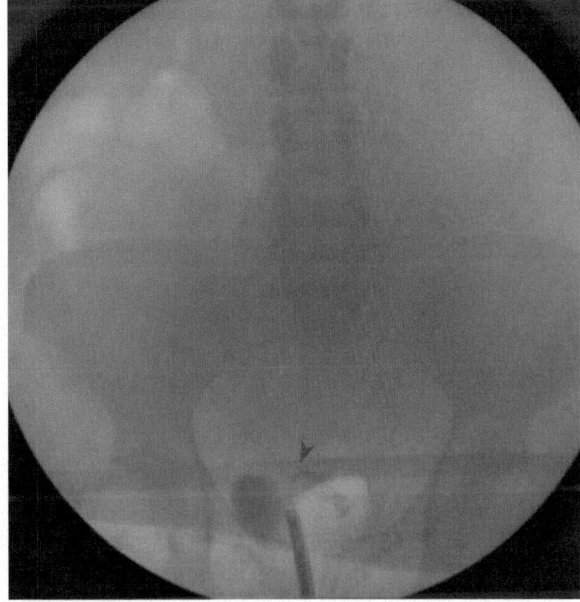

Fig. 14.8 Right retrograde pyelogram shows medial contrast extravasation from the right distal ureter with no contrast opacification proximally. This particular patient was found to have a complete ureteral avulsion which had presented in a delayed fashion

access sheaths up the ureter. Traumatic injuries can also occur during stone fragmentation and during basket retrieval while pulling large stone fragments down the ureter. To minimize ureteral injury during ureteroscopic procedures, we recommend performing a retrograde ureteropyelogram at the beginning of each procedure to help define the anatomy to guide the advancement of wires and sheaths into the collecting system. It is paramount to perform all stone manipulation (fragmentation and retrieval) under direct visualization to minimize the risk of damaging the ureter. Calculi must be fragmented into small enough pieces that can easily fit through the diameter of the ureter and ureteral access sheath without resistance. Most minor ureteral injuries can be managed conservatively by placing an indwelling ureteral stent for 4–6 weeks and performing a retrograde ureteropyelogram at the time of stent removal to ensure that there is no contrast extravasation or residual filling defects. In a recent large systemic review of 2758 pediatric patients who underwent ureteroscopy from 1996 to 2016, the overall complication rate was 11.1% [25]. Clavien I complications included post-op renal colic (0.1%), hematuria (0.1%), urinary tract infections (0.3%), post-op pyrexia (0.2%), and urinary retention (0.03%) [25]. Clavien II/III complications included late ureterovesical junction obstruction (0.02%), stent migration (0.03%), ureteral strictures (0.003%), and intraoperative bleeding/false passage/ureteral perforation/ tear (0.2%) [25]. There were no Clavien IV/V complications and no mortality reported across any of the studies that were reviewed [25].

References

1. Routh JC, Graham DA, Nelson CP. Epidemiological trends in pediatric urolithiasis at United States freestanding pediatric hospitals. J Urol. 2010;184(3):1100–4.
2. Tejwani R, Wang HH, Wolf S, Wiener JS, Routh JC. Outcomes of shock wave lithotripsy and ureteroscopy for treatment of pediatric urolithiasis. J Urol. 2016;196(1):196–201.
3. VanDervoort K, Wiesen J, Frank R, et al. Urolithiasis in pediatric patients: a single center study of incidence, clinical presentation and outcome. J Urol. 2007;177(6):2300–5.
4. Routh JC, Graham DA, Nelson CP. Trends in imaging and surgical management of pediatric urolithiasis at American pediatric hospitals. J Urol. 2010;184(4 Suppl):1816–22.
5. Utangac MM, Daggulli M, Dede O, Sancaktutar AA, Bozkurt Y. Effectiveness of ureteroscopy among the youngest patients: one centre's experience in an endemic region in Turkey. J Pediatr Urol. 2017;13(1):37 e31–6.
6. Assimos D, Krambeck A, Miller NL, et al. Surgical management of stones: American Urological Association/Endourological Society Guideline, PART I. J Urol. 2016;196(4):1153–60.
7. Badawy AA, Saleem MD, Abolyosr A, et al. Extracorporeal shock wave lithotripsy as first line treatment for urinary tract stones in children: outcome of 500 cases. Int Urol Nephrol. 2012;44(3):661–6.
8. Muslumanoglu AY, Tefekli A, Sarilar O, Binbay M, Altunrende F, Ozkuvanci U. Extracorporeal shock wave lithotripsy as first line treatment alternative for urinary tract stones in children: a large scale retrospective analysis. J Urol. 2003;170(6 Pt 1):2405–8.
9. Newman DM, Coury T, Lingeman JE, et al. Extracorporeal shock wave lithotripsy experience in children. J Urol. 1986;136(1 Pt 2):238–40.

10. Ather MH, Noor MA. Does size and site matter for renal stones up to 30-mm in size in children treated by extracorporeal lithotripsy? Urology. 2003;61(1):212–5; discussion 215.
11. Elsobky E, Sheir K, Madbouly K, Mokhtar A. Extracorporeal shock wave lithotripsy in children: experience using two second-generation lithotripters. BJU. 2000;86:851–6.
12. Afshar K, McLorie G, Papanikolaou F, et al. Outcome of small residual stone fragments following shock wave lithotripsy in children. J Urol. 2004;172(4 Pt 2):1600–3.
13. Wadhwa P, Aron M, Seth A, Dogra PN, Hemal AK, Gupta NP. Pediatric shockwave lithotripsy: size matters! J Endourol. 2007;21(2):141–4.
14. Lingeman JE. Extracorporeal shock wave lithotripsy – what happened? J Urol. 2003;169(1):63.
15. El-Nahas A, Awad BE, El-Assmy AM, Abou El-Ghar M, Erkay I, Keneway M, Sheir K. Are there long-term effects of extracorporeal shockwave lithotripsy in paediatric patients? BJU Int. 2013;111:666.
16. Alsagheer G, Mohamed O, Abdel-Kader MS, et al. Extracorporeal shock wave lithotripsy (ESWL) versus flexible ureteroscopy (F-URS) for management of renal stone burden less than 2 cm in children: a randomized comparative study. Afr J Urol. 2018;24(2):120–5.
17. Mokhless I, Marzouk E, Thabet Ael D, Youssif M, Fahmy A. Ureteroscopy in infants and preschool age children: technique and preliminary results. Cent Eur J Urol. 2012;65(1):30–2.
18. Tekgul S, Dogan H, Hoebeke P, et al. Retrograde intrarenal surgery using ureteral access sheaths is a safe and effective treatment for renal stones in children weighing <20. J Pediatr Urol. 2018;14(1):60–1.
19. Gokce MI, Telli O, Akinci A, et al. Effect of prestenting on success and complication rates of ureterorenoscopy in pediatric population. J Endourol. 2016;30(8):850–5.
20. Smaldone MC, Gayed BA, Ost MC. The evolution of the endourologic management of pediatric stone disease. Indian J Urol: IJU: J Urological Soc India. 2009;25(3):302–11.
21. Singh A, Shah G, Young J, Sheridan M, Haas G, Upadhyay J. Ureteral access sheath for the management of pediatric renal and ureteral stones: a single center experience. J Urol. 2006;175(3 Pt 1):1080–2; discussion 1082.
22. Smaldone MC, Cannon GM Jr, Wu HY, et al. Is ureteroscopy first line treatment for pediatric stone disease? J Urol. 2007;178(5):2128–31; discussion 2131.
23. Tan AH, Al-Omar M, Denstedt JD, Razvi H. Ureteroscopy for pediatric urolithiasis: an evolving first-line therapy. Urology. 2005;65(1):153–6.
24. Zhu J, Phillips TM, Mathews RI. Operative management of pediatric urolithiasis. Indian J Urol: IJU: J Urological Soc India. 2010;26(4):536–43.
25. Rob S, Jones P, Pietropaolo A, Griffin S, Somani BK. Ureteroscopy for stone disease in paediatric population is safe and effective in medium-volume and high-volume centres: evidence from a systematic review. Curr Urol Rep. 2017;18(12):92.

Chapter 15
Ureteroscopic Management of Upper Tract Urothelial Carcinoma

Wesley Baas, Andrew Klein, and Bradley F. Schwartz

Introduction

Upper urothelial tract carcinoma (UTUC) is a relatively uncommon class of neoplasm arising from the urothelial lining from the renal calyceal system to the extent of the distal ureterovesical junction. UTUC comprises 5–10% of all urothelial carcinomas and as much as 5–7% of all renal tumors; the rate of incidence has possibly been rising due to improved means of detection [1]. While UTUC shares some common risk factors with urothelial carcinoma of the bladder it is biologically and clinically distinct. UTUC often portends a worse prognosis as it is invasive 60% of the time at diagnosis, compared with 15–25% for bladder cancer [2]. UTUC occurs twice as frequently in males as compared to females and has been linked to exposure to tobacco, aromatic amines, and aristolochic acid. There is also a strong genetic component, as 10–20% of all UTUC are linked to hereditary non-polyposis colorectal carcinoma (HNPCC or Lynch syndrome) [3].

The clinical presentation of UTUC includes gross or microscopic hematuria in 70–80% of cases and flank pain associated with clot or tumor-related hydronephrosis in 20–40% of cases. These local symptoms are not known to influence prognosis. However, constitutional symptoms such as fever, night sweats, fatigue, loss of appetite, weight loss, etc. are associated with metastasis and reduced survival [4]. Localization of disease in the renal pelvis is twice as common compared to disease within the ureter, but 10–20% of cases have multifocal disease, and an additional 20% have concomitant bladder cancer. The incidence of metastatic disease at the time of presentation has been shown to be 7% [3].

UTUC was classically managed surgically with a litany of procedures ranging from segmental ureterectomy for low-grade disease to radical nephroureterectomy

W. Baas · A. Klein · B. F. Schwartz (✉)
Department of Urology, Southern Illinois University School of Medicine,
Springfield, IL, USA
e-mail: bschwartz@siumed.edu

© Springer Nature Switzerland AG 2020   205
B. F. Schwartz, J. D. Denstedt (eds.), *Ureteroscopy*,
https://doi.org/10.1007/978-3-030-26649-3_15

with bladder cuff excision for high-grade disease [4]. Advancements made in the use of flexible ureteroscopic and percutaneous techniques for direct visualization of the entire upper urinary tract have provided clinicians with the ability to biopsy tumor sites and deliver concomitant therapies or interventions [5]. Today, minimally invasive therapy options for UTUC are available depending on the patient's preoperative risk in elective management and/or imperative need of renal sparing treatment.

This chapter will highlight the specific use of ureteroscopic techniques in the diagnosis and management of UTUC.

Diagnosis

A patient presenting to a urology clinic with UTUC often presents because of gross or microscopic hematuria or incidental findings on CT. Computed Tomography Urography (CTU) is the gold standard imaging modality, which has largely replaced standard intravenous pyelograms and renal ultrasound because of improved specificity (93–99%) and sensitivity (67–100%) [6]. CT urography is done in three phases (non-contrast, contrast enhanced, and excretory) [7]. CTU does a poor job of truly staging disease because it is difficult to determine depth of invasion with imaging alone. There are, however, secondary ways of helping predict those with advanced disease. Patients with hydronephrosis on imaging often have advanced disease and poor oncologic outcomes [8]. Enlarged lymph nodes on CTU are also highly predictive of metastatic disease [9]. Downsides to CTU include its inability to be used in patients with renal insufficiency or contrast allergies as well as the fact that radiation doses are quite high given that it is three separate CT scans.

In patients unable to undergo CTU because of iodinated contrast allergy or radiation exposure, magnetic resonance urography (MRU) is a viable alternative. MRU is much the same as CTU in that images are acquired in three phases but is based on magnetic resonance imaging technology which has the advantage of not exposing the patient to radiation. In MRU the contrast is gadolinium-based and can be used in patients with creatinine clearance >30 mL/min. The sensitivity of MRU in diagnosing tumors <2 cm is 75%, which is respectable but still significantly lower than CTU, thus the preference for CTU when possible [10].

Urothelial carcinoma is believed to represent a "field change" disease in which all the urothelial surfaces are prone to neoplasm if there is cancer elsewhere within the urothelium. Because of this, nearly one third of UTUC cases present with synchronous multifocality [11]. As such, all patients diagnosed with UTUC should undergo thorough cystoscopy when staging. There is also a 1–5% risk of concurrent contralateral upper tract involvement, and accordingly, the contralateral side should be evaluated with at least retrograde pyelography during workup [12].

Based off of grade A evidence, the European Association of Urology has recommended urine cytology be performed as part of the standard workup of UTUC once bladder and prostatic urethral UCs have been excluded. They do note, however, that

Fig. 15.1 Example of
ureteroscopic brush biopsy.
(Permission for use granted
by Cook Medical,
Bloomington, Indiana)

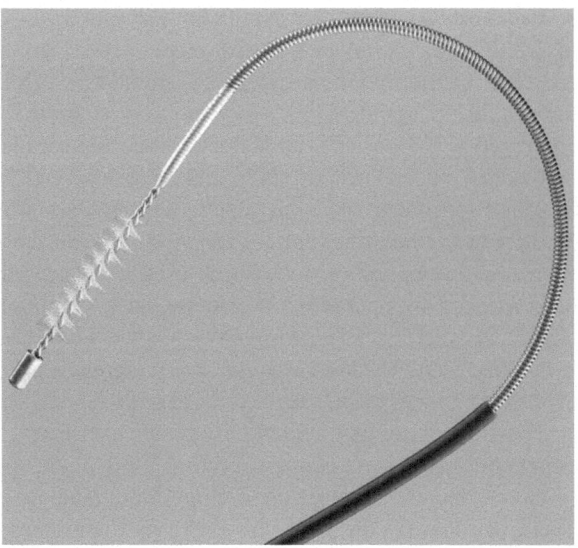

the sensitivity of cytology is lower for UTUC than with bladder cancer and should
be done selectively from each renal pelvis [6]. Selective cytology should be done
before the injection of contrast for retrograde ureteropyelography as exposure to
contrast has been shown to deteriorate cytological specimens [13]. There is also
evidence to suggest that performing a barbotage at the time of ureteroscopy improves
diagnostic yield and was found in one study to identify 91% of cancers compared to
94% for conventional biopsy [14]. Similar to obtaining barbotage cytology is the
use of endoscopic brush cytology (Fig. 15.1). In a small study, Dodd et al. found
that using endoscopic brush cytology resulted in 94% specificity and better
sensitivity than barbotage cytology [15]. It was noted, however, that brush cytology
was not successful in diagnosing dysplasia or carcinoma in situ (CIS). The use of
fluorescence in situ hybridization (FISH) and other molecular tests are not
recommended at this time.

Some clinicians would advocate that treatment can be undertaken with the
diagnosis of UTUC based off of imaging, questioning the necessity of routine
ureteroscopy. Some have raised the theoretical concerns of tumor spread via
pyelovenous or pyelolymphatic backflow as well as the possibility of "seeding" of
the bladder and points distal to the tumor by ureteroscopic manipulation, though
this has largely been disproven [16, 17]. The authors of this chapter feel strongly
that tissue is needed to truly diagnose a patient with UTUC and, as such, ureteroscopy
is routinely performed in our practice.

Ureteroscopy is both diagnostic and potentially therapeutic when done correctly,
which has the advantage of a relatively low degree of invasiveness and can be done
on an outpatient basis. Refinements in optics and the technology of current endoscopes allows urologists to thoroughly examine all aspects of the upper urinary
tracts with improved visualization and lesions can be biopsied and ablated at the
time of diagnosis.

Ureteroscopic biopsy has significantly improved since ureteroscopic management of UTUC was introduced in the 1980s [18]. Despite these improvements, the adequacy of ureteroscopic biopsies is limited by their relatively small size which has resulted in a limited ability to accurately stage UTUC by biopsy. Vashistha et al. compared 118 biopsies with surgical tissue samples and found that ureteroscopic biopsy had a specificity of 100% and a sensitivity of 85.4%. They also found that 87.1% of specimens had concordant grade, but there was only a concordance rate of 58.6% when comparing tumor staging [19]. Because of this, UTUC grade obtained from ureteroscopic biopsy has been used as a surrogate for stage. This has been demonstrated by a number of groups when comparing ureteroscopic biopsy to nephroureterectomy specimens. Low-grade UTUC has been shown to be Ta or T1 at the time of RNU 73–86% of the time, whereas high-grade UTUC is T2 or higher 66% of the time [20, 21].

There are currently a number of options to biopsy a lesion available to the practicing urologist. Most commonly, reusable 3-F cold cup biopsy forceps represent an economic and effective option to biopsy both renal and ureteral lesions (Fig. 15.2). There is currently little data available that compares ureteroscopic biopsy techniques head to head. The best evidence currently comes from Kleinmann et al. in which they retrospectively looked at 504 ureteroscopic biopsies that were performed with either 3-F cold cup biopsy forceps or a 2.4-F stainless steel flat wire basket. They found that diagnosis was successful 63% of the time with forceps compared with 94% with the flat wire basket. These results should be interpreted with caution, however, as the study was retrospective in nature and the authors noted that forceps were preferentially used for smaller, sessile, or non-papillary lesions which by definition will provide less of a sample size and are harder to biopsy [22]. The 2.4-F flat wire basket has the advantage of being able to cut papillary lesions at their stalk and can be used to debulk large tumors. Specifically, a stainless steel flat wire basket

Fig. 15.2 Example of 3-F cold cup biopsy forceps. (Permission for use granted by Cook Medical, Bloomington, Indiana)

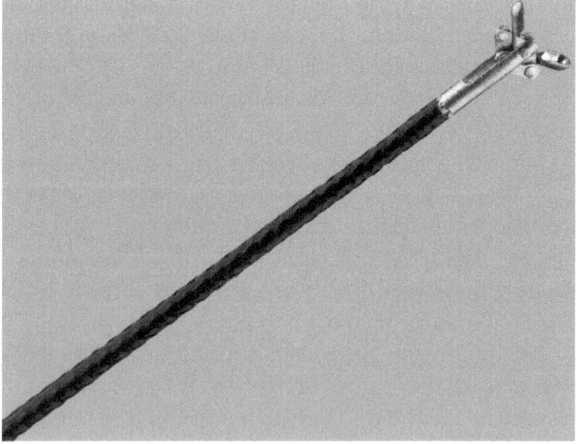

Fig. 15.3 BIGopsy device.
(Permission for use granted
by Cook Medical,
Bloomington, Indiana)

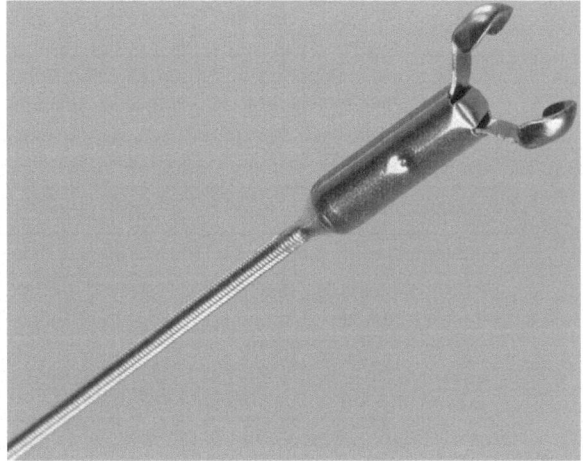

should be used as nitinol baskets commonly used in stone procedures have a tendency to slip off of the tumor [17]. Another option available for biopsy is the BIGopsy™ forceps (Cook ®) (Fig. 15.3). The BIGopsy forceps are 4mm³ in size and provide a sample four times larger than standard 3-F cold cup biopsy forceps. Although it is touted as providing a larger specimen with less architectural distortion of the tissue, the BIGopsy forceps are quite difficult to use as they cannot pass through a standard ureteroscope's working channel. The device has to be back-loaded into the ureteroscope and then advanced along with the ureteroscope through a ureteral access sheath while exposed out of the end of the scope. The large size of the device also takes up a large field of view and is difficult to get significant deflection [23].

The following recommendations were made by the European Association of Urology (EAU) in the 2017 UTUC guidelines in regards to diagnosis (Fig. 15.4) [6]:

1. Perform cystoscopy to rule out a concomitant bladder tumor.
2. Perform CT urography for upper tract evaluation and staging.
3. Use diagnostic ureteroscopy and biopsy only in cases where additional information will impact treatment options.

There are a number of technological advancements in development for the diagnosis and surveillance of UTUC including narrow band imaging (NBI) and photodynamic diagnosis- guided inspection (PDD). These technologies are designed to provide better visualization and improve sensitivity of ureteroscopy. In a small study, narrow band imaging improved the rate of diagnosis of UTUC by 20% [24]. PDD has been reported to have better sensitivity as high as 95.8%. PDD has also shown to have improved ability in detecting CIS and early dysplasia [25]. Despite their promise, these technologies are still in the early phases and have limited evidence, as such they have not reached mainstream popularity [26].

Summary of evidence	LE
The diagnosis of upper tract urothelial carcinoma depends on computed tomography urography and ureteroscopy.	2
Selective urinary cytology has high sensitivity in high-grade tumours including carcinoma *in situ*.	3
Recommendations	GR
Perform urinary cytology as part of a standard diagnostic workup.	A
Perform a cystoscopy to rule out concomitant bladder tumour.	A
Perform a computed tomography urography for upper tract evaluation and for staging.	A
Use diagnostic ureteroscopy and biopsy in cases where additional information will impact treatment decisions.	C
GR = grade of recommendation; LE = level of evidence.	

Fig. 15.4 Summary of evidence and guidelines for the diagnosis of UTUC. (From Roupret et al., Figs. 2, 4, 6, with permission of Elsevier [6])

Management

As examined in the introduction, classically, management of UTUC was limited to radical nephroureterectomy (RNU). Historically, only patients unfit for RNU, those with a functionally or anatomically solitary kidney, or bilateral tumors were considered for minimally invasive treatment options of UTUC. However, with the advancement of technology in the urologist's armamentarium, a number of minimally invasive options for management of UTUC have arisen [27]. These minimally invasive options (namely via ureteroscopic, segmental resections of the ureter, and percutaneous approaches) have been termed nephron-sparing or kidney-sparing surgery (KSS). KSS is an enticing management modality with the goal of preserving the renal unit without compromising oncologic outcomes. Mostly based off of data from conservative therapy of renal cell carcinoma, by preserving the renal unit one could avoid the potential long-term cardiovascular morbidity associated with chronic kidney disease (CKD) [28].

Nephron-sparing options for the treatment of UTUC are broadly separated into segmental ureterectomy, percutaneous, and ureteroscopic approaches. This chapter specifically deals with ureteroscopic management of UTUC. Under the umbrella of ureteroscopy, there are a number of options available to the practicing urologist including cauterization techniques, a variety of lasers, and ureteroscopic resectoscopes.

There is currently no level 1 evidence regarding endoscopic management of UTUC. As discussed by the EAU non-muscle invasive bladder cancer guidelines panel, the currently available data comparing KSS to RNU is both heterogenous and scarce [29]. There are five studies that report oncologic outcomes of URS versus RNU [30–34]. Patients treated with URS were younger, were more unhealthy, and had smaller size and lower-grade UTUC. Despite this heterogeneity, the EAU has released the following recommendations in its guidelines in the management of UTUC in 2017 (Fig. 15.5) [6]:

Recommendations	GR
Offer kidney-sparing management as primary treatment option to patients with low-risk tumours and two functional kidneys.	C
Offer kidney-sparing management in patients with solitary kidney and/or impaired renal function, provided that it will not compromise the oncological outcome. This decision will have to be made on a case-by-case basis, engaging the patient in a shared decision-making process.	C
Offer a kidney-sparing approach in high-risk cancers for distal ureteral tumours and in imperative cases (solitary kidney and/or impaired renal function).	C
Use a laser for endoscopic treatment of upper tract urothelial carcinoma.	C
GR = grade of recommendation.	

Fig. 15.5 EAU Guidelines for kidney-sparing management of UTUC. (From Roupret et al., Figs. 2, 4, 6, with permission of Elsevier [6])

1. KSS should be offered as primary treatment option in patients with low-risk tumors (strong strength rating).
2. Offer KSS in patients with high-risk distal ureteral tumors (weak strength rating).
3. As long as not compromising survival, on a case-by-case basis, KSS should be offered to patients with a solitary kidney and/or impaired renal function (strong).
4. Use a laser for endoscopic treatment of UTUC (weak).

Specific to ureteroscopic of UTUC, the EAU guidelines state that it can be considered as long as the following criteria are met:

1. Laser generation and biopsy forceps are available for use.
2. Both flexible and rigid ureteroscopes are available.
3. The patient is aware earlier second look procedures with closer and more stringent follow-up will be necessary.
4. Complete resection and/or destruction of the tumor is possible.

Unfortunately, there are no guidelines for UTUC from the American Urological Association. There is also no consensus on the ideal nephron-sparing approach used, and the authors would suggest surgical planning on a case-by-case basis. As indicated in the EAU guidelines, patient selection is key, with KSS being ideal for patients with low-grade or low-volume disease or those too unhealthy to undergo RNU. Deciding between a distal ureterectomy, percutaneous, or ureteroscopic approach largely depends on tumor size and location. Large tumors in the renal pelvis/ calyceal collecting system are likely best managed with a percutaneous approach. Smaller-volume tumors throughout essentially the entirety of the collecting system can be managed with a ureteroscopic approach; however, if choosing a ureteroscopic approach, the surgeon must not compromise oncologic outcomes and should be able to deal with all tumors present. The inability to treat a tumor would be an indication to move onto a more aggressive approach.

One of the first ureteroscopic modalities used in the ureteroscopic management of UTUC was the use of electrocautery, including a ureteroscopic resectoscope. One advantage of ureteroscopy with electrocautery and/or the ureteroscopic resectoscope is that the tumor can largely be debulked with cold cup forceps or ureteroscopic basket and provides for a good specimen from the surgery. Electrocautery is also relatively cheap and widely available to the practicing urologists. Despite these advantages, the use of electrocautery has largely fallen out of favor because dispersion of the energy often results in a transmural injury to the urothelium resulting in postoperative stricture, particularly in the thin-walled ureter [35]. There have also been concerns raised about the systemic effects of the absorption of hypotonic irrigation solutions (glycine, sorbitol, or water) as required when using electrocautery, though the authors would argue that the volume of fluid absorbed during ureteroscopy is quite small and this complication is exceedingly rare.

The use of lasers has become a mainstay in the ureteroscopic management of UTUC. In fact, laser ablation/destruction of the tumor is part of the recommendations from the EAU guidelines. There are a number of different types of lasers available to the practicing urologist, each with its own set of advantages and disadvantages.

There is no consensus on the best laser for the treatment of UTUC, but the three most commonly used lasers are the Holmium:YAG (Ho:YAG), neodymium, and thulium lasers.

The most commonly used laser in ureteroscopic management of UTUC is the holmium:YAG laser. Its popularity is likely multifactorial, but the fact that urologists are already familiar with Ho:YAG and facilities own Ho:YAG lasers because of their use in laser lithotripsy for stone is likely a large influence. The Ho:YAG laser emits energy at a wavelength of 2100 nm, which is rapidly absorbed by water. Because of this, the depth of penetration is about 0.4 mm [17]. This shallow depth of penetration allows for concentration of the energy and is believed to lower the risk of stricture and perforation associated with the use of electric coagulators. Ho:YAG can be used on a variety of settings depending on the goal of the operation. Verges et al. have published recommendations of 0.6–1.0 J at a rate of 5–10 Hz, which is similar to the settings used in our practice [17].

Some authors have advocated for the use of the neodymium:YAG (Nd:YAG) laser in the treatment of UTU, but high-quality studies are currently lacking. The Nd:YAG laser produces a wavelength of 1064 nm, which is absorbed by both water and melanin. The absorption depth of the Nd:YAG is 10+ times that of the Ho:YAG laser at about a 4–6 mm depth. Because of its deeper depth of penetration, the Nd:YAG laser is used mostly for renal pelvis tumors and can be used in conjunction with Ho:YAG with the Nd:YAG being optimally used for tumor volume coagulation and the Ho:YAG to remove/ablate the tissue [17]. Verges et al. recommend using the Nd:YAG laser on a 30 W continuous wave setting while sweeping over the tumor and avoiding circumferential usage to prevent ureteral strictures.

The thulium laser, which has widely been used in the treatment of benign prostatic hyperplasia (BPH), has demonstrated efficacy in the treatment of UTUC in a number of small studies. The thulium laser is available in a number of wattages and produces a wavelength similar to holmium at 2010 nm. This is quite close to the peak for absorption in water at 1940 nm. In contrast to the holmium laser which is a pulsed laser, the thulium laser delivers its energy in a continuous wave. While also available in a pulsed fashion, the continuous wave mode theoretically leads to more efficient vaporization and decreases absorption depth (0.2 mm vs 0.4 mm for holmium) [36, 37]. This continuous wave also creates small microbubbles in the surrounding fluid resulting in less tip vibration and, thus, better precision.

The use of thulium laser in the treatment of UTUC was first published by Defidio et al. in 2011 [38]. In their study they found recurrence-free survival to be noninferior compared to holmium, but with the added benefit of increased precision with less bleeding and less mucosal perforation. The most recent study of the thulium laser in the treatment of UTUC comes from Musi et al. [39]. In this study, 42 consecutive patients were enrolled for conservative management of UTUC with thulium laser. The study cohort most consisted of patients with low-grade disease, but regardless, eight (19%) patients had a recurrence and four (9.5%) underwent subsequent nephroureterectomy over a median follow-up period of 26.3 months. Because they experienced no progression or upstaging of disease with no major complications, the authors contend that thulium is a safe and effective minimally invasive option for the treatment of UTUC. The authors of the above study used 150 W and 200 W lasers on a power setting of 10–20 W, which they state has optimal vapocoagulative effects. Two hundred and seventy-two micrometers were used in cases requiring a flexible ureteroscope and 365 µm for rigid ureteroscopy. The authors started at the cranial end of the lesion and worked caudal, stating that this improves visibility. Finally, the authors recommend lowering the power setting to 5 W or increasing the distance between the fiber and the target to improve coagulation.

Surveillance

Similar to bladder cancer, the recurrence rate of UTUC is quite high and requires stringent follow-up. The true recurrence rate of UTUC is difficult to assess, particularly when managed endoscopically, largely because of the lack of currently available evidence, with most studies of endoscopically UTUC not going beyond 50 months of follow-up [40]. Most recurrences happen within 2 years of initial treatment and can occur anywhere within the collecting system, with recurrence within the urinary bladder being the most common [29]. Some authors believe that if followed indefinitely, all patients with UTUC who are treated endoscopically will have a recurrence [40]. As such, it is important when selecting a patient for endoscopic management that he or she is reliable and understand the importance of close, rigorous follow-up.

In its 2017 guidelines, the EAU recommends the following surveillance for patients who underwent KSS for UTUC (Fig. 15.6) [6]:

1. Perform cystoscopy and CT urography at 3 and 6 months following KSS and then annually for 5 years for patients with low-risk tumors. In patients with high-risk tumors, they add urine cytology to the follow-up regimen at the above-noted intervals.
2. Perform ureteroscopy 3 months after KSS in patients with low-risk tumors.
3. Perform ureteroscopy and selective cytology at 3 and 6 months after KSS in patients with high-risk tumors.

How We Do It

As discussed above, there are a number of different ways to manage UTUC. In this section we discuss specifically how we manage UTUC in our practice. This is meant to be a guide for fellow urologists and does not necessarily represent the "best" way, but rather may provide for improvements in your own practice. Figure 15.7 shows a standard treatment algorithm for UTUC.

Summary of evidence	LE
Follow-up is more frequent and stricter in patients who have undergone kidney-sparing treatment compared to radical nephroureterectomy.	3

Recommendations	GR
After radical nephroureterectomy, >5 yr	
Noninvasive tumour	
Perform cystoscopy/urinary cytology at 3 mo, and then annually.	C
Perform computed tomography urography every year.	C
Invasive tumour	
Perform cystoscopy/urinary cytology at 3 mo, and then annually.	C
Perform computed tomography urography every 6 mo for 2 yr, and then annually.	C
After kidney-sparing management, >5 yr	
Perform urinary cytology and computed tomography urography at 3 and 6 mo, and then annually.	C
Perform cystoscopy, ureteroscopy, and cytology *in situ* at 3 and 6 mo, and then every 6 mo for 2 yr, and then annually.	C
GR = grade of recommendation; LE = level of evidence; UTUC = upper urinary tract urothelial carcinoma.	

Fig. 15.6 EAU recommended follow-up for UTUC. (From Roupret et al., Figs. 2, 4, 6, with permission of Elsevier [6])

Starting from presentation, patients often present with microscopic or gross hematuria, for which CTU is performed. Patients also present as consultations for previous imaging findings worrisome for UTUC. It is our practice to obtain a tissue diagnosis on all patients before offering any sort of treatment. We do not obtain cytology preoperatively. Patients are then consented for cystoscopy, bilateral retrograde pyelograms, bilateral ureteroscopy, and possible ureteral/renal pelvis biopsy and fulguration. First a thorough cystoscopy is performed and suspicious areas are biopsied and fulgurated in a standard fashion. Retrograde pyelography is then performed on the contralateral side of the suspected lesion, because as noted earlier, there is a 1–5% risk of having a synchronous contralateral lesion. It is our practice to not perform retrograde pyelography at the beginning of the case on the side of the suspected lesion as the contrast obscures vision and ureteroscopy is to be performed on that side regardless and is much more sensitive than retrograde pyelography. We do, however, inject contrast at the completion of the case to assess for extravasation and to ensure the ureteral stent is placed in the desired location.

To begin the case on the side of the suspected lesion we perform the "no touch technique" in which a wire is not passed before the ureteroscope. In doing so there is no mucosal trauma before we pass the ureteroscope, and thus presumably

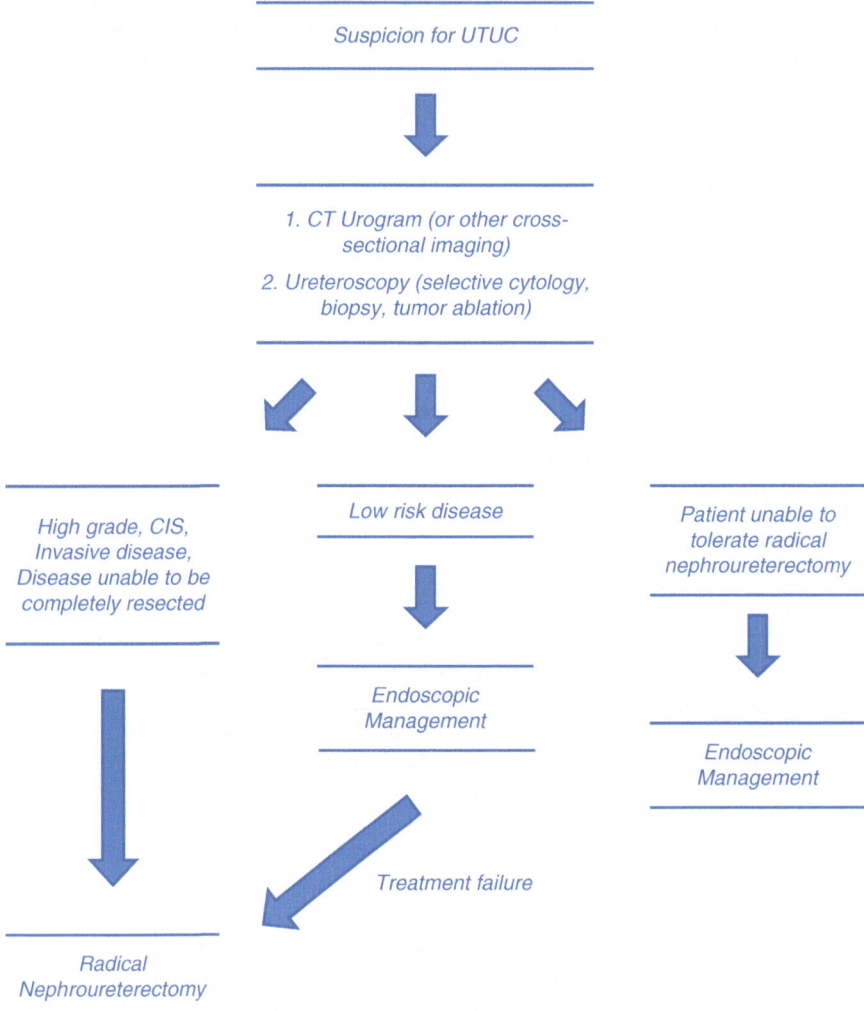

Fig. 15.7 Sample treatment algorithm of UTUC

limiting the possibility of a false positive. Continuous saline irrigation is maintained with the usage of a 60 cc Luer lock syringe affixed to a stopcock and tourniquet tubing. We usually try to drive a flexible ureteroscope through the UO without the assistance of a wire. This is not always possible, and in such cases, we use an angled-tip standard guidewire and pass it a minimal through the ureteroscope to help aid in entering the distal ureter. The entirety of the ureter is then traversed slowly looking for any ureteral lesions. The kidney is then systematically examined as well. Once within the kidney, we often perform barbotage through the working channel of the ureteroscope using normal saline and a 10 cc syringe.

For lesions found within the ureter, a number of options exist. Lesions within the distal ureter may be amendable to using a ureteroscopic resectoscope. The uretero- scopic resectoscope has the advantage of providing a good specimen, but it is quite large in size and usually only goes within the distal ureter. Because it uses electro- coagulative energy, this has a higher risk of causing ureteral strictures and, accord- ingly, should not be done in a circumferential manner. There is also higher risk of ureteral perforation in the thin-walled ureter.

For lesions within the mid to proximal ureter, we try to use a standard 8F semi- rigid ureteroscope. Next to a safety guidewire, we then usually biopsy the lesions multiple times with cold cup biopsy forceps. A 2.4 F flat wire basket works well for papillary lesions which appear to be attached by a stalk. Once debulked by biopsy, the lesion can be further treated either by using a 3F bugbee electrode or via hol- mium laser. Retrograde pyelography is then performed through the ureteroscope, and then a ureteral stent is placed in a standard fashion.

Lesions within the renal collecting system are largely managed the same way as proximal ureteral lesions but must be done through a flexible ureteroscope. Some authors advocate placing a ureteral access sheath if working within the proximal ureter or within the renal collecting system, because it lowers intrarenal pressures and thus allows for better irrigation and theoretically reduces the risk of seeding tumor via pyelovenous and pyelolymphatic backflow. We do not routinely place ureteral access sheaths as we prefer to go via the "no touch technique," but occa- sionally we will place a sheath if debulking a tumor will require multiple passes up into the kidney.

As discussed earlier, in order to manage a patient with UTUC successfully via a ureteroscopic approach, they must be adherent to a stringent surveillance regimen. Deciding on those patients who qualify for ureteroscopic management of UTUC, which again was discussed earlier, should really be done on a case-by-case basis. In our practice, we schedule patients for ureteroscopy for both surveillance and abla- tion every 6 weeks after initial diagnosis until the tumor is completely clear. At the time of those ureteroscopies, we always perform retrograde pyelography on the contralateral side and usually perform barbotage cytology on the side of interest. Once the patient has been cleared of all visible tumor, we then perform ureteroscopy every 3 months for 2 years. If they have a recurrence at any point during that follow- up, the clock resets on the surveillance regimen.

Conclusion

UTUC represents a relatively uncommon neoplasm in which the upper tracts (kid- neys and ureter) are involved with urothelial. Historically, treatment was limited to radical nephroureterectomy. However, a movement has been made to manage UTUC with a nephron-sparing approach, when possible. In this chapter the diagno- sis, management, and surveillance of UTUC using ureteroscopy were discussed. With advancements in technology, the ability of the urologist to manage these tumors in a nephron-sparing fashion is becoming more and more possible. This is particularly fruitful in patients with low-risk disease who, with appropriate follow-up, can still be salvaged with radical nephroureterectomy if they experience recurrences or progression.

References

1. Ploeg M, Aben KK, Kiemeney LA. The present and future burden of urinary bladder cancer in the world. World J Urol. 2009;27(3):289–93.
2. Margulis V, Shariat SF, Matin SF, Kamat AM, Zigeuner R, Kikuchi E, et al. Outcomes of radical nephroureterectomy: a series from the Upper Tract Urothelial Carcinoma Collaboration. Cancer. 2009;115(6):1224–33.
3. Soria F, Shariat SF, Lerner SP, Fritsche HM, Rink M, Kassouf W, et al. Epidemiology, diagnosis, preoperative evaluation and prognostic assessment of upper-tract urothelial carcinoma (UTUC). World J Urol. 2017;35(3):379–87.
4. Mandalapu RS, Matin SF. Contemporary evaluation and management of upper tract urothelial cancer. Urology. 2016;94:17–23.
5. Pan S, Smith AD, Motamedinia P. Minimally invasive therapy for upper tract urothelial cell cancer. J Endourol. 2017;31(3):238–45.
6. Roupret M, Babjuk M, Comperat E, Zigeuner R, Sylvester RJ, Burger M, et al. European Association of Urology Guidelines on upper urinary tract urothelial carcinoma: 2017 update. Eur Urol. 2018;73(1):111–22.
7. Van Der Molen AJ, Cowan NC, Mueller-Lisse UG, Nolte-Ernsting CC, Takahashi S, Cohan RH. CT urography: definition, indications and techniques. A guideline for clinical practice. Eur Radiol. 2008;18(1):4–17.
8. Messer JC, Terrell JD, Herman MP, Ng CK, Scherr DS, Scoll B, et al. Multi-institutional validation of the ability of preoperative hydronephrosis to predict advanced pathologic tumor stage in upper-tract urothelial carcinoma. Urol Oncol. 2013;31(6):904–8.
9. Millan-Rodriguez F, Palou J, de la Torre-Holguera P, Vayreda-Martija JM, Villavicencio-Mavrich H, Vicente-Rodriguez J. Conventional CT signs in staging transitional cell tumors of the upper urinary tract. Eur Urol. 1999;35(4):318–22.
10. Takahashi N, Glockner JF, Hartman RP, King BF, Leibovich BC, Stanley DW, et al. Gadolinium enhanced magnetic resonance urography for upper urinary tract malignancy. J Urol. 2010;183(4):1330–65.
11. Azemar MD, Comperat E, Richard F, Cussenot O, Roupret M. Bladder recurrence after surgery for upper urinary tract urothelial cell carcinoma: frequency, risk factors, and surveillance. Urol Oncol. 2011;29(2):130–6.
12. Fang D, Xiong G, Li X, Kang Y, Zhang L, Zhao G, et al. Incidence, characteristics, treatment strategies, and oncologic outcomes of synchronous bilateral upper tract urothelial carcinoma in the Chinese population. Urol Oncol. 2015;33(2):66.e1–11.
13. Messer J, Shariat SF, Brien JC, Herman MP, Ng CK, Scherr DS, et al. Urinary cytology has a poor performance for predicting invasive or high-grade upper-tract urothelial carcinoma. BJU Int. 2011;108(5):701–5.
14. Malm C, Grahn A, Jaremko G, Tribukait B, Brehmer M. Diagnostic accuracy of upper tract urothelial carcinoma: how samples are collected matters. Scand J Urol. 2017;51(2):137–45.
15. Dodd LG, Johnston WW, Robertson CN, Layfield LJ. Endoscopic brush cytology of the upper urinary tract. Evaluation of its efficacy and potential limitations in diagnosis. Acta Cytol. 1997;41(2):377–84.
16. Hendin BN, Streem SB, Levin HS, Klein EA, Novick AC. Impact of diagnostic ureteroscopy on long-term survival in patients with upper tract transitional cell carcinoma. J Urol. 1999;161(3):783–5.

17. Verges DP, Lallas CD, Hubosky SG, Bagley DH Jr. Endoscopic treatment of upper tract urothelial carcinoma. Curr Urol Rep. 2017;18(4):31.
18. Cho SY. Current status of flexible ureteroscopy in urology. Korean J Urol. 2015;56(10): 680–8.
19. Vashistha V, Shabsigh A, Zynger DL. Utility and diagnostic accuracy of ureteroscopic biopsy in upper tract urothelial carcinoma. Arch Pathol Lab Med. 2013;137(3):400–7.
20. Brown GA, Matin SF, Busby JE, Dinney CP, Grossman HB, Pettaway CA, et al. Ability of clinical grade to predict final pathologic stage in upper urinary tract transitional cell carcinoma: implications for therapy. Urology. 2007;70(2):252–6.
21. Keeley FX, Kulp DA, Bibbo M, McCue PA, Bagley DH. Diagnostic accuracy of ureteroscopic biopsy in upper tract transitional cell carcinoma. J Urol. 1997;157(1):33–7.
22. Kleinmann N, Healy KA, Hubosky SG, Margel D, Bibbo M, Bagley DH. Ureteroscopic biopsy of upper tract urothelial carcinoma: comparison of basket and forceps. J Endourol. 2013;27(12):1450–4.
23. Ritter M, Bolenz C, Bach T, Strobel P, Hacker A. Standardized ex vivo comparison of different upper urinary tract biopsy devices: impact on ureterorenoscopes and tissue quality. World J Urol. 2013;31(4):907–12.
24. Hao YC, Xiao CL, Liu K, Liu YQ, Ma LL. Application of narrow-band imaging flexible ureteroscopy in the diagnosis, treatment and follow-up of upper tract urothelial carcinomas. Zhonghua wai ke za zhi [Chin J Surg]. 2018;56(3):222–6.
25. Osman E, Alnaib Z, Kumar N. Photodynamic diagnosis in upper urinary tract urothelial carcinoma: a systematic review. Arab J Urol. 2017;15(2):100–9.
26. Baard J, Freund JE, de la Rosette JJ, Laguna MP. New technologies for upper tract urothelial carcinoma management. Curr Opin Urol. 2017;27(2):170–5.
27. Audenet F, Traxer O, Yates DR, Cussenot O, Roupret M. Potential role of photodynamic techniques combined with new generation flexible ureterorenoscopes and molecular markers for the management of urothelial carcinoma of the upper urinary tract. BJU Int. 2012;109(4): 608–13; discussion 13–4.
28. Capitanio U, Terrone C, Antonelli A, Minervini A, Volpe A, Furlan M, et al. Nephron-sparing techniques independently decrease the risk of cardiovascular events relative to radical nephrectomy in patients with a T1a-T1b renal mass and normal preoperative renal function. Eur Urol. 2015;67(4):683–9.
29. Seisen T, Colin P, Roupret M. Risk-adapted strategy for the kidney-sparing management of upper tract tumours. Nat Rev Urol. 2015;12(3):155–66.
30. Bin X, Roy OP, Ghiraldi E, Manglik N, Liang T, Vira M, et al. Impact of tumour location and surgical approach on recurrence-free and cancer-specific survival analysis in patients with ureteric tumours. BJU Int. 2012;110(11 Pt B):E514–9.
31. Fajkovic H, Klatte T, Nagele U, Dunzinger M, Zigeuner R, Hubner W, et al. Results and outcomes after endoscopic treatment of upper urinary tract carcinoma: the Austrian experience. World J Urol. 2013;31(1):37–44.
32. Grasso M, Fishman AI, Cohen J, Alexander B. Ureteroscopic and extirpative treatment of upper urinary tract urothelial carcinoma: a 15-year comprehensive review of 160 consecutive patients. BJU Int. 2012;110(11):1618–26.
33. Hoffman A, Yossepowitch O, Erlich Y, Holland R, Lifshitz D. Oncologic results of nephron sparing endoscopic approach for upper tract low grade transitional cell carcinoma in comparison to nephroureterectomy – a case control study. BMC Urol. 2014;14:97.
34. Roupret M, Hupertan V, Traxer O, Loison G, Chartier-Kastler E, Conort P, et al. Comparison of open nephroureterectomy and ureteroscopic and percutaneous management of upper urinary tract transitional cell carcinoma. Urology. 2006;67(6):1181–7.
35. Raman JD, Park R. Endoscopic management of upper-tract urothelial carcinoma. Expert Rev Anticancer Ther. 2017;17(6):545–54.
36. Barbalat Y, Velez MC, Sayegh CI, Chung DE. Evidence of the efficacy and safety of the thulium laser in the treatment of men with benign prostatic obstruction. Ther Adv Urol. 2016;8(3):181–91.

37. Fried NM, Murray KE. High-power thulium fiber laser ablation of urinary tissues at 1.94 microm. J Endourol. 2005;19(1):25–31.
38. Defidio L, De Dominicis M, Di Gianfrancesco L, Fuchs G, Patel A. First collaborative experience with thulium laser ablation of localized upper urinary tract urothelial tumors using retrograde intra-renal surgery. Arch Ital Urol Androl: Organo Ufficiale Soc Ital Ecografia Urol Nefrol. 2011;83(3):147–53.
39. Musi G, Mistretta FA, Marenghi C, Russo A, Catellani M, Nazzani S, et al. Thulium laser treatment of upper urinary tract carcinoma: a multi-institutional analysis of surgical and oncological outcomes. J Endourol. 2018;32(3):257–63.
40. Cutress ML, Stewart GD, Zakikhani P, Phipps S, Thomas BG, Tolley DA. Ureteroscopic and percutaneous management of upper tract urothelial carcinoma (UTUC): systematic review. BJU Int. 2012;110(5):614–28.

Chapter 16
Simulation and Ureteroscopy (URS)

Dima Raskolnikov, Tony Chen, and Robert M. Sweet

Abbreviations

CAD	Canadian dollar
CREST	Center for Research in Education and Simulation Technologies
C-SATS	Crowd-Sourced Assessment of Technical Skills
FFC	Fresh-frozen cadaver
OSATS	Objective Structured Assessment of Technical Skills
TeamSTEPPS	Team Strategies and Tools to Enhance Performance and Patient Safety
TEC	Thiel-embalmed cadaver
VR	Virtual reality

Introduction

Today's endourologists are confronted with a surgical training landscape far different from those of their predecessors. Historically, surgical residency was founded upon the principles of Halsted and the "see one, do one, teach one" model of graduated responsibility [1]. This tradition has been met with modern environmental factors that challenge its sustainability. Work-hour restrictions have led to decreased case volumes for surgical trainees [2]. Public concerns regarding medical errors as a cause of patient harm have led to a more hands-on approach to trainee supervision in the operating room. Even experienced surgeons, years out in practice, need to

D. Raskolnikov · T. Chen
Department of Urology, University of Washington, Seattle, WA, USA

R. M. Sweet (✉)
Department of Urology, University of Washington, Seattle, WA, USA

Department of Surgery, WWAMI Institute for Simulation in Healthcare (WISH), University of Washington, Seattle, WA, USA
e-mail: rsweet@uw.edu

© Springer Nature Switzerland AG 2020
B. F. Schwartz, J. D. Denstedt (eds.), *Ureteroscopy*,
https://doi.org/10.1007/978-3-030-26649-3_16

constantly acquire new technical skills in the face of rapid technological advancements in endourology. With the learning curve for flexible ureteroscopy currently being estimated at approximately 60 cases, surgical simulation is leaned upon to supplement and enhance the traditional surgical training experience [3]. This belief is being increasingly championed by urologic societies including the European Association of Urology Section of Urolithiasis, whose 2017 consensus statement strongly encourages the incorporation of simulation modalities in endourologic training [4].

A simulator is simply any "modality that is designed to represent real conditions" [5]. What can be considered a simulator spans a wide array of platforms and models ranging from physical cadaveric tissue to digital representations. How well a simulator represents real conditions and how useful it may be to achieve a targeted educational or procedural endpoint requires study and validation. Before proceeding to describe the current space of available ureteroscopy simulators, there will be an introductory review of concepts and terminology necessary to understand a simulator's level of fidelity and validity. The technical design and creation of simulator models are beyond the scope of this chapter.

Concepts in Simulation

The evaluation of a simulator comprises assessing for fidelity, reliability, and overall validity. Knowing the keywords and definitions surrounding these concepts is necessary in order to understand the literature surrounding simulator testing.

Fidelity

The concept of fidelity describes the degree of faithfulness to an intended construct. Ureteroscopy simulators are often described in terms of low or high fidelity, but this is an oversimplification. There are several domains of fidelity that are not mutually inclusive or exclusive of each other: *anatomic, tissue, physiologic, and affective fidelity*. Anatomic fidelity describes how well the simulator replicates the physical structures of interest, such as length and caliber of the ureter or the size and orientation of the renal calyces or presence of anatomic landmarks. On the other hand, tissue fidelity speaks to how well the physical behaviors and characteristics of human tissue are replicated, such as the elasticity or coefficient of friction of the ureter. Physiologic fidelity relates to the degree to which a model represents a physiologic state or process [6]. Affective fidelity describes how well a simulation can engage a participant into suspending his or her disbelief that the procedure or scenario is a simulation [7]. A simulator may simultaneously have both high- and low-fidelity domains. For example, an extracorporeal membrane oxygenation machine can be considered to have high physiologic fidelity for the process of replicating physiologic gas exchange but completely lacks anatomic or tissue fidelity of the human heart and lung.

Validity

The decision upon whether to use a simulation-based educational tool or curriculum is related directly to its ability to achieve a given set of educational goals/objectives. This is done through gathering *validity evidence*. Historically, validity was described within a framework that included terms such as construct validity, criterion validity, and content validity. This was based on 1966 recommendations by the American Psychological Association, the American Educational Research Association, and the National Council on Measurement in Education. This framework was updated several times, most recently in 2014. Highlights of the significant changes will be reviewed in subsequent sections. Unfortunately, existing publications related to validity for ureteroscopy was heavily designed and based upon on historical definitions. It is thus important to know both the historical and updated validity definitions.

Historical Validity Terminology

Validity was previously divided into subjective and objective metrics, defined by the types of data used to assess them. *Subjective validity* relies on survey response data and includes *content validity*, which is how comprehensively the intended construct is represented as judged by experts and *face validity* which is how well a simulator appears to replicate its intended construct on a more superficial level.

Objective validity, divided into *construct* and *criterion validity*, used structured scoring metrics to assess a simulator's validity, such as the Objective Structured Assessment of Technical Skills (OSATS) format. Construct validity was often defined as a simulator's ability to discern between classifications of perceived skill, such as "novice and an expert." *Criterion validity*, which relates new and previous simulators, can be subdivided into *concurrent validity*, which benchmarks the simulator's assessments against the existing "gold standard," and *predictive validity*, which evaluates the simulator's ability to correlate with future performance [8].

Updated Validity Terminology

With the 2014 update, validity terminology has shifted away from the abovementioned framework. The current definition of validity is "the degree to which evidence and theory support the interpretation of simulator data/scores for measuring a certain construct," where a construct is "the concepts or characteristics that a simulator is designed to measure" [9]. This reflects the belief that simulator validation is a perpetual process of hypothesis-driven evidence gathering and also that construct validity is of main importance. The updated guidelines refer to five sources of validity evidence including *content, response processes, internal structure, relations with other variables, and consequences*. Content evidence evaluates the appropriateness of the simulator's educational content and learning objectives to the intended construct. Response processes evidence ensures learners and evaluators are in agreement with respect to the intended construct and evaluation metrics. Internal structure evidence describes the appropriateness and reliability of individual simulator components with the overall intended construct. Relations with other variables evidence evaluates how the simulator scores statistically against varying rubrics or models. Consequences evidence assesses how the simulator's assessments may be used to impact the learner or society as a whole [10]. Taken together, the new validity terminology is a holistic approach to simulator validation and takes into account the principle that varying purposes, learning objectives, and learner audiences will naturally require different simulators—a nuance that was lost in the previous validity terminology. Knowing the historical terminology is necessary to understand the methods and results of existing simulation evidence, but understanding modern validity theory is necessary to move the field of simulation forward.

Reliability

Reliability deserves special mention and is a measure of the reproducibility of the effects or outputs of a training system and is considered a critical part of the abovementioned "internal structure" aspects of validity [10]. Reliability is depicted as an r-value correlation coefficient between 0 and 1, and acceptable reliability values depend upon the application, but for the most part, $r \geq 0.8$ is desirable for highstakes assessment. The reproducibility of a simulator's results or effects across varying factors includes test-retest reliability for different versions of examination, inter-station reliability for different tasks or stations within a simulation, and interrater reliability for reproducibility across different observers. Test-retest reliability describes how consistent a simulator's effects on a subject is, whereas inter or intraobserver reliability describes the consistency of interactions between the simulator and designated observers or evaluators [8, 11].

Simulation Models

Driven by educational learning objectives, curriculum and model developers have taken a variety of approaches to create training strategies to meet the training and assessment needs for ureteroscopic procedures. Each approach has its own unique set of strengths and limitations. Not only must the platforms be practical, they must also take into account ethical and financial considerations that might limit widespread deployment. A variety of approaches to simulation curriculum and model development has thus emerged. For the purpose of comparison, these models may be grouped into those based on human cadavers, animal models, benchtop models, and virtual reality. Some have validity evidence simply for the model itself (old validity theory), while others have validity evidence as part of a curriculum designed around a well-defined construct (modern theory). As we describe these systems and you consider the evidence provided, it is important to take note of this difference.

Human Cadavers

Despite advances in both materials sciences and computer processing technology, human cadavers remain the gold standard for ureteroscopy simulation platforms due to their high tissue and anatomic fidelity [12]. However, they also have some of the highest barriers to scalability. These competing factors are well demonstrated by the existing simulation literature. Ahmed et al. reported the results of a comprehensive endourological training program developed by the British Association of Urological Surgeons that was based on fresh-frozen cadaver (FFC) models [13]. The authors enrolled 81 residents in a 3-day training program, with 2 trainees allocated to each FFC simulator along with an expert endoscopist for supervision. The residents completed training modules which covered core upper tract endoscopic skills including flexible and semirigid ureteroscopy. After completion, trainee and faculty participants assessed the curriculum on an evaluation survey. All respondents rated the simulators >3/5 on a Likert scale on measures of fidelity and validity, noting that the curriculum is particularly useful for learning anatomy, steps of an operation, and fostering transferrable surgical skills. While this study is notable for its relatively large size, it also highlights the challenges of FFCs-based simulators. The authors commented that the program cost was £17,150, nearly all of which was supported by a combination of delegate fees and sponsorship. If implemented widely, the current cost of procuring and storing FFCs at a ratio of 1:2 trainees is likely prohibitive, even when excluding the opportunity cost of faculty needed to supervise each station. In addition, FFCs are variable and lack standardization, which challenges the validity of the use of FFCs for assessment.

Huri et al. evaluated a training curriculum that included both FFC simulators and those based on Thiel-embalmed cadavers (TEC) [14]. Twelve urologists without prior endoscopic experience underwent a flexible ureteroscopy course using these models. Before and after course completion, participants performed a standardized set of tasks intended to simulate treatment of a renal calyceal stone. After simulator training, all participants demonstrated statistically significant improvements in task completion times. At the end of the course, fluoroscopy did not reveal anatomic damage to any cadaver. All ureteroscopes maintained functional integrity as well. While this study was neither designed nor powered to detect differences between FFC- and TEC-based simulators, the authors noted that both models offered high fidelity. They also noted that cadaveric models offer a bloodless field, absence of respiratory variation, and decreased ureteric tone. Each of these characteristics could potentially be construed as an advantage or disadvantage, depending on the learning objectives of the simulation activity.

Lastly, Mains et al. reported the results of an inaugural "Master Class in Flexible Ureteroscopy," a 2-day training program utilizing TEC simulators to teach flexible ureteroscopy [15]. Eight trainees underwent a training program under the supervision of expert endoscopists, with focused training on three available TEC simulators. Participants completed qualitative questionnaires after simulation training. Results demonstrated high degrees of simulator fidelity and validity, as well as subjectively high durability.

Collectively, these three studies robustly demonstrate the relative strengths and weaknesses of cadaveric simulation curricula for ureteroscopy. Anatomic and tissue fidelity are both high, suggesting that TEC- and FFC-based simulators may be most appropriate for teaching specific aspects of ureteroscopy that depend on these specific properties. On the other hand, resource constraints, the need for subjective evaluation of skills, and the lack of standardization inherent to these models may limit their appropriateness for widespread use. Capital costs may be particularly prohibitive outside of university settings where cadavers are widely used for other types of educational programming.

Animal Models

Comparative studies of porcine and human renal anatomy have demonstrated many similarities, both with respect to vasculature and the structure of the collecting system [16]. For this reason, porcine animal models have offered a compelling platform for urological simulation. Soria et al. developed a training curriculum that combined the use of non-biologic simulators, biologic simulators, and a live porcine model for retrograde intrarenal surgery [17]. The authors enrolled 60 urologists without ureteroscopic experience in a 2-day course that culminated in endoscopic stone treatment in a porcine animal model of bilateral nephrolithiasis. A questionnaire was then used to evaluate what would now include content aspects of validity, which was completed by both trainees and their instructors. The porcine simulator was rated as having favorable face, content, and construct validity using the old validity terminology. Most trainees improved their endoscopic skills by >40% as measured by a structured checklist. The authors noted that this multifaceted approach to simulation in ureteroscopy was well received, with the strongest potential role for in vivo porcine models for additional mastery in those who had developed basic ureteroscopic skills.

Strohmaier provided one of the earliest descriptions of an ex vivo porcine model that could be used for urological simulation [18]. Building on this work, Hu et al. developed a ureteroscopy simulator using isolated porcine kidneys and ureters that were purchased from a local slaughterhouse [19]. Twenty urologists were assigned to flexible ureteroscopy tasks, which were then graded on time and skill by experienced evaluators. After training on the simulator, task completion time significantly decreased, and a greater number of trainees attained a subjective "pass" rating. Though this study is limited in its generalizability due to a nonstandard grading scheme, it does demonstrate that an anatomically relevant ex vivo simulator can be locally purchased without significant procurement or storage costs.

As with FFC models, animal models lack standardization and require subjective evaluation limiting assessment capabilities. While further research is necessary to elucidate the effects of ureteroscopy simulation on porcine cadavers, this modality may offer an appealing degree of fidelity without introducing many of the limitations inherent to human FFC/TEC simulators.

Benchtop Models

While human- and animal-based simulation models have inherently high fidelity, synthetic benchtop models introduce their own unique advantages. Several benchtop ureteroscopy simulators are thus now commercially available. Broadly, these trainers may be categorized as those that augment the user experience with virtual reality (VR) and those that do not. Unlike the cadaveric simulator space, benchtop models also benefit from a greater number of validation studies evaluating their relative efficacy.

Non-virtual Reality-Based Simulators

The Uro-Scopic Trainer (Limbs & Things, UK) is a physical model that incorporates the pelvis, urethra, bladder, ureters, and collecting system, allowing for simulation of either flexible or semirigid ureteroscopy (Fig. 16.1). Matsumoto evaluated 17 urology residents in endoscopic task completion using this model [20]. The residents were asked to perform ureteroscopy and remove a simulated mid-ureteral stone within the Uro-Scopic Trainer, both before and after completing a didactic session followed by supervised practice on the Uro-Scopic Trainer. Simulation resulted in significant improvement in performance measured on a global rating scale, checklist, and task completion time. Interobserver reliability in these measurements was high. It should be noted that some of these gains were realized after just the didactic session alone. However, the authors concluded that a combined didactic and practical curriculum utilizing the Uro-Scopic Trainer is an effective way to help prepare resident for operative ureteroscopy.

The Scope Trainer (Mediskills, UK) is another benchtop simulator that features an expandable bladder, normal length ureters, and two kidneys with renal pelves and calyces. Brehmer initially evaluated 14 urologists with a mix of endoscopic experience in task-specific skills which they performed on both live patients and the Scope Trainer [21]. All participants considered the simulator to be representative of live flexible ureteroscopy, suggesting high content validity. Construct validity was also demonstrated, as those participants with subspecialty endourological training scored significantly higher than the rest of the cohort when evaluated on a task-specific

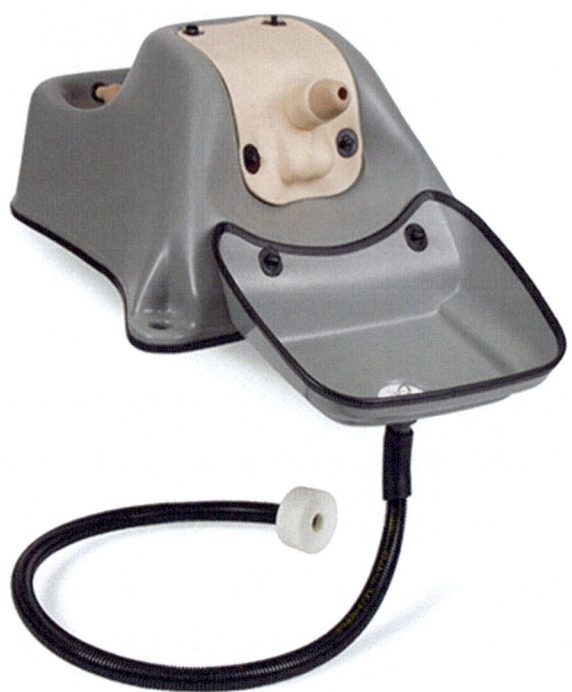

checklist. Brehmer then explored the ability of the Scope Trainer to improve dexterity for semirigid ureteroscopy [22]. Using a validated OSATS protocol [23], his group evaluated 26 urology residents in semirigid ureteroscopy skills after a focused training course on the benchtop model. Trainees demonstrated a statistically significant improvement in scores and reported increased familiarity with the procedure.

The Center for Research in Education and Simulation Technologies (CREST) developed an endoscopic urinary tract model (Simagine Health, USA) that was the first to utilize 3D printing techniques for urologic models. Organosilicate models were made with intraluminal tissue-analogous textures to simulate the human renal collecting system (Fig. 16.2). This benchtop model was initially piloted by Kishore et al. with a cohort of residents at their own institution that demonstrated good validity evidence, but it wasn't blinded [23]. It was subsequently "taken on the road" by Argun et al. to evaluate residents in a blinded three institutional study of various core ureteroscopic skills using a similar OSATS for endourology evaluation tool [24]. Refinements to the tool were provided by evaluating validity evidence of items of the pilot study. This curriculum/model has high construct and internal validity, and the model has been used at multiple AUA and industry-sponsored hands-on courses since.

White et al. examined validity evidence for the Adult Ureteroscopy Trainer (Ideal Anatomic Modeling, USA), a benchtop model that was created with rapid

Fig. 16.2 The CREST
ureteroscopy trainer.
(Courtesy of Simagine
Health, USA)

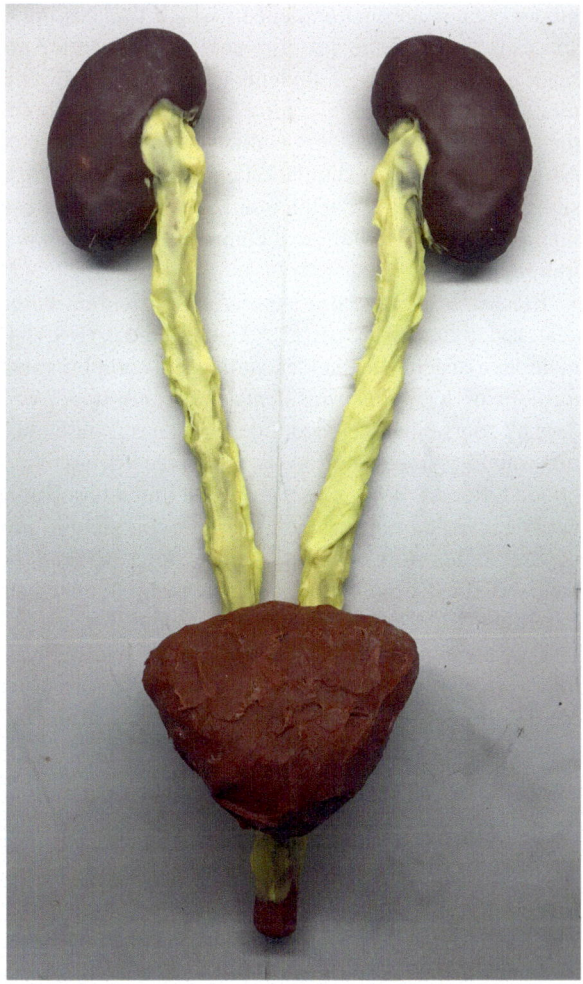

prototyping based on the collecting system of a patient with recurrent nephrolithiasis [25]. A mix of 46 resident and faculty urologists were asked to perform ureteroscopy and basket manipulation of a lower pole stone in the Trainer while supervised by an experienced endourologist. Afterwards, participants completed a questionnaire to evaluate their experience. Results demonstrated robust face, content, and construct validity, as well as high fidelity. Other groups have replicated this process in creating phantoms of the human kidney with intact collecting systems using 3D printing [26].

Villa et al. described the Key-Box (Porgès-Coloplast, France), a benchtop model that is unique in that it does not seek to model significant anatomic or tissue fidelity [27]. Instead, it is composed of a set of maze-like boxes that are designed to be traversed with a flexible ureteroscope. Instead of reproducing human anatomy, the model creates an environment in which trainees are forced to navigate complex spaces to facilitate the dexterity necessary for future ureteroscopy in humans. Villa randomized 16 medical students to either a 10-day training period with this new model or a non-training control [28]. The endoscopic skills of both groups were then assessed by an expert endourologist using a scale developed by Matsumoto [29]. The group with simulation experience scored significantly higher in all measures, including task completion time. The authors concluded that despite its low fidelity, the Key-Box offers a compelling starting point for benchtop ureteroscopy training.

Blankstein described a simulation curriculum based on a ureteroscopy trainer designed by Cook Medical (Cook Medical, USA) [30]. This benchtop model includes a distensible bladder, simple and complex calyceal systems, and a modeled tortuous ureter. Fifteen residents at various stages of training were enrolled in a 2-week course that included didactic lectures, individualized feedback, and simulation training. Trainee performance was recorded on video and then reviewed by two blinded experts. When compared to an initial baseline assessment, postcourse evaluations revealed improvements in task completion times and overall performance scores. Scores correlated with trainee ureteroscopy experience, and 80% of participants rated the benchtop model as realistic. Collectively, the simulator was felt to have high face, content, and construct validity.

The advantages of all of these models and their associated curricula are their relatively low-cost, standardized nature. Portability and usability vary widely among the systems described above. They, like the biologic systems, still require subjective means of assessment.

Virtual Reality-Based Simulators

The URO Mentor (Symbionix, Israel) sought to enhance benchtop model simulator design by augmenting the user's experience with a virtual reality (VR) component. Initially described by Michel, the simulator is composed of a computer workstation, proprietary software, and a mannequin with associated cystoscopes and ureteroscopes (Fig. 16.3) [31]. These tools not only allow trainees to simulate a variety of endourological procedures, but the system also captures performance data, potentially reducing the high cost of expert supervision needed for conventional benchtop models. Watterson et al. randomized 20 novice trainees to either no training or individualized instruction on the URO Mentor [32]. Before and after intervention, the simulated endoscopic skills of the two groups were assessed both subjectively by blinded observers and objectively by data collected through the simulator. Post-testing revealed significant improvements in all measurements in the training group, with high correlation between the simulator and blinded observer ratings. Though encouraging, such results must be interpreted in light of their limited generalizability, since performance on a simulator is not necessarily generalizable to operative skill.

Fig. 16.3 The URO
Mentor simulator.
(Courtesy of 3D Systems,
USA)

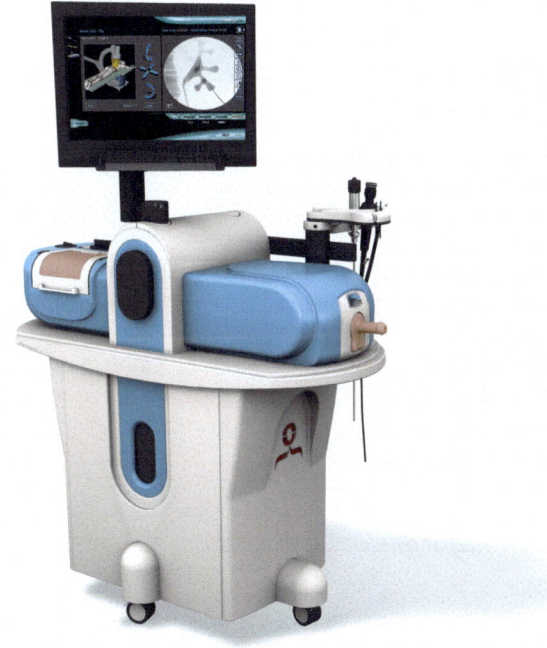

Since that initial report, multiple other groups have examined for validity evidence for the URO Mentor. Wilhelm et al. evaluated 21 medical students in simulated proximal ureteral stone manipulation, with or without training on the URO Mentor [33]. This group's results largely mirrored the results of the Watterson trial [32]. Jacomides et al. performed a similar study, though enrolled a mix of medical students, junior, and senior residents, all of whom underwent simulation training over several sessions [34]. Post-intervention assessment revealed a benefit for all groups, with medical students demonstrating the greatest degree of improvement. In light of resource constraints, simulation time may be most effective if focused on those with the least endourological experience.

Ogan et al. measured the effect of URO Mentor simulation with respect to subsequent human cadaveric ureteroscopy for both medical students and residents [35]. Trainees were evaluated at baseline on the URO Mentor, underwent 5 h of supervised simulator training, re-evaluated on the URO Mentor, and then performed diagnostic ureteroscopy on a human cadaver while supervised by experienced endourologists. Interestingly, post-training URO Mentor and cadaveric ureteroscopy performance scores correlated strongly for medical students, but not for residents. In the resident group, cadaveric simulation scores more closely correlated with resident postgraduate year level. The authors speculated that VR-based measurements may not be the most appropriate tools for measuring performance of experienced operators, like those residents who had volunteered for their study. They noted that the high cost (approximately $60,000) of the URO Mentor platform may be potentially offset by reductions in operative time.

Knoll et al. compared the performance of experienced and inexperienced urologists during simulated treatment of a lower calyceal stone, also on the URO Mentor simulator [36]. Performance was graded on completion time, stone contact time, complications, and treatment success. Of the 20 participants, those with <40 and >80 previous flexible ureteroscopy cases had statistically significant differences in performance, suggesting robust construct validity. In a larger study, Dolmans et al. asked 89 urologic trainees and faculty to perform endoscopic manipulation of a distal ureteral stone using the URO Mentor [37]. Afterwards, the participants completed a questionnaire about their experience. Of the respondents, 25% rated the realism of the URO Mentor ≥3.5 on a 5-point scale. While 82% felt that it was a useful educational tool, 73% reported that they would purchase the URO Mentor "if financial means were available" [37]. Advantages of the system are standardization and objective means of assessment. Poor force-feedback, inaccurate tool-tissue responses, and cost/unit represent downsides.

Cross-Platform Comparisons

Given the challenges inherent to validating a ureteroscopy simulation platform in isolation, it is hardly surprising that even less data exists to support meaningful cross-platform comparisons. However, that data which does exist is informative. Misha et al. compared the effects of simulation training using two conventional benchtop simulators – the Uro-Scopic Trainer and the Endo-Urologie-Modell (Karl Storz, Germany) – to training with the VR-based URO Mentor [38]. Twenty-one urologists without ureteroscopic experience rotated through all three simulators, each time being graded on endoscopic performance by expert endoscopist. At the end of the day, they completed an evaluation questionnaire. Interestingly, no difference was seen in the degree of improvement that the urologists experience from one station type to another. Participants did, however, rate the URO Mentor experience as having the highest face validity, but given the subjects were without Ureteroscopic experience, this diminishes the impact of such a determination. For example, participants often noted that the URO Mentor offered an opportunity to simulate the challenge posed by respiratory variation.

Chou et al. recruited 16 first year medical students to undergo didactic training on ureteroscopy, followed by randomization to either focused simulator practice with the Uro-Scopic Trainer or with the URO Mentor [39]. Two months later, the participants performed an endoscopic mid-ureteral stone procedure on an ex vivo kidney/ureter model, which was assessed by an expert endoscopist. No statistically significant difference was detected between the two groups, suggesting that didactics followed by training on either platform may be similarly effective.

Matsumoto has explored trainee performance on ureteroscopy simulation in a variety of settings. In a 2002 study, this group randomized 40 fourth year medical students to a didactic session, training with the Uro-Scopic Trainer, or training with a low-fidelity model [29]. The low-fidelity model was constructed from a Penrose drain, a cup, molded latex, and two straws, with a total production cost of $20 CAD. Afterwards, the participants were graded by blinded examiners on their ability to basket extract a mid-ureteral stone. Despite the $3,700 CAD cost of the Uro-Scopic Trainer, students assigned to that group performed no better than those who have used the low-fidelity simulator. Both of these groups scored higher than those who received the didactic session alone. In a later study, Matsumoto evaluated the ability of 16 residents to extract a distal ureteral stone using the URO Mentor [40]. This performance was then compared to their ability to complete a similar task using the Uro-Scopic Trainer. Those trainees with more experience scored higher than their junior colleagues, and for both groups, the performance was comparable across platforms.

Crowdsourcing

Even more recent technological innovations have introduced new opportunities for improvement in surgical simulation. Dai et al. described the role of crowdsourced feedback for surgical education, leveraging platforms like Amazon Mechanical Turk [41]. Crowdsourcing involves the use of a large cohort of non-experts to perform a specific task, like evaluating technical performance. In their analysis of the existing surgical literature, crowd and expert evaluations correlated closely. Non-expert evaluation was also faster and more cost-effective. Conti et al. explored this possibility for ureteroscopic simulation in particular [42]. In their study, the video recordings of 30 residents performing ureteroscopic stone treatment were submitted to the Crowd-Sourced Assessment of Technical Skills (C-SATS, Inc., Seattle, WA) platform for crowd-based assessment. The videos were also scored by faculty endourologists blinded to resident level of training. Both groups used a previously validated evaluation tool intended for ureteroscopy. Not only did the crowd-sourced evaluations fail to correlate with expert evaluations, the expert evaluations themselves had poor interobserver reliability. The authors conclude that video-only evaluation of ureteroscopic skill may be inappropriate. On the other hand, the study similarly highlighted one of the main advantages of the crowd: while expert evaluation turnover ranged from 1 to 9 weeks, crowd workers completed 2,488 evaluations in 36 h.

Nontechnical Skills (NTS)

Nontechnical skill describes a set of behaviors that include cognitive skills, social skills, and personal resource factors that collectively enhance interprofessional collaboration, teamwork, and miscommunication prevention. With a 2013 *Journal of Patient Safety* study concluding that between 210,000 and 400,000 deaths per year in the United States are due to preventable errors such as communications breakdowns, NTS' impact on patient care is increasingly being studied [43]. Communication skills are critical in the operating room during ureteroscopy, as basketing and guide-wire handling are often dependent on the surgeon and assistant working together. The potential demand for reducing the surgeon's reliance on an assistant for stone basketing has led to the marketing of technologies like the Lithovue Empower (Boston Scientific, USA) single-surgeon basketing device. However, the role of the assistant will likely persist in the near future, and the ability of the surgeon to have the skillset necessary to efficiently work in a team environment is indispensable. To this end, nontechnical skill-based literature within urology is in its infancy, but a study by Brunkhorst et al. has demonstrated that incorporating NTS training within a curriculum has measurable benefits [44]. Additional focus and training in this general area are needed, and some of the groundwork has been established by the US Agency for Healthcare Research and Quality, which has developed a program entitled Team Strategies and Tools to Enhance Performance and Patient Safety TeamSTEPPS®, an evidence-based curriculum which seems to improve teamwork and communication between professionals in healthcare environments [45].

Future Directions

Simulation in ureteroscopy moving forward will no doubt benefit from the burgeoning of technological advancements that will enable higher-fidelity virtual and augmented reality and lower-cost higher-quality models. It is crucial that with increasing integration of simulation into ureteroscopy training, the field addresses some of the inherent limitations in the existing scientific literature. The updated validity paradigm requires many existing simulators to be reassessed and to have additional validity evidence gathered with a focus on gathering validity evidence around intended use with intended populations. Additional studies with participant demographics appropriate to the intended simulator end-user are needed (i.e., a simulator validated with senior medical students cannot have its conclusions applied to residents or attendings). Studies are also needed to translate simulator and training performance to improved patient outcomes to help justify the resource investment. Governing bodies and specialty societies will be well-positioned to assume the responsibilities of creating, standardizing, implementing, and gathering validity evidence of simulation curriculum, as evidenced by the Netherlands already implementing a progressive program of formal, national-level training curricula [46]. Finally, there is a growing a trend towards outsourcing assessments to crowd-sourced human evaluators or automated means of assessment with embedded data-driven sensors in physical models and/or VR models to reduce the growing burden of expert assessment [41].

Conclusions

While simulation does not replace the need for first-hand ureteroscopy experience, the available technologies and curricula seek to augment the acquisition of skills in this surgery. A wide range of simulation modalities have been described with varying ranges of fidelity each with unique benefits and drawbacks. Having a good understanding of modern validity evidence theory, the intended learner audience, and how a particular simulator may fit into such a construct is necessary to guide the appropriate simulator choice. As the field of simulation in ureteroscopy matures, the authors expect formal and standardized curricula incorporating both technical and nontechnical skills to become increasingly adopted. Technology will continue to mature to bring more cost-effective higher-fidelity simulator models to this future-looking discipline.

References

1. Reznick RK, MacRae H. Teaching surgical skills – changes in the wind. N Engl J Med. 2006;355(25):2664–9.
2. Chikwe J, de Souza AC, Pepper JR. No time to train the surgeons. BMJ. 2004;328(7437):418–9.
3. Quirke K, Aydin A, Brunckhorst O, et al. Learning curves in urolithiasis surgery: a systematic review. J Endourol. 2018;32(11):1008–20.
4. Ahmed K, Patel S, Aydin A, et al. European Association of Urology Section of Urolithiasis (EULIS) consensus statement on simulation, training, and assessment in urolithiasis. Eur Urol Focus. 2018l;4(4):614–20. https://doi.org/10.1016/j.euf.2017.03.006. Epub 2017 Mar 31.
5. Cambridge Dictionary.
6. Talbot TB. Balancing physiology, anatomy and immersion: how much biological fidelity is necessary in a medical simulation? Mil Med. 2013;178(10S):28–36.
7. Volante M, Babu SV, Chaturvedi H, et al. Effects of virtual human appearance fidelity on emotion contagion in affective inter-personal simulations. IEEE Trans Vis Comput Graph. 2016;22(4):1326–35.
8. McDougall EM. Validation of surgical simulators. J Endourol. 2007;21(3):244–7.
9. American Educational Research Association, American Psychological Association, and National Council on Measurement in Education. Standards for educational and psychological testing. Washington, DC: American Educational Research Association; 2014.
10. Noureldin YA, Sweet RM. A call for a shift in theory and terminology for validation studies in urologic education. J Urol. 2017;2017:3–6.
11. Cook DA, Zendejas B, Hamstra SJ, Hatala R, Brydges R. What counts as validity evidence? Examples and prevalence in a systematic review of simulation-based assessment. Adv Health Sci Educ Theory Pract. 2014;19(2):233–50.
12. Anastakis DJ, Regehr G, Reznick RK, et al. Assessment of technical skills transfer from the bench training model to the human model. Am J Surg. 1999;177(2):167–70.
13. Ahmed K, Aydin A, Dasgupta P, Khan MS, McCabe JE. A novel cadaveric simulation program in urology. J Surg Educ. 2015;72(4):556–65.
14. Huri E, Skolarikos A, Tatar İ, et al. Simulation of RIRS in soft cadavers: a novel training model by the Cadaveric Research On Endourology Training (CRET) Study Group. World J Urol. 2016;34(5):741–6.

15. Mains E, Tang B, Golabek T, et al. Ureterorenoscopy training on cadavers embalmed by Thiel's method: simulation or a further step towards reality? Initial report. Cent Eur J Urol. 2017;70(1):81–7.
16. Pereira-Sampaio MA, Favorito LA, Sampaio FJB. Pig kidney: anatomical relationships between the intrarenal arteries and the kidney collecting system. Applied study for urological research and surgical training. J Urol. 2004;172(5 I):2077–81.
17. Soria F, Morcillo E, Serrano A, et al. Development and validation of a novel skills training model for retrograde intrarenal surgery. J Endourol. 2015;29(11):1276–81.
18. Strohmaier WL, Giese A. Porcine urinary tract as a training model for ureteroscopy. Urol Int. 2001;66(1):30–2.
19. Hu D, Liu T, Wang X. Flexible ureteroscopy training for surgeons using isolated porcine kidneys in vitro endourology and technology. BMC Urol. 2015;15(1):1–4.
20. Matsumoto ED, Hamstra SJ, Radomski SB, Cusimano MD. A novel approach to endourological training: training at the Surgical Skills Center. J Urol. 2001;166(4):1261–6.
21. Brehmer M, Tolley DA. Validation of a bench model for endoscopic surgery in the upper urinary tract. Eur Urol. 2002;42(2):175–80.
22. Brehmer M, Swartz R. Training on bench models improves dexterity in ureteroscopy. Eur Urol. 2005;48(3):458–63.
23. Kishore TA, Pedro RN, Monga M, Sweet RM. Assessment of validity of an OSATS for cystoscopic and ureteroscopic cognitive and psychomotor skills. J Endourol. 2008;22(12):2707–12.
24. Argun OB, Chrouser K, Chauhan S, et al. Multi-institutional validation of an OSATS for the assessment of cystoscopic and ureteroscopic skills. J Urol. 2015;194(4):1098–105.
25. White MA, DeHaan AP, Stephens DD, Maes AA, Maatman TJ. Validation of a high fidelity adult ureteroscopy and renoscopy simulator. J Urol. 2010;183(2):673–7.
26. Adams F, Qiu T, Mark A, et al. Soft 3D-printed phantom of the human kidney with collecting system. Ann Biomed Eng. 2017;45(4):963–72.
27. Villa L, Somani BK, Sener TE, et al. Comprehensive flexible ureteroscopy (FURS) simulator for training in endourology: the k-box model. Cent Eur J Urol. 2016;69(1):118–20.
28. Villa L, Şener TE, Somani BK, et al. Initial content validation results of a new simulation model for flexible ureteroscopy: the key-box. J Endourol. 2017;31(1):72–7.
29. Matsumoto ED, Hamstra SJ, Radomski SB, Cusimano MD. The effect of bench model fidelity on endourological skills. J Urol. 2002;167(March):1243–7.
30. Blankstein U, Lantz AG, John D'A, Honey R, Pace KT, Ordon M, Lee JY. Simulation-based flexible ureteroscopy training using a novel ureteroscopy part-task trainer. J Can Urol Assoc. 2015;9:331–5.
31. Michel MS, Knoll T, Köhrmann KU, Alken P. The URO Mentor: development and evaluation of a new computer-based interactive training system for virtual life-like simulation of diagnostic and therapeutic endourological procedures. BJU Int. 2002;89(3):174–7.
32. Watterson JD, Beiko DT, Kuan JK, Denstedt JD. A randomized, prospective blinded study validating the acquisition of ureteroscopy skills using a computer based virtual reality endourological simulator. J Urol. 2002;168(5):1928–32.
33. Wilhelm DM, Ogan K, Roehrborn CG, Cadeddu JA, Pearle MS. Assessment of basic endoscopic performance using a virtual reality simulator. J Am Coll Surg. 2002;195(5):675–81.
34. Jacomides L, Ogan K, Cadeddu JA, Pearle MS. Use of a virtual reality simulator for ureteroscopy training. J Urol. 2004;171(1):320–3.
35. Ogan K, Jacomides L, Shulman MJ, Roehrborn CG, Cadeddu JA, Pearle MS. Virtual ureteroscopy predicts ureteroscopic proficiency of medical students on a cadaver. J Urol. 2004;172(2):667–71.
36. Knoll T, Trojan L, Haecker A, Alken P, Michel MS. Validation of computer-based training in ureterorenoscopy. BJU Int. 2005;95(9):1276–9.

37. Dolmans VEMG, Schout BMA, de Beer NAM, Bemelmans BLH, Scherpbier AJJA, Hendrikx AJM. The virtual reality endourologic simulator is realistic and useful for educational purposes. J Endourol. 2009;23(7):1175–81.
38. Mishra S, Sharma R, Kumar A, Ganatra P, Sabnis RB, Desai MR. Comparative performance of high-fidelity training models for flexible ureteroscopy: are all models effective? Indian J Urol. 2011;27(4):451–6.
39. Chou DS, Abdelshehid C, Clayman RV, McDougall EM. Comparison of results of virtual-reality simulator and training model for basic ureteroscopy training. J Endourol. 2006;20(4):266–71.
40. Matsumoto ED, Pace KT, Honey RJDA. Virtual reality ureteroscopy simulator as a valid tool for assessing endourological skills. Int J Urol. 2006;13(7):896–901.
41. Dai JC, Lendvay TS, Sorensen MD. Crowdsourcing in surgical skills acquisition: a developing technology in surgical education. J Grad Med Educ. 2017;9(6):697–705. https://doi.org/10.4300/JGME-D-17-00322.1. Review.
42. Conti SL, Brubaker W, Chung BI, et al. Crowd sourced assessment of ureteroscopy with laser lithotripsy video feed does not correlate with trainee experience. J Endourol. 2018;33(1):end.2018.0534.
43. James J. A new, evidence based estimate of patient harms associated with hospital care. J Patient Saf. 2013;9(3):122–8.
44. Brunckhorst O, Shahid S, Aydin A, et al. Simulation-based ureteroscopy skills training curriculum with integration of technical and non-technical skills: a randomized controlled trial. Surg Endosc. 2015;29(9):2728–35.
45. Weld LR, Stringer MT, Ebertowski JS, et al. TeamSTEPPS improves operating room efficiency and patient safety. Am J Med Qual. 2016;31(5):408–14.
46. de Vries AH, Schout BMA, van Merriënboer JJG, et al. High educational impact of a national simulation-based urological curriculum including technical and non-technical skills. Surg Endosc Other Interv Tech. 2017;31(2):928–36.

Chapter 17
Robotics and Ureteroscopy

Jens J. Rassweiler, Marcel Fiedler, Nikos Charalampogiannis, Ahmet Sinan Kabakci, Remzi Sağlam, and Jan-Thorsten Klein

Summary

Recently developed robotic devices may significantly compensate for ergonomic deficiencies of FURS. In 2008, Mihir Desai reported the first robotic flexible ureteroscopy using the Sensei-Magellan system designed for cardiology. However this project has been discontinued.

The Avicenna Roboflex™ consists of the console and the manipulator of flexible ureterorenoscope. The console provides an adjustable seat with armrests and two joysticks to manipulate the endoscope; the right wheel enables deflection similar to the hand-piece of any standard ureterorenoscope. The left joystick allows rotation as well as advancing and retracting the scope. First clinical studies could demonstrate safe and effective application of the device with significant improved ergonomics for the surgeon. Nevertheless, future studies are necessary to evaluate the final role of robotic FURS.

J. J. Rassweiler (✉) · M. Fiedler · N. Charalampogiannis
Department of Urology, SLK Kliniken Heilbronn, University of Heidelberg, Heilbronn, Baden-Württemberg, Germany
e-mail: jens.rassweiler@slk-kliniken.de

A. S. Kabakci
Department of Urology, SLK Kliniken Heilbronn, University of Heidelberg, Heilbronn, Baden-Württemberg, Germany

Department of Bioengineering, Hacettepe University, Ankara, Turkey

R. Sağlam
Department of Urology, Medicana International Hospital, Ankara, Turkey

J.-T. Klein
Department of Urology, Medical School Ulm, University of Ulm, Ulm, Germany

© Springer Nature Switzerland AG 2020   239
B. F. Schwartz, J. D. Denstedt (eds.), *Ureteroscopy*,
https://doi.org/10.1007/978-3-030-26649-3_17

Introduction

Since the end of the last century, minimally invasive surgery replaced open surgery for multiple indications accomplished by a continuous improvement of video-endoscopic technology, implementation of physical principles and even the introduction of robot-assisted surgery [1–3]. However, this represents an ongoing process: at the end of the last century, extracorporeal shock wave lithotripsy (ESWL) dominated therapeutic strategies by eliminating open surgery and decreasing the use of endourologic techniques, such as ureteroscopy (URS) and percutaneous nephrolithotomy (PCNL). Subsequently especially retrograde intrarenal surgery (RIRS) has gained significant importance [4–6].

This was enabled by the continuous improvement of the endourological armamentarium with miniaturization of the instruments [7, 8]. However, flexible ureteroscopy (FURS)/retrograde intrarenal surgery is limited by ergonomic deficiencies during stone manipulation, laser disintegration or extraction of fragments, which may become cumbersome mainly when treating multiple stones or larger renal calculi and may even lead to orthopaedic problems among urologists [9, 10]. Based on the positive experience with master-slave systems in laparoscopic surgery and recently also in cardiology and interventional radiology, several groups focused on the usefulness and further development of such robotic devices for RIRS/FURS to overcome most of such methodological obstacles (Table 17.1).

In this chapter, we want to focus on actual developments of robot-assisted flexible ureteroscopy including technical evolutions in video endoscopy, endoscopic armamentarium, and intraoperative navigation [11–15].

Historical Update of Development of Robotic Surgical Devices

Such new developments require a short historical review of robotic devices for laparoscopic surgery, which revolutionized video-endoscopic surgery particularly in urology (Table 17.1). Already in 1996, Buess and Schurr et al. [16] developed the ARTEMIS-System and presented the first experimental results, when successfully performing a telesurgical laparoscopic cholecystectomy in an experimental model (Fig. 17.1a). However, despite various promising experimental trials in abdominal and cardiac surgery, the device never made it beyond the experimental state.

Based on the voice-controlled camera-arm AESOP, the ZEUS System (Computer motion Inc., Goleta, CA, USA) has been developed and used for cardiac surgery and gynaecological procedures [17]. The ZEUS System (Fig. 17.1b) was based on the combination of a control unit and three tele-manipulators. Three separate robot arms were transported on small carts. The arms were mounted by hand on the rails of the operating table. The surgeon was seated on an open console with a high-backed chair with armrests, handling the instrument controllers. The most impressive

Table 17.1 Overview on the most important robotic devices in surgery

Device	Description	Comment
Robodoc	Automated drilling of the shaft for hip prosthesis based on CT	Clinical problems (pain)
Caspar	Automated drilling for hip prosthesis based on CT	No more in clinical use
Probot	Automated resection of the prostate based on TRUS	No more in clinical use (only prototype)
Neuro-arm	Master-slave system with open console for neurosurgery	Developing company does not exist anymore
AESOP	Voice-controlled camera-arm for laparoscopy	Developing company does not exist anymore
ARTEMIS	Master-slave system with open console for laparoscopy	Only experimental
ZEUS	Master-slave system with open console for laparoscopy	Developing company does not exist anymore
da Vinci	Master-slave system with closed console for laparoscopy	Still used in the fourth generation of device
Sensei-Magellan	Master-slave system for angiography and cardiology	Not suitable for endourology (i.e. FURS)
Avicenna Roboflex	Master-slave system with open console for flexible ureteroscopy	Still used in the third improved version
Focal one	Automated system to perform transrectal HIFU	Still used in the third improved version
Aquabeam	Automated system to perform TURP (Aquablation) based on TRUS	First clinical trials
Monarch	Master-slave system with game-pad for bronchoscopy	First clinical cases

demonstration with ZEUS represented the transatlantic laparoscopic cholecystectomy (Lindbergh-procedure) pioneered by Marescaux [18].

Parallel to ZEUS, the da Vinci Surgical system (Intuitive Surgical, Sunnyvale, United States) was introduced initially also designed for robot-assisted coronary artery surgery [19]. In 2000, Binder pioneered the first robot-assisted radical prostatectomy in Frankfurt followed by other European groups [20–22]. In 2001, Menon et al. achieved the breakthrough in urologic surgery establishing a full-working clinical programme [23]. Subsequently, FDA approved the use of the system for prostatic surgery. The da Vinci 2000 addressed most ergonomic problems of classical laparoscopy sufficiently, such as limited depth perception, eye-hand coordination and range of motion by introducing the Endo-wrist™ technology. da Vinci provided a closed console offering a 3D-CCD-video-system with in-line view. The cable-driven instruments with up to seven DOF and loop-like handles enabled an ergonomic working position due to the clutch mechanism [24] and instruments with 7° of freedom. In the last decade, the company introduced further elaborated systems, such as da Vinci SI, X and XI (Fig. 17.1c, d), which nowadays represent a very high standard [24–27].

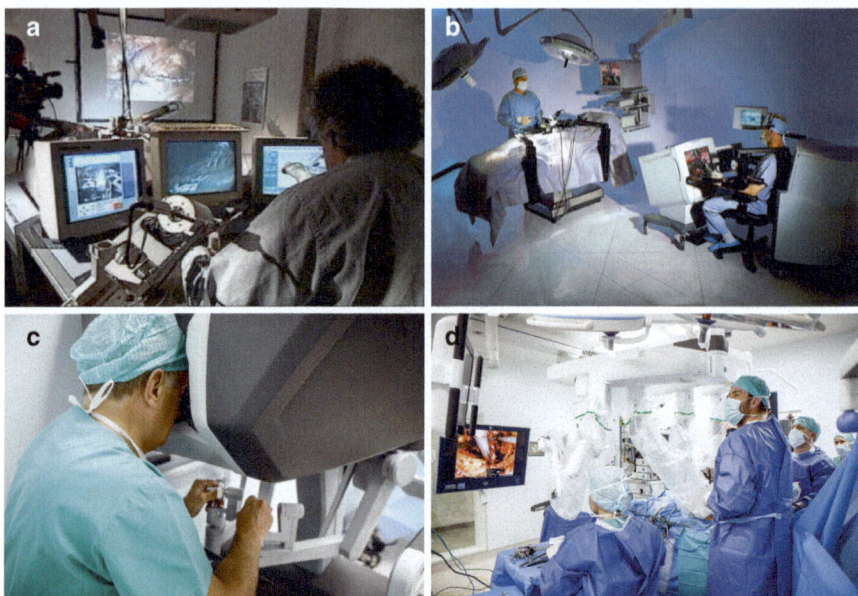

Fig. 17.1 History of robotic devices for laparoscopic surgery. (**a**) *ARTEMIS:* first master-slave system used experimentally (G. Buess, German Nuclear Research Centre, Karlsuhe, Germany). Open console, 3D video technology with polarizing glasses. (**b**) *ZEUS:* first clinically used robotic system for laparoscopic coronary artery revascularization. Open console, instruments with only 5° of freedom (DOF). 3D video technology with helmet or 2D video. (**c**) *dA Vinci XI:* console of last generation of robotic system for interdisciplinary use. In-line view with 3D HD video technology, 7 DOF for all instruments. (**d**) *dA Vinci XI:* four-arm system, telescope can be inserted via every port access. OR table (Trumpf Medical) can be moved without undocking of the robot. Integration of the robot in new OR-1 system (Karl Storz). (Figure 1a, b from Rassweiler et al. [30], with permission of Springer Nature)

The Ergonomic Deficiencies of Flexible Ureteroscopy

The surgeon usually stands and has to control fluoroscopy and the laser device by a foot-pedal, while fixing the position of the endoscope with one hand and deflecting/rotating it with the other hand (Table 17.2). Additionally, the assistant needs to insert the laser fibre or any accessory instrument (basket, N-gage) and then activate it according to the surgeon's demand. During this process the surgeon and assistant have a very limited working space. Thus the aim of a robotic device should mainly act also as a master-slave system trying to help the surgeon by offering an ergonomic working position and alleviating the manipulation of the endoscope without increasing the risk of damaging the urogenital system.

Table 17.2 Ergonomic requirements for classical flexible ureterorenoscopy (FURS) during intrarenal stone management

Operative manoeuvre	Extremity used	Action by
Insertion of ureteroscope	Fingers of both hands (at glans and instrument)	Surgeon
Deflection of ureterscope	Hand holding hand-piece	Surgeon
	Thumb at handle	
	Fingers at meatus	
Rotation of ureterscope	Hand holding hand-piece	Surgeon
	Fingers of the other hand at meatus	
Fluoroscopy	Right foot (foot switch)	Surgeon (radiotechnician)
Movement of table/C-arm	Right foot (foot switch)Hand (manually)	Radiotechnician (surgeon, assistant)
Irrigation		
By syringe	Hand	Nurse/assistant
By mechanic device	Foot	Nurse/assistant (surgeon)
By pump	Finger activation (button)	Nurse/technician
Laser lithotripsy		
Insertion of fibre	Fingers at ureteroscope	Nurse/assistant
Laser settings	Finger (button)	Nurse/technician
Activation	Right foot (foot switch)	Surgeon
Use of basket/grasper		
Insertion	Fingers at ureteroscope	Nurse/assistant
Manipulation	Hand and thumb	Surgeon
Closure	Fingers at handle	Nurse/assistant

From Rassweiler et al. [30], with permission of Springer Nature

Historical Development of Master-Slave Systems for Flexible Ureteroscopy

The development of robotic master-slave systems was not only limited to laparoscopy (Table 17.1). Also for neurosurgery, NOTES, interventional radiology, cardiology and endourology, several robotic devices have been developed [28–31].

Sensei-Magellan System

In 2008, Desai et al. [12] first reported a robotic flexible ureteroscopy using the Sensei-Magellan system (Hansen Medical, Mountain View, USA) designed for cardiology and angiography. This device has different components: an open console providing a chair with armrest and a joystick to control the movement of the inserted catheter. The console offers two screens for fluoroscopic and endoscopic images. The robotic arm is driven by electronic motors to manipulate the flexible catheter. The electronic rack contains computer hardware, power supplies and video distribution units (Fig. 17.2a).

The robotic flexible catheter system consists of an outer catheter sheath (14/12F) and inner catheter guide (12/10F). For robotic FURS, a 7.5F fibre-optic flexible ureteroscope was inserted and fixed in the inner catheter guide. Thus, remote manipulation of the catheter system manoeuvres the ureteroscope tip (Fig. 17.2b). The tip of the outer sheath was positioned at ureteropelvic junction to stabilize navigation of inner guide inside the collecting system (Fig. 17.2c). In this system, the ureteroscope is manipulated only passively, which proved to be a problem, because the robotic arm was mainly designed for interventional radiology (Table 17.3; Fig. 17.2d). Consequently, this project has been discontinued after the first 18 treated [11–13].

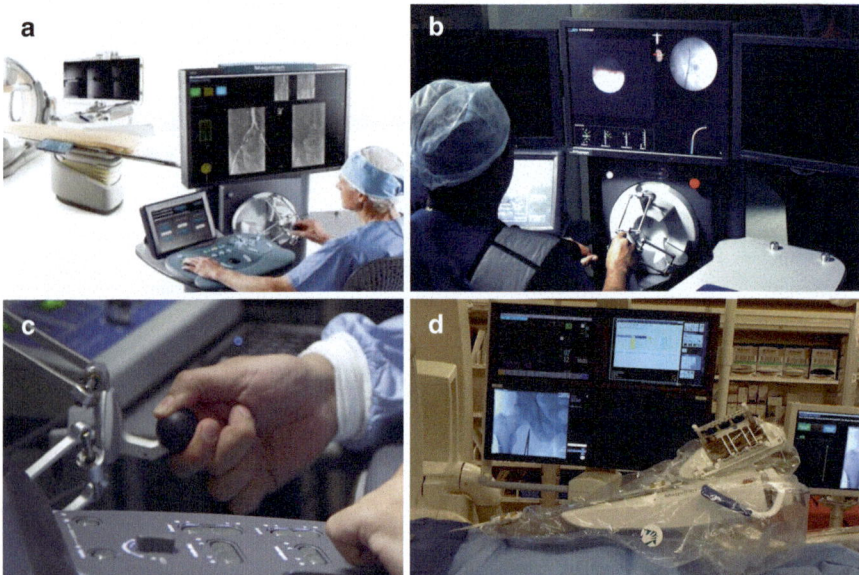

Fig. 17.2 Sensei-Magellan system (Hansen Medical, Mountain View, United States). (**a**) Master-slave system designed for angiography and transvascular cardiologic interventions. (**b**) Open console with the joystick analog endoscopic and fluoroscopic image during robotic flexible ureteroscopy. (**c**) Joystick at the console controls the deflection and rotation of the inner sheath. (**d**) Robotic arm covered with sterile drape mounted to the operating table (here during angiography). (Figure 2a, b from Rassweiler et al. [30], with permission of Springer Nature)

Table 17.3 Comparison of ergonomic features of Sensei™ and Roboflex™

Functions	Sensei	Roboflex
Seat	Adjustable saddle-type seat	Adjustable seat
	No arm rest	With integrated arm rest and foot-pedal
Imaging	Console with integrated	Console with integrated
	Fluoroscopy and endoscopic image screens	Endoscopic image screen
	Animation of position of catheter-tip (3D navigation)	Animation of position of ureteroscope in collecting system
Insertion of ureteroscope	Indirect insertion of inner sheath (scope glued to the sheath)	Fine-tunable by left joystick with numeric display of horizontal movement
Deflection of ureteroscope	Indirect deflection by the inner sheath based on single joystick (omega-force dimension)	Fine-tunable deflection via wheel for right hand with display of grade and direction of deflection
Rotation of ureterscope	Indirect rotation by the inner sheath (scope glued to the sheath)	Fine-tunable by sophisticated left joystick
Irrigation	No irrigation system included	Integrated irrigation pump activated by touchscreen
Laser lithotripsy	No function for laser fibre integrated	Integrated control of laser fibre by touchscreen
		Activation by foot-pedal
Use of basket/ grasper	No function for basket or grasper integrated	No function for basket or grasper integrated

From Rassweiler et al. [30], with permission of Springer Nature

Roboflex Avicenna Prototype

Since 2010, ELMED (Ankara, Turkey) is working on a robot specifically designed for FURS [14]. Roboflex Avicenna was continuously developed to perform flexible ureteroscopy providing all necessary functions for FURS [15]. The prototype consisted of a small console with an integrated flat screen and two joysticks to move the endoscope, which is held by the hand-piece of the robotic arm (manipulator). This basic designed has not changed; however, several significant improvements have been accomplished during further development including size and design of the function screen, design of the joysticks to control rotation and deflection of endoscope, fine adjustment of deflection of endoscope and range of rotation of the manipulator (Table 17.3). Actually, Roboflex Avicenna represents the only robot, especially developed for flexible ureteroscopy [21, 32]. The device has CE mark since 2013, and FDA approval is pending.

Monarch

In March 2018 Monarch Platform was used in a clinical case of robotic bronchos-copy for the first time [31]. The system utilizes the common endoscopy procedure to insert a flexible robot into hard-to-reach places inside the human body (Table 17.1). A doctor trained on the system uses a video game-style controller to navigate inside, with help from 3D models. Like in the Sensei-Magellan system, the technology is based on the robotic control of an external tube using two robotic arms (one for the outer and one for the endoscope) also to advance and retract the endoscope. However, the Monarch Platform also enables the additional movement of the flexi-ble scope to reach small distal branches of the bronchial system. An irrigation sys-tem is integrated. Another main feature of the device represents the integration of CT imaging to guide the biopsy. Of course, the same technology might be used for flexible ureteroscopy in the near future.

Clinical Experience with Avicenna Roboflex

Since we have significant experience with Avicenna Roboflex based on a close col-laboration with developing company and clinical partner in Ankara, Turkey, we want to focus more in detail on this robotic system [32].

Design of the Device

The robot consists of an open console and the manipulator of the flexible ureterore-noscope. The *manipulator* drives the flexible ureteroscope using its own mechanics (Fig. 17.3a). For this purpose the hand-piece of scope has to be attached directly to an especially designed master plate of the manipulator (Fig. 17.3b). Micromotors move the steering lever of the hand-piece for deflection with several ranges of motion. The robotic arm enables bilateral rotation, advancement and retraction of the ureteroscope. Additionally the height of the robotic arm can be adjusted accord-ing to the patient's size. Actually, there are three exchangeable master plates avail-able for three flexible digital ureteroscopes (Karl Storz Flex X2; Olympus URF-V2; Wolf Cobra/Viper digital).

All functions of the robotic arm are controlled at the console providing an inte-grated adjustable seat with two armrests and two integrated foot-pedals for activa-tion of fluoroscopy and the laser lithotripter via a pneumatic pedal controller (Fig. 17.3c). The control panel at the console is used by touchscreen functions. The integrated HD monitor displays the endoscopic image and all information about the position of ureteroscope in the collecting system (Fig. 17.3d). All main manoeuvres to navigate the flexible endoscope can be fine-tuned at the control panel, such as horizontal movement (= insertion/retraction of the endoscope) with a range of

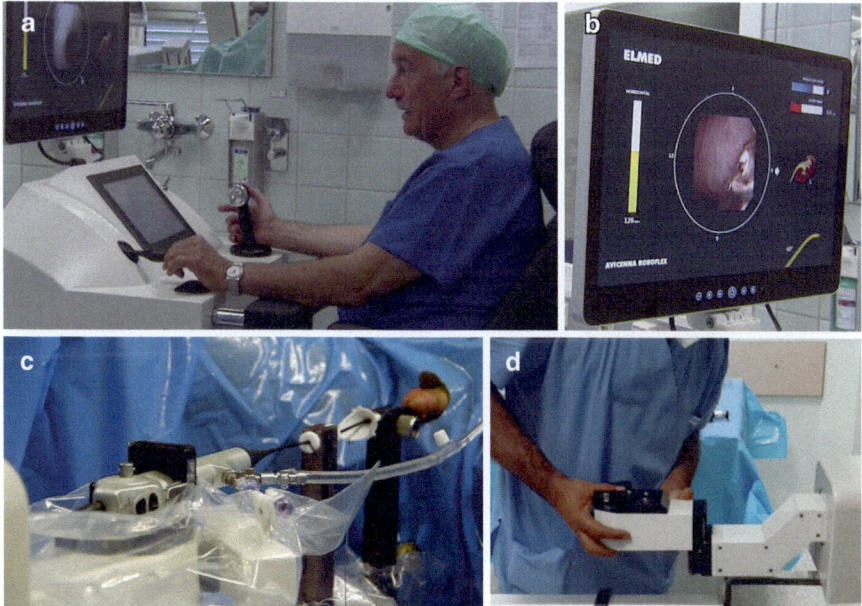

Fig. 17.3 Avicenna Roboflex System (ELMED, Ankara, Turkey). (**a**) Robotic arm with the hand-piece of a digital flexible ureteroscope (Flex XC, Karl Storz, Tuttlingen, Germany) fixed in the master plate and the flexible part supported by one or two stabilizers before entering the access sheath. (**b**) Exchange of the master plate (i.e. when using a disposable device). (**c**) Open console with sophisticated left-hand joystick for rotation and insertion/retraction and fine-tuned right-hand wheel for deflection. Touchscreen functions for laser activation, irrigation, and fine-tuning of movements. (**d**) Integrated screen with display of digital endoscopic image and graphic information about axis and deflection of endoscope. (Fig. 3a–**c** from Rassweiler et al. [30], with permission of Springer Nature)

150 mm, bilateral rotation (220° to each side) and deflection of the scope (262° to each side). For this purpose the left hand controls a specifically developed horizontal joystick, whereas the right hand uses a wheel for deflection. All numeric parameters of endoscope navigation are displayed on the control panel and the HD-screen. The deflection can be adjusted to European as well as US settings. Additionally, the infusion speed of the irrigation fluid can be adjusted together with a motorized insertion and retraction of laser fibre.

Operative Technique

During the procedure the robotic arm is covered by a sterile plastic drape which is accomplished parallel to the anaesthesia of the patient. We have standardized our technique using routinely a 12/14F access sheath with hydrophilic coating (35 to 45–55 cm; Flexor parallel, Cook-Medical, Daniels Way, USA) enabling placement a safety guide wire (Expert Nitinol wire 0.35i×150 cm, IMP, Karlsruhe, Germany) parallel to the sheath. Position of the access sheath should be 1 cm below the UPJ (Fig. 17.4a), to

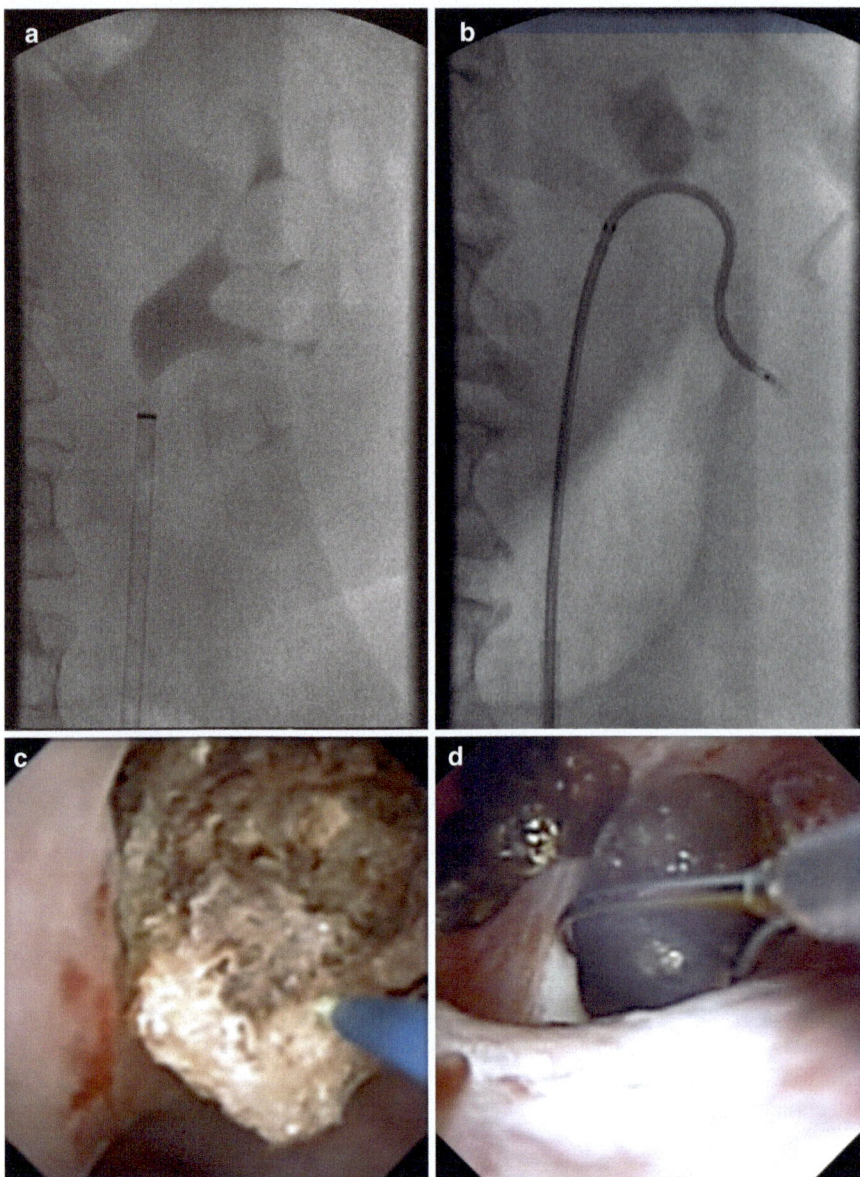

Fig. 17.4 Stone treatment during robot-assisted flexible ureteroscopy. (**a**) Fluoroscopy before the procedure (Siemens Lithoskop, Erlangen, Germany). The access sheath has to be positioned 1 cm below the ureteropelvic junction to minimize the risk of injury to the endoscope during deflection. (**b**) Fluoroscopy during laser lithotripsy to verify the position of the endoscope. (**c**) Digital endoscopic image (3× magnification) during lithotripsy using dusting mode (Holmium-YAG laser; 0.5 J, 15 Hz). (**d**) Endoscopic image during fragment extraction using N-Gage basket (Cook-Medical, Daniels Way, USA). The robot separates the assistant from the surgeon. (Figure 4a–c from Rassweiler et al. [30], with permission of Springer Nature)

allow enough flexibility of the ureteroscope. After arranging the position of seat and armrest by activating the memorized setting of each surgeon, the ureteroscope is inserted manually into the access sheath and fixed by one or two stabilizers (Fig. 17.3a). The definitive placement of the manipulator depends on the side of the stone and the size of the patient. Then the brakes of the manipulator are locked.

The endoscope is placed at the distal end of the access sheath with a horizontal value of 50 mm. Short-term digital fluoroscopy is used to determine the actual localization of stone and instrument (Fig. 17.4b). Once the endoscope has reached the renal pelvis, the scope needs to be rotated according to the axis of the kidney. Then, a systematic inspection of the entire collecting system is carried out. When the stone is visualized, the endoscope needs to be retracted and straightened slightly (<70°) to guarantee safe insertion of the laser fibre. Optionally Roboflex™ provides a memory function to guide the scope to its previous place once the laser fibre is inserted and the tip visualized endoscopically. However, with increasing experience there was no need to use this function.

Basically, any Holmium-YAG laser can be used, but we strongly recommend a laser, which allows application of higher frequencies on low energy level such as Lumenis Pulse 120 (Lumenis, Yokneam, Israel) or Sphinx Jr. (LISA laser products, Katlenburg, Germany) with adequate small-calibre laser fibres (200–270 μ-fibre; Slimline™, Rigifib™). Laser-induced lithotripsy is initiated preferably aiming at pulverization or "dusting" of the stone (0.5 J, 15 Hz) by meander-like movement of the tip of the laser fibre in the range of millimetres (Fig. 17.4c). The smaller fibre size allows sufficient bending of scope without deteriorating the efficacy of stone dusting or fragmentation (1.2 J, 10 Hz). Once fragmentation is progressing, increase of energy might be helpful to apply the "pop-corn effect" or better "Jacuzzi effect" for fine disintegration of the fragments similar to intracorporeal shock wave lithotripsy with a stable position of the laser fibre at the neck of the calyx (Fig. 17.4d).

If necessary, introduction of tip-less baskets or other forceps-like devices (i.e. N-gage™, Cook) for retrieval of fragments is performed. Here, the separation of the surgeon at the console from the assistant at the bed-side is very helpful (Fig. 17.4d). Once the fragment is entrapped, the endoscope is driven back. Herein, the numeric demonstration of position of the tip of the endoscope along the horizontal axis is very helpful to anticipate, when the fragment will reach the distal end of the access sheath. When the fragment is pulled into the sheath, the assistant disconnects the ureteroscope from the distal stabilizer and extracts the stone. The endpoint of the treatment represents a stone-free status based on endoscopic inspection respectively remaining stone dust or fragments less than 2 mm. Then, the access sheath is retrieved under endoscopic inspection and a double J-stent placed. We usually introduce the stent with a string taped to the Foley catheter to be extracted the following morning.

Clinical Studies

The clinical introduction of the device was accomplished according to the IDEAL-system (idea, development, evaluation, assessment, long-term study) for the stages in surgical innovation [33]. First studies with the prototypes in Ankara were able to prove safety of the device [14]. Next step represented a proctored multicentric study, where seven experienced surgeons treated 81 patients (mean age 42, range 6–68) with renal calculi (mean volume 1296 +/− 544, range 432–3100 mm³) in an observational study (IDEAL stage 2) proctored by the urologist (R.S.) being involved in development and clinical introduction of the device [15]. In this study the positive impact of Roboflex™ on ergonomics could be verified by use of a validated questionnaire (Table 17.4).

The efficacy of the device in a real-life scenario was evaluated in a multicentric phase-2 study at two European centres (Ankara, Heilbronn) collecting data from 266 patients [32]. We could again prove safety and efficacy of the system, but of course comparing our results with the initial study, docking time of the robot was longer (4 vs. 1 min), whereas time to visualize the stone was similar (4 vs. 3.7 min). According to the larger stone volume (1620 vs. 1300 mm³), the console time was longer (96 vs. 53 min). Moreover, we were able to demonstrate that we could safely and successfully apply all modern techniques and protocols of flexible URS, such as laser dusting, using pop-corn/Jacuzzi effect and extraction of larger fragments [17]. In this setting, Avicenna Roboflex™ proved to be robust with only two cases of technical failure requiring conversion to classical FURS. The radiation exposure for the surgeon can be significantly reduced. In conclusion, we were able to integrate the device easily in our daily routine.

Recently, Geavlete et al. [34] present a phase-3 study comparing robot-assisted versus classical FURS in 132 patients. Treatment time (51 vs. 50 min.) and fragmentation time (37 vs. 39 min.) were similar, but stone-free rate (92.4 vs. 89.4%) favoured the robotic approach (Table 17.5).

Discussion

Robotic Assistance for Endourology

During the last 15 years, robot-assisted surgery has gained an established and irreversible role in urologic laparoscopic surgery [20, 24, 26]. Just in the year 2016, installations of da Vinci systems increased by 21% to more than 2500 units worldwide, and robotic procedures leaped by 25% to more than 450,000, mainly performed in urology, gynaecology and visceral surgery [35]. The main advantages of robot-assisted surgery include significant improvement of ergonomics, which enabled the widespread application of laparoscopic techniques with acceptable learning curves.

Table 17.4 Comparison of ergonomics of conventional versus robot-assisted flexible ureteroscopy using a validated questionnaire

(a) Experience of surgeons								
Surgeon	1	2	3	4	5	6	7	Mean
Initials	B.E.	A.Y.M	K.S	R.S.	Z.T.	J.R	O.T.	
Age (years)	51	52	50	67	40	59	46	52,14
FURS-experience (years)	16	7	10	5	5	16	15	10,57
FURS-work load (h/week)	10	12	15	7	10	6	18	11,14

(b) Classical FURS								
Surgeon	1	2	3	4	5	6	7	Mean
Complaints (0–5)	Classical FURS	Classical FURS	Classical FURS	Classical FURS	Classical FURS	Classical FURS	Classical FURS	
Musculoskeletal pain	3	3	3	3	3	3	1	2.71
Neck pain	3	2	2	2	2	3	1	2.14
Shoulder stiffness	5	3	3	4	2	3	1	3.00
Arm pain	5	3	3	4	3	3	1	3.14
Forearm pain	5	3	3	3	3	4	1	3.14
Elbow stiffness	5	2	2	2	2	4	2	2.71
Hand pain	3	3	3	3	4	4	2	3.14
Wrist stiffness	3	4	4	3	3	4	1	3.14
Finger numbness	1	2	2	1	3	3	2	2.00
Back pain	3	1	1	2	3	3	1	2.00
Leg pain	2	2	2	2	3	4	2	2.43
Eye strain	0	2	2	2	3	2	1	1.71
Total score	38	30	30	31	34	40	16	31,3*

(c) Robotic FURS								
Surgeon	1	2	3	4	5	6	7	Mean
Complaints (0–5)	Robot-assisted FURS	Robot-assisted FURS	Robot-assisted FURS	Robot-assisted FURS	Robot-assisted FURS	Robot-assisted FURS	Robot-assisted FURS	Mean
Musculoskeletal pain	0	1	0	0	0	0	0	0,14
Neck pain	0	0	0	0	1	1	0	0,29
Shoulder stiffness	2	0	0	1	0	0	0	0,43
Arm pain	2	1	1	1	0	0	0	0,71
Forearm pain	2	1	1	0	0	0	0	0,57
Elbow stiffness	2	0	0	0	0	0	0	0,29
Hand pain	2	0	0	0	1	1	1	0,71
Wrist stiffness	0	0	0	0	1	0	1	0,29
Finger numbness	0	1	1	1	1	1	1	0,86
Back pain	0	0	0	0	0	1	0	0,14
Leg pain	0	0	0	0	0	2	0	0,29
Eye strain	0	1	1	0	2	1	1	0,86
Total score	10	5	4	3	6	7	4	5,6*

From Saglam et al. [15], with permission of Elsevier

$*p < 0.01$

Table 17.5 Comparison of clinical studies of robotic flexible ureteroscopy

Parameters	Desai et al. (2011)	Saglam et al. (2014)	Geavlete et al. (2016)	Rassweiler et al. (2018)
Robotic device	Sensei (Hansen Medical)	Roboflex – prototype 2 (ELMED)	Roboflex – prototype 2 (ELMED)	Roboflex – final design (ELMED)
No. of patients	18 (12 males)	81 (56 males)	67 (27 males)	266 (176 males)
Stone size	10 (5–15) mm	13 (5–30) mm	21 (11–36) mm	14 (5–30) mm
Multiple stones	3 (16.7%)	52 (64.2%)	23 (34.3%)	192 (72.2%)
Total operating time	91 (60–130) min	74 (40–182) min	51 (38–103) min	96 (59–193) min
Robot docking	7 (4–18) min	1 (0.5–2) min	n.a.	4 (1–29) min
Console time	41 (21–70) min	53 (23–153) min	37 (27–86) min	65 (16–174) min
Stone localisation	9 (1–36) min	4 (2–8) min	n.a.	4 (1–12) min
Intraoperative complications	0	1 (1.2%) failure of device	0%	2 (0.7%) failures of device
Complete stone disintegration	17 (94.4%)	79 (96.2%)	65 (98.5%)	258 (96.9%)

From Rassweiler et al. [30], with permission of Springer Nature
n.a. not available

The use of robotic master-slave systems has not been limited to laparoscopic surgery. There are other examples from gastroenterology, cardiology, interventional radiology, neurosurgery and endourology [28–32]. In endourology the first clinical applications tried to modify the Sensei-Magellan system designed for cardiovascular intervention to perform robot-assisted flexible ureterorenoscopy [11–13]. In this system, the surgeon sits in front of an open console manipulating a steerable flexible tube usually used for transvascular intra-cardiac interventions by use of a joystick (Fig. 17.2a). The remote manipulation system (Omega X, Force Dimension, Nyon, Switzerland) manoeuvres the outer and inner sheath of the device. To manipulate a flexible ureteroscope, the instrument tip had to be glued to the inner guide. This means that the ureteroscope could be manipulated only passively and its own deflection mechanics were not used. Such a system might be very useful for transvascular robotic atrial fibrillation ablation or any catheter-based angiographic procedure, but it proved to be insufficient for FURS [11–13, 32].

The new Monarch™ system (Auris, USA) has been pushed significantly recently. It was developed for bronchoscopy, but the company sees also applications for other flexible endoscopes (i.e. FURS/RIRS) in the near future [31]. Interestingly, the device seems to work based on some principles like the Sensei-Magellan™ without using the mechanics of the bronchoscope. The only difference is that the surgeon does not use a joystick but controls the device via a handheld keyboard similar to computer games. The two arms have an integrated cable-driven system with small wheels similar to the da Vinci device. This enables flexible movement of the tips of either the inner or outer sheath. Approximation of the arms results in advancement of the inner sheath. There are no specific functions (i.e. movement and activation of the laser fibre) integrated. Thus it remains unclear whether Monarch will be really useful for robot-assisted flexible ureteroscopy.

Important Features for Robotic FURS

Avicenna Roboflex has been developed specifically for FURS /RIRS. For robot-assisted flexible ureteroscopy, specific technological features are of importance, such as chip at the tip video technology of the digital endoscope, easy manipulation of the endoscope and activation of the laser and fluoroscopy. Roboflex uses the mechanical functions of the endoscope by digital control of the movement of the hand-piece. Such a system needs to be versatile. The exchangeable master plates enable the use of different kinds of digital ureteroscopes including disposable devices. Also any holmium-YAG laser lithotripter can be used, and the laser-control device takes any laser fibre. The main advantage of this concept represents the fact that all new developments of flexible ureteroscopes including video technology, mechanics or the working channel can be immediately implemented.

Particularly, the two joysticks for navigation of the ureteroscope have been significantly improved during the developmental phase (Table 17.5). Any necessary movement (insertion, retraction, rotation, deflection) can be fine-tuned according to the clinical situation. The range of rotation (210° in each direction = 420°) is beyond the human manual capabilities during classical FURS (max. 120°). During robot-assisted deflection, 10° of movement with the wheel results in 3° deflection of the tip compared to 60° by manual use with the thumb of the same endoscope.

Learning Curve of Robotic FURS

Surgical robots are mainly introduced to improve ergonomics of minimally invasive surgery. This can result in a shorter learning curve of the procedure and also improve the quality and outcome of the procedure. One third of urologists have reported on hand-wrist and other ergonomic problems during classical FURS [9, 10], which was reflected by the recently published validated questionnaire comparing classical versus robot-assisted FURS [15]. Avicenna Roboflex™ provided a suitable platform improving ergonomics significantly (Table 17.4).

After only short introduction at the training model, all seven surgeons were able to perform robotic-assisted FURS safely and in a reasonable time frame compared to their own published series of classical FURS [36, 37]. Also in the second study involving more surgeons, the learning curve was short (maximal five cases). Of course, retrograde intrarenal surgery is less complicated compared to laparoscopic radical prostatectomy, particularly in case of small stones, which can be extracted by use of a nitinol basket. On the other side, the introduction of the device provides a safe and non-exhausting environment for the surgeon. Based on this we were able to extend the indication of FURS/RIRS to larger intrarenal calculi resulting in the decrease of extracorporeal shock wave lithotripsy and percutaneous nephrolithotomy [32]. This means also a significant reduction of radiation exposure to patients and surgeons [38, 39].

Impact on the Lifetime of the Endoscope

Suboptimal ergonomics may be one of the reasons for imperfect performance of FURS mainly in complicated cases resulting in the need of second sessions and frequent repair of the endoscopes. Carey et al. [40] reported an 8.1% damage rate at a single tertiary centre with a 40 to 48 uses before the initial repair of new flexible ureteroscopes. The main reason for repair was errant laser firing (36%) and excessive torque (28%). Theoretically, the functions included in Roboflex™ such as insertion of laser fibre only in straight position of scope using a memory function, step-wise motorized advancement of laser fibre and force-controlled (maximal 1 N/ mm^2) deflection of scope should contribute to a longer lifetime of ureterorenoscopes. However, the use of the device in a real-life scenario demonstrated various factors of breakage of an endoscope, such as inadequate handling during sterilization and cleaning of the instrument or technical failure of the chip. Not all of them can be avoided by use of the robot. Moreover the hygienic safety criteria have become much more stringent. The use of Cidex sterilization is no more allowed. Thus, minimal leakage of the working channel may require complete repair exchange of the scope. On the other side, Roboflex™ proved to be very robust in clinical routing requiring only one exchange of the master plate after more than 300 cases.

Limitations of the Device: Cost Discussion

Obviously, there has been always criticism against the use of a robot for FURS. This concerns the issue of unnecessary costs, a robotic hype and the final efficacy of the device [38]. It is evident that the main strength of the robot is to facilitate stone disintegration and extraction, where during classical FURS most ergonomic limitations are present (Table 17.2). Therefore, it is not surprising that in a recent in vitro study using a simple model for endoscopic navigation, no significant differences between the techniques could be demonstrated [38]. A possible limitation of the device may be the lack of tactile feedback. Similar to our experiences with da Vinci robot, lack of tactile feedback did not prove to be problematic during performance of robotic FURS mainly based on superior image quality of the used digital endoscope.

However, similar to classical FURS, one has to follow certain guidelines: (i) we recommend to place a guide wire parallel to the sheath, (ii) the ureteroscope should not be preloaded with a laser fibre when entering the collecting system and (iii) the access sheath should be placed 1 cm below the UPJ (Fig. 17.4a). The surgeon can always observe on the screen or console in which direction and how many degrees the endoscope is deflected. This has to be in accordance to the endoscopic image to minimize the risk of damage to the mucosa and/or instrument.

Like with all surgical robots, there is the discussion about costs [41]. Possible financial revenues for robotic systems include longer durability of the endoscope, shorter operating times, less secondary procedures. Actually there is no demand from patients like with the da Vinci system for radical prostatectomy. The ergonomic advantages and reduced radiation exposure for the surgeon should be considered, but similar to the other robotic systems have no financial benefit. On the other side, unlike da Vinci, the Avicenna Roboflex represents a single investment without resulting in further costs (i.e. for instruments). Also adequate reimbursement of FURS /RIRS in relationship to PCNL may help the distribution of the device. Future studies have to focus more on these issues.

Conclusions

Despite its increased application, FURS may represent a challenging technique particularly in complicated cases. Robotic systems have been developed and tested. Avicenna Roboflex™ provides a suitable, safe, and robust platform for robotic FURS with significant improvement of ergonomics. However, future studies are necessary to evaluate the final role of robotic FURS (IDEAL stage 3).

References

1. Rassweiler JJ, Knoll T, Köhrmann KU, McAteer JA, Lingeman JE, Cleveland RO, Bailey MR, Chaussy C. Shock wave technology and application: an update. Eur Urol. 2011;59:784–96.
2. Rassweiler JJ, Teber D. Advances in laparoscopic surgery in urology. Nat Rev Urol. 2016;13:387–99.
3. Rassweiler J, Binder J, Frede T. Robotic and telesurgery: will they change our future. Curr Opin Urol. 2001;11:309–20.
4. Monga M, Dretler SP, Landman J, Slaton JW, Conradie MC, Clayman RV. Maximizing ureteroscope deflection: "play it straight". Urology. 2002;60:902–5.
5. Beiko DT, Denstedt JD. Advances in ureterorenoscopy. Urol Clin North Am. 2007;34:397–408.
6. Preminger GM, Tiselius HG, Assimos DG, Alken P, Buck AC, Gallucci M, Knoll T, Lingeman JE, Nakada SY, Pearle MS, Sarica K, Türk C, Wolf JS Jr, American Urological Association Education and Research, Inc; European Association of Urology. 2007 Guideline for the management of ureteral calculi. Eur Urol. 2007;52:1610–31.
7. Wright AE, Rukin NJ, Somani BK. Ureteroscopy and stones: current status and future expectations. World J Nephrol. 2014;3:243–8.
8. Rassweiler J, Rassweiler MC, Klein J. New technology in ureteroscopy and percutaneous nephrolithotomy. Curr Opin Urol. 2016;26:95–106.
9. Elkoushy MA, Andonian S. Prevalence of orthopedic complaints among endourologists are common and their compliance with radiation safety measures very important. Endourology. 2011;25(10):1609–13.

10. Healy KA, Pak RW, Cleary RC, Colo-Herdman A, Bagley D. Hand and wrist problems among endourologists are very common. Endourology. 2011;25(12):1905–20.
11. Aron M, Haber GP, Desai MM, Gill IS. Flexible robotics: a new paradigm. Curr Opin Urol. 2007;17(3):151–5.
12. Desai MM, Aron M, Inderbir SG, Pascal-Haber Ukimura O, Kaouk JH, Stahler G, Barbagli O, Carlson C. Flexible robotic retrograde renoscopy: description of novel robotic device and preliminary laboratory experience. Urology. 2008;72:42–6.
13. Desai MM, Grover R, Aron M, Ganpule A, Joshi SS, Desai MR, Gill IS. Robotic flexible ureteroscopy for renal calculi: initial clinical experience. J Urol. 2011;186:563–8.
14. Saglam R, Kabakci AS, Koruk E, Tokatli Z. How did we designed and improved a new Turkish robot for flexible ureterorenoscopy. J Endourol. 2012;26(suppl1):A275. (MP44-12).
15. Saglam R, Muslumanoglu AY, Tokatlı Z, et al. A new robot for flexible ureteroscopy: development and early clinical results (IDEAL Stage 1–2b). Eur Urol. 2014;66:1092–100.
16. Schurr MO, Buess G, Neisius B, Voges U. Robotics and telemanipulation technologies for endoscopic surgery. A review of the ARTEMIS project. Surg Endosc. 2000;14:375–81.
17. Reichenspurner H, Damiano R, Mack M, et al. Use of the voice-controlled surgical system ZEUS for endoscopic coronary bypass grafting. J Thorac Cardiovasc Surg. 1999;118:11–6.
18. Marescaux J, Leroy J, Gagner M, et al. Transatlantic robot-assisted telesurgery. Nature. 2001;413:379–80.
19. Mohr FW, Falk V, Diegeler A, Autschbach R. Computer-enhanced coronary artery surgery. J Thorac Cardiovasc Surg. 1999;117:1212–5.
20. Binder J, Kramer W. Robotically assisted laparoscopic radical prostatectomy. BJU Int. 2001;87:408–10.
21. Abbou CC, Hoznek A, Salomon L, Olsson LE, Lobontiu A, Saint F, Cicco A, Antiphon P, Chopin D. Laparoscopic radical prostatectomy with a remote controlled robot. J Urol. 2001;165:1964–6.
22. Rassweiler J, Frede T, Seemann O, Stock C, Sentker L. Telesurgical laparoscopic radical prostatectomy. Eur Urol. 2001;40:75–83.
23. Menon M, Shrivastava A, Tewari A, et al. Laparoscopic and robot assisted radical prostatectomy: establishment of a structured program and preliminary analysis of outcomes. J Urol. 2002;168:945–9.
24. Leal Ghezzi T, Campos Corleta O. 30 years of robotic surgery. World J Surg. 2016;40:2550–7.
25. Rassweiler JJ, Autorino R, Klein J, Mottrie A, Goezen AS, Stolzenburg JU, Rha KH, Schurr M, Kaouk J, Patel V, Dasgupta P, Liatsikos E. Future of robotic surgery in urology. BJU Int. 2017;120:822–41.
26. Rassweiler JJ, Goezen AS, Rassweiler-Seyfried MC, Liatsikos E, Bach T, Stolzenburg JU, Klein J. Robots in urology: an analysis of present and future devices. Urologe A. 2018;57:1075–90.
27. Territo A, Gausa L, Alcaraz A, Musquera M, Doumerc N, Decaestecker K, Desender L, Stockle M, Janssen M, Fornara P, Mohammed N, Siena G, Serni S, Sahin S, Tuğcu V, Basile G, Breda A. The European experience on robot-assisted kidney transplantation: minimum of one-year follow-up. BJU Int. 2018;122:255–62.
28. Harris SJ, Arambula-Cosio F, Mei Q, Hibberd RD, Davies BL, Wickham JE, Nathan MS, Kundu B. The Probot – an active robot for prostate resection. Proc Inst Mech Eng H. 1997;211:317–25.
29. Sutherland GR, Maddahi Y, Gan LS, Lama S, Zareinia K. Robotics in the neurosurgical treatment of glioma. Surg Neurol Int. 2015;6(Suppl 1):S1–8.
30. Rassweiler J, Fiedler M, Charalampogiannis N, Kabakci AS, Saglam R, Klein JT. Robot-assisted flexible ureteroscopy: an update. Urolithiasis. 2018;46:69–77.
31. https://www.geekfence.com/2018/03/24/monarch-is-a-new-platform-from-surgical-robot-pioneer-frederic-moll/.
32. Klein JT, Fiedler M, Kabakci AS, Saglam R, Rassweiler J. Multicenter phase II study of the clinical use of the Avicenna Roboflex URS robot in robotic retrograde intrarenal surgery. J Urol. 2016;195(Suppl):116 A. (abstract No. PD 18-08).

33. Proietti S, Dragos L, Emiliani E, Buttice S, Talso M, Baghdadi M, Villa L, Doizi S, Giusti G, Traxer O. Ureteroscopic skills with and without Roboflex Avicenna in the K-box^R simulator. Cent Eur J Urol. 2017;70:76–80.

34. Geavlete P, Saglam R, Georgescu D, Multescu R, iordache V, Kabakci AS, Ene C, Geavlete B. Robotic flexible ureteroscopy versus classis flexible ureteroscopy in renal stones: initial Romanian experience. Chirurgia. 2016;111:326–9.

35. Williams S, Swanson C. Bull vs. bear: Intuitive Surgical, Inc. Stock http://www.fool.com/investing/general/2014/10/06/bull-vs-bear-intuitive-surgical-inc-stock.aspx.

36. Akman T, Binbay M, Ugurlu M, Kaba M, Akcay M, Yazici O, Ozgor F, Mumlumanoglu AY. Outcomes of retrograde intra-renal surgery compared with percutaneous nephrolithotomy in elderly patients with moderate-size kidney stones: a matched-pair analysis. Urolithiasis. 2013;

37. Erkurt B, Caskurlu T, Atis G, Gurbuz C, Arikan O, Pelit ES, Altay A, Erdogan F, Yildirim A. Treatment of renal stones with flexible ureteroscopy in preschool age children. J Endourol. 2012;26:625–9.

38. Hellawell GO, Mutch SJ, Thevendran G, Wells E, Morgan RJ. Radiation exposure and the urologist: what are the risks? J Urol. 2005;174:948–52.

39. Kim KP, Miller DL, Berrington de Gonzalez A, Balter S, Kleinerman RA, Ostroumova E, Simon SL, Linet MS. Occupational radiation doses to operators performing fluoroscopically-guided procedures. Health Phys. 2012;103:80–99.

40. Carey RI, Gomez CS, Maurici G, Lynne CM, Leveillee RJ, Bird VG. Frequency of uretero-scope damage seen at a tertiary care center. J Urol. 2006;176:607–10.

41. Caddedu JA. Comment on Saglam R, Muslumanoglu AY, Tokatlı Z, et al. A new robot for flexible ureteroscopy: development and early clinical results (IDEAL Stage 1–2b). Eur Urol. 2014;66:1092–100; J. Urol 2015; 193:1277.

Index

The manufacturer's authorised representative in the EU is Springer
Nature Customer Service Centre GmbH, Europaplatz 3, 69115 Heidelberg,
Germany. If you have any concerns regarding our products, please
contact ProductSafety@springernature.com

Printed and bound by CPI Group (UK) Ltd, Croydon, CR0 4YY

29/04/2026

02099451-0012